U0231714

美国针灸立法汇编

美国南部地区针灸立法汇编

Collection of Acupuncture Laws in the Southern United States of America

（汉英对照）

总顾问

刘保延　沈远东

主　编

桑　珍　杨宇洋　宋欣阳　张博源

上海科学技术出版社

内 容 提 要

针灸于19世纪上半叶传入美国，在20世纪70年代"针灸热"的影响之下，开始在美国流行。针灸在美国流行的五十多年间，经历了三次热潮，完成了法律本土化、教育本土化、职业本土化和医学属性本土化四个层次的本土化，广泛应用于变态反应性疾病、糖尿病、艾滋病、肿瘤、高血压、肥胖症、戒毒、戒酒、戒烟、化疗或手术后发生的恶心和呕吐等领域。美国47个州及华盛顿特区都在州议会法中专章规定了针灸师执业法律制度，广泛涉及针灸与东方医学的概念、针灸师的准入条件、教育培训、执业规范、行业组织管理和惩戒规则等内容。

本书为美国南部十州针灸立法汇编，包括阿肯色州、北卡罗来纳州、佛罗里达州、肯塔基州、路易斯安那州、密西西比州、南卡罗来纳州、田纳西州、西弗吉尼亚州、佐治亚州，从针灸人员的法律地位、准入与注册、日常管理机构、职业道德、惩戒报告等方面展开介绍。希望本书的出版能为中医药政策和法律的制定者、中医药政策和法制研究者以及高等院校、科研机构中医药学科的研习者们提供参考和借鉴。

图书在版编目（ＣＩＰ）数据

美国南部地区针灸立法汇编 = Collection of Acupuncture Laws in the Southern United States of America：汉英对照 / 桑珍等主编；刘保延，沈远东总顾问. -- 上海：上海科学技术出版社，2025.1
（美国针灸立法汇编）
ISBN 978-7-5478-6569-9

Ⅰ. ①美… Ⅱ. ①桑… ②刘… ③沈… Ⅲ. ①针灸学－立法－汇编－美国－汉、英 Ⅳ. ①D937.122.16

中国国家版本馆CIP数据核字(2024)第050912号

美国南部地区针灸立法汇编：Collection of Acupuncture Laws in the Southern United States of America（汉英对照）
总顾问　刘保延　沈远东
主　编　桑　珍　杨宇洋　宋欣阳　张博源

上海世纪出版(集团)有限公司
上海科学技术出版社　出版、发行
（上海市闵行区号景路159弄A座9F－10F）
邮政编码 201101　www.sstp.cn
上海展强印刷有限公司印刷
开本787×1092　1/16　印张 29.25
字数 500 千字
2025 年 1 月第 1 版　2025 年 1 月第 1 次印刷
ISBN 978－7－5478－6569－9/R・2979
定价：258.00 元

编委会名单

丛 书 前 言

　　针灸是我国历代劳动人民及医学家在长期与疾病作斗争中创造和发展起来的一种医学,具有悠久的历史。它是以中医理论为指导,运用针刺和艾灸防治疾病的一门临床学科。针灸具有适应证广、疗效明显、操作方便、经济安全等优点,数千年来深受广大劳动人民的欢迎,对中华民族的繁衍昌盛作出了巨大的贡献。

　　几千年来,针灸不仅对我国人民的保健事业作出重大贡献,而且很早就流传到国外,成为世界医学的重要组成部分,并产生积极而深远的影响。根据世界卫生组织统计,目前有113个成员国认可使用针灸,其中29个成员国设立了相关法律法规,20个成员国将针灸纳入医疗保险体系。针灸的神奇疗效引发全球持续的"针灸热"。针灸推拿等治疗手段成为奥运会运动员们缓解伤痛的新时尚。我国援外医疗队采用针灸、推拿、中药以及中西医结合方法治疗了不少疑难重症,挽救了许多垂危病人的生命,得到受援国政府和人民的充分肯定。不少国家先后对针灸进行了立法,成立了针灸学术团体、针灸教育机构和研究机构。

　　从20世纪70年代开始,世界卫生组织就积极地向全世界推广针灸,在多国设立针灸培训机构,支持创建世界针灸学会联合会,发布了针灸治疗的适宜病症、针灸经穴定位、从业人员培训指南等一系列国际标准,努力推进针灸的国际化与标准化进程。伴随着针灸的全球化应用,针灸针的国际贸易也逐年增长。2011年5月,国际标准化组织/中医药技术委员会(ISO/TC 249)在第二次荷兰海牙年会上,决议成立专门的工作组承担针灸针的国际标准研制工作,由中国专家担任召集人的职位。《ISO 17218:2014 一次性使用无菌针灸针》于2014年2月3日正式出版,成为首个在传统医药领域内由中国主导发布的ISO国际标准。截至目前,ISO/TC 249已发布了7项针灸针的国际标准,为针灸的国际化推广应用作出了积极的贡献。

　　针灸于19世纪上半叶传入美国,在20世纪70年代"针灸热"的影响之下,开始在美国流行。针灸在美国流行的五十年间,经历了三次热潮,完成了法律本土化、教育本土化、职业本土化和医学属性本土化四个层次的本土化。起初,针灸在美国主要用于治疗疼痛症状,后来也广泛应用于变态反应性疾病、糖尿病、艾滋病、各种肿瘤、高血压、肥胖症、戒毒、戒酒、戒烟、化疗或手术后发生的恶心和呕吐、不孕症、性功能不全、神经衰弱、紧张综合征、网球肘、肌纤维组织炎、中风后遗症、骨性关节炎、美容、体外受精、血液病、哮喘等领域。针灸在美国的发展并没有昙花一现,而是入乡随俗,遍地开花。美国的医疗改革给低成本针灸提供了全新的发展契机。中医针灸疗法针对很多病症可以采取非手术的保守疗法,成本低廉,疗效显著。迄今为止,美国 50 个州除了南达科他州、亚拉巴马州、俄克拉何马州 3 个州没有专门的针灸立法之外,其余 47 个州及华盛顿特区都在州议会法中专章规定了针灸师执业法律制度,广泛涉及针灸与东方医学的概念、针灸师的准入条件、教育培训、执业规范、行业组织管理和惩戒规则等内容。

"美国针灸立法汇编"丛书编委会经过两年多的信息搜集,资料整理分析,将美国 47 个州针灸法律英文文本进行了收集、翻译、校对和法律评析,重点展示美国各州现行针灸法律制度的全貌。本丛书共 5 册,按照新英格兰地区、中西部地区、西部地区、南部地区、西南部地区划分。每一区域立法均从针灸人员的法律地位、准入与注册、日常管理机构、职业道德、惩戒报告等方面展开介绍。希望本丛书的出版能为中医药政策和法律的制定者、中医药政策和法制研究者以及高等院校、科研机构中医药学科的研习者们提供参考和借鉴。由于时间仓促、经验不足,可能存在不严谨之处,望广大读者朋友不吝指正。

编　者
2023 年 3 月

目　录

阿 肯 色 州

阿肯色州针灸法[①]

第一节　总　　则

第 17–102–101 条　简称

本章应当被称为《阿肯色州针灸服务法》。

第 17–102–102 条　定义

下列定义适用于本章：

(1)"针灸"系指插入、操作和摘除针灸针,以及在身体特定部位使用其他方式和步骤,通过控制和调节患者的能量流动与平衡和患者的功能来恢复和维持健康,进而预防、治疗或纠正痼疾、疾病、损伤、疼痛,或其他状态或紊乱,但针灸不得被视为手术。

(2)"针灸师"系指根据本章获得执照在本州从事针灸和相关技术的人,包括"执业针灸师""认证针灸师""针灸医师"和"东方针灸医师"。

(3)"委员会"系指阿肯色州针灸及相关技术委员会。

(4)"整脊疗法医师"系指根据阿肯色州整脊疗法法案(第 17–81–101 条及其后各条)获得执照的人。

(5)"艾灸"系指在身体特定部位热敷,或使用加热的针灸针,以预防、治疗或纠正痼疾、疾病、损伤、疼痛或其他病症。

(6)(A)"相关技术"系指使用所有相关的针灸诊断和治疗技术(东方的、传统的和现代的)通过控制和调节能量的流动和平衡以及患者的功能来恢复和维持健康,进而预防或纠正痼疾、疾病、损伤、疼痛,或其他病症的独特的基本保健系统。

(B)如本条第(6)款所述,"相关技术"包括但不限于针灸、艾灸或其他加热方式、拔罐、磁疗、冷激光、电针(包括皮肤电活动评估)、冷敷、离子泵线、生活方式咨询(包括一般膳食指南)、推拿,配合针灸、呼吸和功法技巧的按摩,以及在美国合法和在售的中草

---

① 　根据《阿肯色州法典注释版》第 17 卷第 3 编第 102 章"针灸师"译出。

药的推荐。"相关技术"包括但不限于推拿,但不得涉及脊柱或脊柱外关节的操作、活动或调整。

第 17－102－103 条　资金处置

（a）（1）本章授权的所有费用均为阿肯色州针灸及相关技术委员会的财产,并应提供给阿肯色州针灸及相关技术委员会的财政部,以便按照本章的规定进行处理。

（2）在财经年度结束时,委员会财政部的任何盈余应保留在财政部,并可在随后的年份中用于本协议规定之目的。

（b）委员会收到的所有资金应存入委员会指定的金融机构,并用于完成本章目的和委员会在本章下的职责,包括但不限于:

（1）出版和发行阿肯色州针灸实践法案,第 17－102－101 条及其后各条。

（2）出版及年度发行执业针灸师名录。

（3）调查违反本章规定的行为。

（4）采取行动强制遵守本章规定。

（5）因其依照本章规定的行为而对其提起的诉讼进行抗辩。

第 17－102－104 条　虚假广告

（a）第 17－102－102(4)中界定的人不得以任何具有误导性、欺诈性、欺骗性或不实性的方式寻求赞助或宣传赞助。

（b）根据本节规定,对于第 17－102－102(2)中界定的针灸师,如不称自己为执业针灸师、认证针灸师、针灸医师或东方针灸医师,则构成虚假广告。

（c）根据本章获得执照或认证的人不得自称是医生或医师。

（d）如有违反本节的行为,则可以根据第 17－102－309(a)(4)采取纪律处分。

第 17－102－105 条　公共卫生与健康

（a）针灸师在进行针灸治疗时只能使用预先消毒过的器具。在针灸实践中使用"U"形针是违法的。

（b）卫生措施包括:

（1）在处理针灸针和不同患者之前,应使用肥皂、水或其他消毒剂洗手。

（2）在插入针灸针之前,应使用酒精或其他杀菌溶液彻底擦拭穿透区域的皮肤。

（c）如未通过国家认可的洁针技术课程,任何人不得从事针灸实践及相关技术。

第 17－102－106 条　对违反行为的诉讼

根据阿肯色州针灸及相关技术委员会的要求和授权,阿肯色州的检察官有责任对其管辖范围内发生的违反本章规定的犯罪行为提起诉讼,直至最终判决。

第 17－102－107 条　重新命名为第 17－102－205 条

第 17－102－108 条　重新命名为第 17－102－206 条

第 17－102－109 条　重新命名为第 17－102－103 条

第 17－102－110 条　重新命名为第 17－102－106 条

第二节　针灸及相关技术委员会

第 17－102－201 条　委员会的创建、成员、委任

（a）（1）阿肯色州针灸及相关技术委员会成立。委员会由五名经州长委任为正式成员的人士及一名由州长委任为当然成员的人士组成。

（2）委员会的三名正式成员应为合格针灸师。

（3）（A）应当委任两名正式成员代表公众，其不得在本辖区或任何其他司法管辖区从事针灸和相关技术的工作，也不得退休于受规管的职业，或与其有任何经济利益关系。

（B）公众成员须经参议院确认。

（C）公众成员应当为有表决权的正式成员，但不得参与考试评分。

（4）（A）当然成员必须是根据阿肯色州医疗实践法案第 17－95－201 及其后各条，第 17－95－301 条及其后各条，第 17－95－401 条及其后各条获得执照的医师，其有权获悉所有委员会会议的情况并参与委员会的审议。

（B）但是，当然成员无表决权，不得担任委员会的高级职员，也不得作为处理事务所需的法定人数或多数票。

（5）（A）从 2010 年 10 月开始，该委员会应每两年向众议院公共卫生委员会、福利委员会和劳工委员会以及参议院公共卫生委员会、福利委员会和劳工委员会提交一份书面报告。

（B）根据第 17－102－205 条的要求，报告应包含一份 2009 年至 2010 年 10 月及之后的核证副本，涵盖自上次报告以来期间的所有委员会会议记录。

（C）该报告应包含对委员会职能的全面评估，包括但不限于员工和办公场所是否充足，以及众议院公共卫生委员会、福利委员会、劳工委员会、参议院公共卫生委员会、福利委员会和劳工委员会可能要求的任何其他信息，以使上述部门能够向州长提出建议，即委员会是否应继续存在，或是否应根据州长发布的公告解散和废除。

（b）（1）委员会最初的正式成员须由州长委任，交错任期如下：

（A）一名成员的任期应在一年后届满。

（B）一名成员的任期应在两年后届满。

（C）一名成员的任期应在三年后届满。

（2）根据 1999 年第 536 号法案任命的两名额外成员中，一名任期两年，另一名任期三年。

（3）最初的委员会当然成员的任期为三年。

（4）继任者任期为三年。

（5）未届满任期的空缺应当由州长委任填补。

（6）委员会成员应任职至其继任者被委任并合格为止。

（c）州长可出于任何理由将任何正式成员从委员会中除名，只要证明吊销或撤销其针灸及相关技术执照是正当的。

（d）在过去两年内担任或曾经担任过受委员会审核学校的教员的人，不得在委员会任职。

第 17-102-202 条　委员会成员——资格

（a）阿肯色州针灸及相关技术委员会的每位成员应为美国公民、本州居民，并且在开始执行该办公室的职责之前，须作出《阿肯色州宪法》为州官员所订明的誓言，并须将该誓言送交州务卿存档，而州务卿须随即向每名获如此委任的人颁发委任证书。

（b）每名正式成员还应毕业于著名的针灸或东方医学学院或研究所，并通过国家针灸与东方医学认证委员会认证。

第 17-102-203 条　委员会成员——责任

阿肯色州针灸及相关技术委员会的任何成员在其任期内或之后，均不应为其作为成员履行职责时的任何官方行为所造成的损害承担责任。因此而提出的任何诉讼，一经提出，应在不损害原告利益的情况下予以驳回，费用由原告承担。

第 17-102-204 条　委员会组织——会议

（a）阿肯色州针灸及相关技术委员会应在 1997 年 8 月 1 日起六十日内召开会议，并从其成员中选出一名主席、一名部长和一名财务总监，任期由委员会规定。

（b）（1）委员会有责任每六个月定期召开一次会议。

（2）阿肯色州针灸及相关技术委员会主席或阿肯色州针灸及相关技术委员会秘书可根据委员会任意两名正式成员的要求，随时召开委员会特别会议。

（3）三名正式成员构成委员会任何会议的法定人数。

（c）委员会应根据自己的规则决定向成员发出会议通知和其他事项的时间和方式。

（d）委员会的任何行动均须经委员会全体成员（当然成员除外）多数赞成票通过。

第 17-102-205 条　委员会会议记录

（a）阿肯色州针灸及相关技术委员会部长应保存会议记录和所有申请执照的人员的记录以及阿肯色州针灸及相关技术委员会的行动记录。

（b）部长还应记录所有获得委员会颁发执照的针灸师的姓名、地址和执照号码，以及执照续期、吊销和撤销的记录。

第 17-102-206 条　委员会的义务和权力

（a）（1）阿肯色州针灸及相关技术委员会有权支付其在履行职能时认为必要或适当的任何费用。

（2）本节规定的所有支出应从阿肯色州针灸及相关技术委员会收取的费用和罚款中扣除。

（b）阿肯色州针灸及相关技术委员会有权：

（1）制定适当的规章制度，以履行本章规定的阿肯色州针灸及相关技术委员会的职责。

（2）起诉和应诉。

（3）加盖"阿肯色州针灸及相关技术委员会"字样的公章。

（4）（A）提供部长证书。

（B）经盖章的阿肯色州针灸及相关技术委员会部长的证书应被州法院接受，作为阿肯色州针灸及相关技术委员会会议记录的最佳证据，并且同样根据本章的要求，被州法院接受为对任何人颁发执照或不颁发执照的最佳证据。

（5）（A）通过、发布并修订符合法律的规则，以使阿肯色州针灸及相关技术委员会能够实施本章的规定。

（B）在本法生效之日起三十日内，阿肯色州针灸及相关技术委员会应颁布新规则以取代以下现有规则：第一编、第二编、第三编、第四编、第五编、第六编。

（C）本法案生效日期后的所有拟议规则，均应由阿肯色州医学委员会根据《阿肯色州行政程序法》第25－15－201条及其后各条以书面方式批准，但须先提交至立法会行政规则小组委员会。

（6）记录阿肯色州针灸及相关技术委员会的所有程序、收入和支出。

（7）为申请人设立执照考试标准、组织考试或委托他人组织考试。

（8）（A）出于本章所述的任何原因颁发、拒绝、续期、吊销或撤销针灸和相关技术的执照。

（B）除本章另有规定外，阿肯色州针灸及相关技术委员会对在阿肯色州允许何人可从事针灸及相关技术有专属管辖权。

（9）根据本章实施纪律处分程序。

（c）（1）在履行阿肯色州针灸及相关技术委员会的职责时，阿肯色州针灸及相关技术委员会可对阿肯色州针灸及相关技术委员会司法管辖区内的任何事项进行宣誓和收集证言，并发出传票，从而强制相关人员出席阿肯色州针灸及相关技术委员会会议，以审查阿肯色州针灸及相关技术委员会的任何待决事实或情形，以便阿肯色州针灸及相关技术委员会采取行动。

（2）阿肯色州针灸及相关技术委员会发出的所有传票均应按照法律规定的法院传票送达方式进行送达，所有以此方式送达的人应服从传票，否则将承担不服从法院传票的法律规定的处罚。

第17－102－207条　重新命名为第17－102－307条

第17－102－208条　重新命名为第17－102－308条

第17－102－209条　重新命名为第17－102－309条

第17－102－210条　重新命名为第17－102－310条

第17－102－211条　重新命名为第17－102－311条

第三节　执　　照

第17－102－301条　执照要求

为保障生命和健康，在本州有偿或者无偿地从事针灸及相关技术活动者，均应当按照本章规定提交有关证据，证明其有执业资格或获得执照。

第17－102－302条　2013年8月16日被2013年法案及第1147号法案废除

第17－102－303条　违法实践-处罚-禁令

（a）除本章另有规定外，对未经本章规定取得执照的任何人而言，以下行为是违法的：

（1）从事或教唆从事针灸及相关技术；或

（2）使用任何标志、卡片或装置来表明此人是针灸师。

（b）除本章另有规定外，任何人如未事先获得本章规定的执照或以其他方式的许可而尝试从事本章所界定的针灸及相关技术，即构成轻罪。一经定罪，应处一千美元以上、五千美元以下罚款，或处县监狱中一个月以上、十一个月以下监禁，或两罪并罚。每日应构成一项单独的罪行。

（c）在阿肯色州针灸和相关技术委员会或该委员会的任何成员提起的诉讼中，或者在被指控非法行医发生的县或被告居住的县或在珀拉斯凯县提起的诉讼中，具有一般衡平法管辖权的本州法院有权禁止非法从事针灸及相关技术。颁发禁令并不能使违反本章规定的任何人免于刑事诉讼，但禁令救济应当作为刑事诉讼责任的补充。

第 17‑102‑304 条　申请‑费用‑资格

（a）（1）除非已通过考试并被认定具有阿肯色州针灸及相关技术国家委员会通过的规则中规定的必要资格，否则任何人均不得获得针灸执照及相关技术的执照。

（2）（A）根据本章规定在阿肯色州进行针灸及相关技术执业执照的申请，应采用委员会提供的表格并以书面形式向阿肯色州针灸及相关技术委员会的部长提出。

（B）申请书应由申请人亲自签署，并在有权主持宣誓的官员面前确认。

（3）在申请人有资格参加考试之前，应向委员会提供以下充分证据：

（A）已顺利完成至少六十个学期学分的学时，其中包括科学领域的至少三十个学期学分的学时。

（B）已完成针灸及相关技术课程，并已按照本节所述获得委员会批准的机构颁发的证书或文凭。该计划中接受的培训不得少于四个学年，并且应包括至少八百学时的受监督的临床实践。

（b）在批准针灸及相关技术机构之前，委员会应确定该机构符合职业教育标准。这些标准应规定机构：

（1）将至少四个学年的学习计划作为毕业的前提。

（2）符合委员会批准的国家审核机构的最低要求。

（3）要求参加经过严格监督的临床或实习计划。

（4）仅在亲自上课和就诊后，方可授予针灸及相关技术证书，文凭或学位。

（c）为获得参加考试资格，申请人还必须：

（1）年满二十一岁。

（2）是美国公民或合法居民。

（3）未在任何其他州被吊销或撤销针灸执照及相关技术的执照，也未因任何原因被列入察看状态。

（4）未犯过第 17‑3‑102 条所列的重罪。

（5）不能习惯性使用麻醉剂、毒品或幻觉制剂。

（d）委员会可收取以下费用：

（1）首次申请执照费，费用不超过两百五十美元。

（2）笔试和实践考试费，不包括国家认可的考试的费用，费用不超过三百五十美元。

（3）两年一次的执照续期费，费用不超过四百美元。

（4）执照到期后，延迟续期三十日以上，但不迟于一年，该滞纳金不超过一百美元，不包括任何其他费用。

（5）互惠许可，费用不超过七百五十美元。

（6）年度继续教育提供者注册，费用不超过两百美元。

（7）支付所有合理和必要的行政费用。

（e）（1）（A）如申请人已获批，则应当接受考试。

（B）申请人通过考试的，不退还任何费用，并应根据本章向申请人颁发针灸执照及相关技术执照。

（C）申请人已获批但未出席考试的，不应退还其任何费用，但申请人应有资格参与之后考试。

（D）已获批申请人考试不及格，不得退还其任何费用，由委员会酌情决定是否有资格之后进行重新考试，每一门不及格的科目需支付五十美元的考试费用，最高不超过一百五十美元。

（2）申请人未获批的，应将申请书和一半考试费退还给申请人，并明确说明不予批准的原因。

第 17－102－305 条　考试

（a）考试应采用英语及书面形式，考试应包括以下科目：

（1）解剖学及生理学。

（2）病理学。

（3）诊断。

（4）卫生、卫生设备及消毒技术。

（5）针灸及相关原理、实践和技术。

（6）中草药学。

（b）阿肯色州针灸及相关技术委员会应每年至少举行一次考试，并应当将所有考试的日期和时间以书面形式通知所有申请人。如委员会认为国家考试足以使医师有资格获得本州执照，则可采用国家认可的考试。

（c）委员会应当向每一位已向委员会提交申请并获得委员会批准，且已支付所需费用申请人颁发执照，并且申请人还必须：

（1）通过委员会考试，每科分数不低于百分之七十；或

（2）在国家认可的考试中取得及格分数。

第 17－102－306 条　执照展示

根据本章获得执照的人应当将其执照张贴在其执业地点的显著位置。

第 17－102－307 条　执照续期

每名持证人须缴付每两年一次的执照续期费用，并符合本章所规定的继续教育要求。在执照有效期届满后一年内未续期的，不得续期，也不得恢复、补发或者恢复续期，但符合下列条件的，可以申请领取新的执照：

（1）符合阿肯色州针灸及相关技术委员会的所有现行标准。

（2）参加并通过考试，并支付所有相关费用，如同首次申请执照一样。

第 17－102－308 条　继续教育

（a）阿肯色州针灸及相关技术委员会不得将任何从事针灸和相关技术实践的人员的执照续期，除非持证人向委员会提供出席获委员会批准的一个或多个上两年度继续教育学时不少于二十四学时的证据。

（b）居住在州外的持证人应遵守继续教育的要求。

（c）提供虚假或伪造的出席教育课程的证据，应视为吊销或撤销执照的原因。

第 17－102－309 条　纪律处分－理由－委员会诉讼

（a）执照申请人或执业针灸师的以下行为，应构成阿肯色州针灸及相关技术委员会可采取本条（b）款规定的纪律处分的理由：

（1）企图以贿赂、欺诈或欺骗手段获得、取得或续期针灸执照及相关技术执照。

（2）在任何司法管辖区内，对与针灸实践及相关技术的实践能力直接相关的罪行已认罪或不抗辩，或已被裁定有罪。

（3）以他人的名义做广告、执业或试图执业。

（4）在针灸和相关技术的服务中作出具有欺骗性的、不真实性或欺诈性的陈述。

（5）由于疏忽、习惯或其他原因导致精神障碍、不合适行为或不称职行为。

（6）习惯性地放纵或对成瘾性毒品、违法毒品、酗酒上瘾。

（7）在针灸和相关技术的实践中存在不专业的行为。

（8）在提交与患者健康或福利有关的保险表格、文件或信息时实施欺诈或欺骗；或

（9）故意或反复违反本章任何规定或委员会的任何规则或命令。

（b）当委员会认定任何人犯有本条（a）款所述的任何行为时，其有权：

（1）拒绝向违法者颁发执照。

（2）撤销或吊销违法者的执照。

（3）限制违法者的犯罪行为。

（4）对每项罪名或单独的违法行为处以不超过五千美元的行政罚款。

（5）纠正违法者；或

（6）将违法者列入一段时间的察看期，并服从委员会规定的条件。

（c）委员会不得恢复针灸师的执照或安排向其视为不合格的人员颁发执照，直至委员会确信其已遵守最终命令中规定的所有条款和条件，并且能够安全地从事针灸及相关技术。

（d）根据本节进行的纪律处分程序应按照《阿肯色州行政程序法》第 25－15－201 条及其后各条进行。

第 17－102－310 条　豁免行为

本章的任何内容均不得解释为禁止或要求有关内外科、整脊疗法医师、骨病、牙科、足病学、验光、基督教科学、理疗、美容、推拿疗法或本州现行或未来颁布的法律所定义的任何医疗技术分支的执照。这些专业或治疗方式的特权和实践不受本规则的限制、约束、扩大或任何改变。

第 17－102－311 条　免责条款

（a）本章并不限制、干扰或阻止任何其他级别的执业卫生保健专业人员在其州许可委

员会允许的情况下从事针灸和相关技术。

（b）然而,整脊疗法医师在完成由整脊疗法医师教育委员会认证大学的针灸教育课程后,可以将针灸作为整脊疗法医师训练的一部分。

（c）按摩治疗师在完成拔罐疗法的教育课程后,可以将拔罐疗法作为按摩疗法的一部分。

第 17‒102‒312 条　处方药

第 17‒102‒102(2)规定的针灸师不得处方、分发或施用第 20‒64‒503 条中界定的处方药。

第 17‒102‒313 条　注射

第 17‒102‒102(2)规定的针灸师不得实施注射。

阿肯色州针灸行政法[①]

第　一　节

A. 定义：下列定义适用于本法案中诸条例。

1. "法案"系指《阿肯色州针灸行政法》,如《阿肯色州法典》第 17‒102‒101 及其后各条所示。

2. "针灸"系指在身体上插入、操作及摘除针灸针,以及在身体特定部位使用其他方式来控制和调节患者的能量流动和平衡,以及预防、治疗或缓解痼疾、疾病、损伤、疼痛或其他病症,从而恢复和维持机体健康。针灸不应被视为外科手术。

3. "针灸师"系指在阿肯色州根据该法案获得从事针灸及相关技术实践许可的人,包括执业针灸师,缩写为"L.Ac."。

4. "申请人"系指向阿肯色州针灸及相关技术委员会提交执照申请的人。

5. "委员会"系指阿肯色州针灸及相关技术委员会。

6. "临床经验"系指针灸和相关技术专业达到毕业的要求后,该法案中定义的针灸及其相关技术的实践。一年的临床经验应符合国家针灸与东方医学认证委员会（NCCAOM）的要求。

7. "机构"系指教授针灸及其相关技术专业的学校,经针灸及东方医学教育审核委员会（ACAOM）认证,且根据《阿肯色州法典》第 17‒102‒304(b)条,已获得委员会批准。

8. "持证人"系指根据该法案获得执照的个人,根据本规则第一节 A.3.定义为针灸师。根据该法案第 17‒102‒311 条获得豁免的人不得获得执照,也不得使用"持证"这一描述性术语在阿肯色州的针灸实践中。

9. "艾灸"系指在身体的特定部位使用热敷或使用加热的针灸针,以预防、治疗或缓解

---

① 　根据《阿肯色州行政法典》第 7 卷第 37 编第 1 章"阿肯色州针灸及相关技术委员会规则"译出。

痼疾、疾病、损伤、疼痛或其他病症。

10."办公室"系指用于提供针灸和相关技术实践的实体设施。

11."相关技术"系指中国和亚洲传统医疗技术中使用的技术，第一节B条规定的执业范围中所述的除针灸外，包括中草药。

12."规则"系指根据该法案颁布的有关针灸师、申请人、教育计划、教育机构和该法案所涵盖的一切事项的规章制度。

13."受监督的临床实践"系指根据 NCCAOM 的定义，在适当的监督下观察和应用针灸及其相关技术在实际治疗中的应用。

14."监督"系指对受培训人员或从事临床实践的人员直接进行的协调、指导和持续评估过程，应由委员会批准的针灸及相关技术研究所指定的讲师或导师提供。

B.执业范围：阿肯色州的针灸和相关技术实践是一个独特的初级卫生保健系统，其目标是通过控制和调节人的能量流动平衡以及功能来预防、治疗或缓解任何疾病、损伤、疼痛或其他病症，从而恢复维持健康。针灸及其相关技术包括中国/亚洲医疗技术的所有传统和现代诊断、治疗方法。针灸师的执业范围应包括但不限于：

1.评价和管理服务。

2.检查和诊断测试。

3.安排放射学、实验室或其他诊断测试。

4.利用针、艾灸或其他加热形式，低温、光线、激光、声音、振动、磁力、电流、拔火罐、放血、吸力、压力、离子泵或其他装置或方式刺激身体的穴位或区域。

5.物理治疗的方法和技术，包括推拿、刮痧、指压、按摩及其他针灸及相关技术附带的按摩。

6.治疗性运动、呼吸技巧、冥想，使用生物反馈和其他利用颜色、光线、声音、电磁能等的治疗方式。

7.膳食和营养咨询以及使用治疗性食品、饮料和膳食补充剂。

8.推荐在美国合法和市售的任何中草药、西医草药或如维生素、矿物质、酶、氨基酸、营养补充剂和腺素等药物。

9.关于身体、情感和精神生活方式平衡的咨询。

C.但在阿肯色州的针灸实践不得涉及：

a.对脊柱或脊柱外关节的操纵、移动或调整。

b.开具、分发、注射或使用根据《阿肯色州法典》第20-64-503条定义的任何药物或处方药。

第 二 节

A.1 委员会的构成和职责：除该法案规定的职责外，应：

1.随时召开特别会议。特别会议通知应在特别会议前至少二十四小时向委员会成员、要求通知的媒体和所有其他有关方面发出。

2.按委员会所订定的时间表定期举行会议。定期会议通知应在定期会议前至少三日向委员会成员、媒体和所有要求通知这种会议的有关各方发出。

3. 保存所有已获批的教育计划的档案。

4. 保存所有持证人和临时持证人的档案。

5. 颁发教育计划和教育机构批准证书。

6. 根据该法案的规定,下放其部长职责。

7. 如任何委员会成员连续三次缺席定期会议,且未出席任何期间特别会议时,通知州长。

8. 在每年五月举行的第一次委员会会议上选举出主席、秘书和财务主管。

9. 根据《阿肯色州法典》第 17－102－108 条,履行职责并行使规则授予它的其他权利,或行使合理的法定权力和职责中隐含的其他权力,以及为履行本法案下的职责而合理地行使需要的其他权力。

A.2 公开记录:根据《阿肯色州信息自由法》和《阿肯色州行政程序法》,委员会保存的所有记录应供公众查阅。

B. 委员会会议

(a)定期会议。委员会每六个月至少举行一次会议,可更频繁地举行会议。

(b)特别会议。根据主席或秘书应委员会任何两名正式成员的要求,委员会可在任何时间召开特别会议。

(c)法定人数。委员会法定人数由出席任何会议的三名委员会正式成员组成。为确定法定人数,当然成员不得被视为正式成员。

(d)投票。委员会采取的任何正式行动,均须获得委员会正式成员多数赞成票,即五名正式成员中的三名。对任何官方行动的表决不得包括当然成员的表决。

C. 出台规则

委员会可通过必要的规章制度,以开展其事务并根据法案履行其职责。所有规章制度都应根据《阿肯色州行政程序法》的规定予以采纳。在向阿肯色州立法委员会行政法规委员会提交任何拟议的规章制度之前,该规则应得到阿肯色州医疗委员会的书面批准。

除委员会提议的规章制度外,利害关系方还可呈请委员会根据《阿肯色州行政程序法》修改或增补规章制度。委员会应在其下次定期会议上审议这项书面请求。

第 三 节

A.1 总则

所有有关执照的代理行动都应遵守《阿肯色州针灸服务法》,第 17－102－101 以及第 25－15－201 条及其后各条(若适用)。

A.2 保存当前地址的要求

所有持有阿肯色州针灸及相关技术委员会颁发的执照的人都必须向委员会提供资料,以便委员会能够保持联系,并提供投诉和/或听证会的通知。持证人须在更改业务地址和/或住址后十个工作日内,向委员会发出书面通知。听证通知书通过挂号邮件寄往委员会存档的最新地址。

A.3 首次执照申请

（a）根据该法案及本规章制度的条文,委员会不得向不合格者颁发执照。

（b）所有申请人必须为二十一岁及以上的美国公民和/或合法居民,没有在其他州有任何暂停或吊销的针灸及相关技术的执照,没有因任何原因而被列入察看期,没有被判《阿肯色州法典》第17-3-102条所列重罪,没有习惯使用麻醉剂、药物或幻觉制剂。

（c）每名申请人必须提供一份由申请人签署的陈述书,以及一份经公证人核实的签署书,说明其:

（1）曾在任何其他州获得针灸和相关技术的执业执照,或因任何原因被吊销或受察看;以及

（2）曾被判有《阿肯色州法典》第17-3-102条所列任一重罪。

A.4 每名申请针灸及有关技术执业执照的人,均须按照委员会所提供的现行表格提出申请。所有申请必须以英文填写。

（a）所需物品。每份申请须附有:

1. 第三节 C 条中指明的执照申请费用。

2. 由申请人签署的公证表格,授权向委员会公布有关申请人及其执照资格的补充信息,包括但不限于教育背景、犯罪背景调查、成绩单、证书和教育机构认证信息。

（b）核实:申请人受教育程度的核实范围应包括:

1. 经认证的教育机构出具的证明申请人已完成针灸及相关技术课程的证书或文凭的核证副本。

2. 申请人的成绩单的正式副本,应由申请人收到证书或文凭的认可教育机构直接送交委员会,须核实申请人是否达到所需的学术及临床教育毕业要求,并指明每门学科所完成的科目及学时。

（c）充足的文件:委员会应确定这些文件是否足够支持执照申请。委员会可自行决定,要求任何申请人提供进一步的文件、资格证明和/或要求面谈,以确定其资格。

B. 授权表格

委员会须提供授权执照申请及续期所需的表格。授权表格可无须经委员会准许复制,但不得由任何准持证人以任何方式更改或改动。委员会须向任何公众人士或任何准持证人提供授权表格。可以书面形式,或以电话方式向委员会办公室,或向委员会秘书索取表格。

C.1 执照规定

（a）教育规定:每名申请人须提供充分证据,证明其已完成获批的四年制针灸及相关技术教育计划,并已从根据 C.1.(a)1 批准的学院取得该获批的教育计划的证书或文凭。按照ACAOM 要求,该计划必须包括一项中草药教学。

（1）获批的教育机构及计划。为使委员会决定某机构符合专业教育标准,该机构必须规定至少四学年的学习计划,而该计划必须符合针灸及东方医学教育审核委员会（ACAOM）的教育水平和标准或委员会认为合理的其他标准,并要求学生参加一个受监督的临床或实习计划,包括至少八百学时受监督的临床实践,并只在学生参加课程和诊所后才颁发证书、文凭或学位。外国机构的申请人应提供可证明该机构和项目符合相同或者更高标准的文件。

（2）前提条件：顺利完成大学教育，获得不少于六十个学期学分，包括在相关科学领域至少三十个学期学分，包括但不限于生物学、化学、解剖学、生理学和心理学。

（b）考试要求

申请人须通过委员会批准的国家认可的东方医学或针灸和中草药考试。

C.2 费用：根据《阿肯色州法典》第 17 - 102 - 304（d）（1）-（7）项的规定，委员会须就下列事项收取费用：

（a）初始/互惠许可申请，定为二百五十美元。

（b）每两年一次许可续期或原始和互惠许可，定为四百美元。

（c）延迟续期（除申请费外），定为一百美元。

（d）继续教育提供者一次性注册费，定为二百美元。

（e）行政支持费（年），定为一百美元。

D. 互惠许可：

（a）资格要求。申请互惠许可的申请人应在美国另一司法管辖区持有实质相似的执照。

（1）若其他州的执照与阿肯色州执照实质相似，要求申请人通过 NCCAOM 以下科目的考试或另一州的许可资格要求申请人通过 NCCAOM 以下科目的考试中的任何一种：

i. 东方医学；或

ii. 针灸和中草药。

（2）申请人应持有信誉良好的职业执照。

（3）申请人不得因下列原因被撤销执照：

i. 不诚实的行为；或

ii. 违反法律、规则或道德规范。

（4）申请人不得持有在美国司法管辖区内被吊销或察看期执照。

（b）所需文件。申请人应提交一份完全签署的申请表、所需费用和下述文件。

（1）证明申请人执照来自另一个与阿肯色州实质相似的司法管辖区，申请人应提交以下信息：

i. 该州现行有效执照的证明。委员会可在线或通过电话核实该信息。

ii. 申请人已通过 NCCAOM 东方医学或针灸和中草药考试的证明。委员会可在线或通过电话核实该信息。

（2）为了证明申请人没有如第三条.D.（a）（3），因不诚实或违反法律、规则或道德而被撤销执照，并且申请人没有持有第三条.D.（a）（4）要求的吊销或察看状态的执照，申请人应向委员会提供：

i. 申请人目前或曾经获得执照的所有州的名称。

ii. 申请人目前或曾经获得执照的每个州出具的信誉良好或其他信息的信函，证明申请人没有因第三条.D.（a）（3）所列的原因被撤销执照，也没有持有第三条.D.（a）（4）所述的吊销或察看状态的执照。委员会可在线或通过电话核实该信息。

（c）临时执照。

（1）委员会应在收到申请、所需费用和第三条.D.（b）（1）.i.和 ii.要求的文件后立即颁发临时执照。证明申请人持有另一个司法管辖区的，与阿肯色州执照实质相似的具有信誉良好的执照。

（2）申请人应提交一份完整的申请表以及所有必需的剩余文件，以获得执照。

（3）临时执照的有效期至少为九十日，或直到委员会对申请作出决定为止，以先到者为准。

E. 针灸戒毒专家

（a）戒毒专家应向委员会注册，提供以下任一证明：

（1）完成国家针灸戒毒协会（NADA）认证课程的核证副本；或

（2）另一州针灸戒毒专家的有效认证（或注册或执照）证明。

（b）针灸戒毒专家只能在获得阿肯色州针灸及相关技术委员会执照的针灸师的监督下执业。

（c）针灸戒毒专家只能使用 NADA 的五点耳穴戒毒疗法治疗药物滥用，并不得以任何其他方式提供治疗。

F. 来自没有针灸执照的州的针灸执照申请人

（a）申请人来自不颁发针灸执照的州应在针灸和相关技术领域具有足够的能力。

（b）所需文件。

（1）申请人须提交一份已完全签署的申请表及所需费用。

（2）作为申请人在针灸及相关技术领域具有足够能力的证明，申请人应提供申请人已通过 NCCAOM 东方医学或针灸和中草药考试的证明。委员会可在线或通过电话核实该信息。

G. 军事执照

（a）（1）"自动执照"系指在个人未满足《阿肯色州法典》第 17 章或本规则规定的职业执照要求的情况下颁发职业执照。

（2）本款所称"退伍老兵"系指在非不光彩的情况下被解除现役的美国武装部队前成员。

（b）委员会应授予在美国另一个司法管辖区持有基本同等执照并且有下述情况的个人自动执照：

（1）驻扎在阿肯色州的现役军人。

（2）退伍老兵退伍后一年内申请执照者；或

（3）第三条.G.(b)(1)或(2)规定的人的配偶。

（c）委员会应在收到以下所有文件后授予此类自动执照：

（1）支付初始许可费。

（2）个人在另一州持有基本同等的执照证明。

（3）证明申请人是第三条.G.(b)(1)、(2)或(3)规定的合格申请人的证据。

H. 执照前犯罪背景调查

（a）根据 2019 年第 990 号法案，个人可呈请在获得执照前确定个人的犯罪记录是否会取消其获得执照的资格。

（b）个人必须从委员会取得执照前犯罪背景调查申请表。

（c）委员会的工作人员会在合理的时间内以书面形式对已完成的申请表作出决定。

（d）委员会工作人员的答复将说明作出该决定的原因。

（e）委员会工作人员对申请表作出的所有决定将由个人所提供的信息决定。

（f）不得对委员会工作人员就发执照前犯罪背景调查申请作出的决定提出上诉。

（g）委员会将保留一份申请表和答复的副本，并在正式申请过程中进行审查。

I. 豁免请求

（a）如果个人被判定犯有《阿肯色州法典》17－3－102（a）项中所列的罪行，在《阿肯色州法典》17－3－102（e）项中永久取消资格的罪行除外，如果以下人员提出豁免请求，委员会可基于定罪情况取消潜在申请人资格或吊销其执照：

（1）受影响的执照申请人；或

（2）持有被撤销执照的个人。

（b）委员会可在考虑以下事项后批准豁免，包括但不限于：

（1）犯罪时的年龄。

（2）犯罪的周边环境。

（3）犯罪的持续时间。

（4）犯罪后的工作经历。

（5）犯罪后的雇佣证明。

（6）犯罪后的品德证明。

（7）违法行为与职业执照的关联性。

（8）其他证明申请人取得执照不会对公众健康或安全构成威胁的证据。

（c）申请人如提出豁免申请，必须以书面形式提出，并随附已填妥的申请表及费用。

（d）委员会将作出书面决定，并说明作出该决定的理由。

（e）根据本条规定，对裁决的上诉应遵守《行政程序法》第25－15－201条及其后各条。

第　四　节

A.1 执照续期：每一位执照续期申请人必须提供一份声明，说明其自申请执照或自上次申请执照续期以来，是否：

（a）曾在任何与针灸及有关技术的执业有关的司法管辖区，或曾在执照续期申请人获发执照、核证、注册或在法律上承认执业的任何其他卫生保健专业中，受到任何纪律处分；和

（b）曾被判定在任何司法管辖区犯有任一《阿肯色州法典》第17－3－102条所列重罪。

任何执照续期申请人，如受到第三节 A.1 条内任何诉讼或法律程序约束，均会受到纪律处分，包括拒绝申请、吊销或撤销执照。

A.2 执照期限：执照有效期为1月1日至第二年的12月31日。新执业针灸师须获取执照，且在执照首次颁发日期后的第二年的12月31日续期。如执照在此日期前仍未续期，执照即为到期，而持证人在符合续期规定前不得继续执业。委员会应在12月1日之前向持证人发出续期通知。

A.3 执照续期:除本法案或本条例另有规定外,或依据其他州法律,委员会收到执业针灸师续期申请后,应将其执照续期两年,该续期申请应包括《阿肯色州法典》第17－102－308条和本规则第四节B条中所要求的任何继续教育文件,及第三节C.2条规定的两年期执照续期费用。

A.4 逾期执照续期:

(a)每名持证人应缴付两年一次的执照续期费用,并符合法案及本条例所指明的继续教育要求。在执照期满后三十日的宽限期内(12月31日),不需要加收滞纳金。如执照逾期三十日至一年,则须评估逾期续期费用,而持证人应符合续期的所有规定。执照到期后,不得进行针灸及相关技术的实践。

(b)符合《阿肯色州法典》第17－1－107条规定的条件,并能证明该个人通过了适用的考试,且成绩足以在发放初始执照时获得执照,为了重新获得执照,提供可接受的继续专业教育(CPE)学时数的完成证明,计算方法为持证人持有待恢复注册或无效执照的年数的十二倍,但不超过六十学时。

A.5 到期执照:持证人在执照到期后,不得进行针灸及相关技术的实践,直至根据第四节A.3及第四节A.4续期执照。

B.1 继续教育:委员会不应续期持证人的执照,除非持证人向委员会提交证据,证明在上一个两年期期间内参加不少于二十四学时委员会认可的教育课程或继续教育课程,应包括为卫生保健专业人员开设的心肺复苏术(CPR)课程,并视为所需二十四学时继续教育中的两学时。

不得连续两年重修获批的继续教育课程以获得学分。与针灸或相关技术的教学课程证明可用于最多四个继续教育学时,但须经委员会批准。

B.2 委员会可接受其批准课程或NCCAOM批准课程的学时作为有效的继续教育学时,但文件内须包含:提供者的联系信息,课程信息(包括任何相关的NCCAOM参考),和正式印章或签名。

(a)如该课程尚未获NCCAOM或委员会批准继续教育,持证人应向委员会提交关于该课程的资料,包括赞助或展示该课程的人或组织、该课程所涵盖主题的大纲及该课程的时间。

(b)委员会应就所有提交审批的继续教育课程做出及时答复。如在申请人提交邮戳后六十日内,委员会并没有以书面形式明确否定该申请人提交,该项提交应获批准。

(c)批准继续教育提供者的申请须以个别课程为基础,提供者申请人须负责获取和向委员会提交适当的信息及费用。

(d)如委员会拒绝批准申请执照续期所需的任何课程,申请人有额外九十日以取得所需学时,在此期间申请人可继续执业。如未能在上述九十日内取得适当的学时,执照不予续期。

第 五 节

A. 驳回申请听证程序

(a)如委员会做出初步裁定拒绝执照申请,委员会将以书面形式通知申请人拒绝的理由或依据。申请人如被委员会拒绝颁发执照,可就该项决定提出上诉,并要求在全体委员会席前就该项申请进行听证。申请人应在接获拒绝通知后三十日内,以书面向委员会提出上诉。

（b）委员会须在就拒绝执照而提出上诉后三十日内,就该项申请举行听证会。在上诉听证会至少二十日前,以书面形式通知申请人听证会日期、时间及地点。

（c）委员会及申请人须在听证会前不迟于十日披露所有他们拟传唤为证人的姓名、地址及电话号码,并须提供一份双方各自愿作为证据的证物清单。

（d）申请人不得在听证会举行前就与申请或上诉有关的任何事项与委员会任何成员进行联系,而委员会成员亦不得违反《阿肯色州行政程序法》或《阿肯色州信息自由法案》进行联系。

（e）在听证会中,申请人应有机会通过证词或文件、盘问所有证人,并传召证人陈述证据,供委员会考虑是否批准或拒绝申请人的执照。

（f）委员会的听证受《阿肯色州行政程序法》管辖,而委员会在其程序中不受《阿肯色州证据规则》或《阿肯色州民事诉讼规则》的约束。然而,本条例可作为审裁官的听证指导。委员会主席应就在听证会期间提出的所有动议以及所有证据和程序事项做出裁决。委员会可委任一名公正的听证官来主持或协助委员会。

（g）委员会不得向不合格者颁发执照,除非委员会确信申请人已遵守该法案及本条例所列的所有条款、条件及规定,并确信申请人有能力安全地和道德地从事针灸及相关技术的实践。

（h）如申请人被拒绝颁发执照,则不得再申请执照,直至满足下列任一项:

（1）被拒绝颁发执照之日起满一年的;或

（2）申请人的证书和/或资格的情况或事实发生重大变化的。

B.1 投诉和纪律处分程序

（a）投诉可由任何人通过电话、书面或当面向任何委员会成员或委员会代表提出。委员会应准备投诉表格。该表格可在委员会办公室或委员会秘书获得。书面投诉表应提交给委员会以启动审查程序。如果投诉以电话方式提出,投诉表格应邮寄给投诉人。

（b）委员会秘书须备存一份书面记录,记录接获的所有投诉的日期、投诉人的姓名、地址及电话号码、投诉对象（答辩人）的姓名、提出投诉的方法（例如电话、信件、宣誓式书面投诉等）,以及委员会指示的其他相关资料。

（c）针灸师须让每名患者签署一份具有以下信息的表格:所有执业针灸师都受《阿肯色州法典》第17-102-101条及其后各条,以及阿肯色州针灸及相关技术委员会（ASBART）的规则管辖。患者可以联系 ASBART 进行咨询或投诉。

B.2 受理投诉程序

（a）一旦收到书面签署的投诉,或委员会在会议上因多数成员投票并发起的书面投诉,如委员会有合理根据相信该投诉已违反或正在违反其颁布的法案或条例,则委员会秘书须:

1. 记录收到任何由委员会或任何其他各方提出的投诉的日期。

2. 确定答辩人是否获得委员会批准在阿肯色州从事针灸及相关技术实践,或是否是执照申请人。

3. 分配一个投诉编号并创建一个单独的文件。投诉编号应从投诉提交年度的最后两位数字开始,依次进行编号(例如：11－001)。

4. 在收到投诉之日起七个工作日内,向申诉人发送收到投诉的书面确认书。

(b) 在委员会接获投诉后七个工作日内,以挂号邮件的方式向答辩人提供该投诉的副本及就该投诉相关的所有文件。答辩人也应收到书面形式通知委员会已就该投诉展开调查,答辩人可向委员会提交与该投诉相关的文件。

(c) 在投诉调查期间及在该事项解决前,双方均不得与委员会任何成员联系。

B.3 投诉的审查

(a) 委员会将审查所有针对持证人或申请人发出的书面并签署的投诉文件。

(b) 答辩人应有至少二十个日历日的时间以提供就该投诉的书面答复,并应告知答辩人须提供的所有文件及证物,以支持答辩人的立场。

(c) 如委员会决定需要进一步资料,委员会可发出传票,或雇用调查员、专家或其他能提供必要服务的人员,以协助处理及调查该投诉。

(d) 在调查完成后,委员会将编写一份初步调查结果的书面摘要。摘要不得指明任何当事人姓名,而应指明案件编号,直至该问题确定举行听证会为止。委员会应在举行听证会前,向申诉人及答辩人提供调查结果的副本。

(e) 如委员会认为其不具有司法管辖权,或如委员会确实具有司法管辖权,但发现并未违反规定,则会以书面通知申诉人及答辩人。这封信须给出该案件不能接受调查和/或采取行动的理由(例如,由于法律的限制,或投诉的性质是费用纠纷,或没有违反该法案或规则),或认为该投诉可以提交到另一个机构。委员会的信将于委员会做出决定之日起三十日内送交申诉人和答辩人。这封信将说明委员会的行动和决定的理由,并由主席签署。

B.4 委员会听证会

(a) 根据第五节 B.3(e),除非委员会驳回该投诉,否则上述投诉须安排在全体委员会前进行听证。该事项应仅提及案件编号,并应根据《阿肯色州行政程序法》的规定提出。

(b) 答辩人应在听证会拟定日期至少三十日前收到通知。申诉人也应当收到听证通知副本。听证通知应当对答辩人提出足够详细的指控,以便充分披露和告知违反该法案和该条例的行为。

(c) 答辩人可就听证会通知书自愿提交答辩书。任何对指控的书面答复必须在投诉进行听证会的日期十日前提交委员会。

(d) 答辩人可就通知和投诉放弃听证。放弃听证权利必须是以书面形式,由答辩人签署,并提交至委员会。

(e) 委员会可随时与持证人签订和解协议,作为解决投诉的手段。任何提议的和解协议,必须由委员会在有资格投票的人的多数票表决通过后批准,并必须在持证人或申请人明知而有意放弃其听证会权利后,得到另一方批准。

(f) 依据《阿肯色州法典》第 17－102－206(c)项和《阿肯色州法典》第 17－80－102 条,委员会获权发出传票。

(g) 在任何听证会上,委员会可委任一名公正的听证官主持或协助委员会。

B.5 纪律处分程序

（a）各方须在听证会前不少于十日,互相披露拟在听证会中传唤证人的所有人的姓名、地址及电话号码,并须提供一份双方各自愿作为证据的证物清单。如果对方未拥有所列出的任何证据的副本,则拟提供证物的一方应在提供书面证物清单时提供其副本。

（b）答辩人不得在委员会发出听证会通知后,就任何事项与委员会任何成员进行联系,而委员会成员亦不得违反《阿肯色州行政程序法》或《阿肯色州信息自由法案》进行单方面联系。

（c）在听证会中,任何一方均可提供证据,通过证词或文件,盘问证人及传唤证人。

（d）委员会的听证会受《阿肯色州行政程序法》的约束,其程序不受《阿肯色州证据规则》或《阿肯色州民事诉讼程序规则》的约束。然而,本条例可作为审裁官的听证指导。委员会主席或其委任的听证官员须就在听证会期间提出的所有动议以及所有证据及程序事项做出裁定。

（e）持证人被发现有任何行为触犯本法案,或违反委员会的命令,或违反本条例,委员会可施加以下制裁:

1. 拒绝向申请人颁发执照。

2. 撤销或者吊销持证人的执照。

3. 限制持证人执业。

4. 对持证人的每项罪名或单独罪行判处不超过五千美元的行政罚款。

5. 谴责持证人;或

6. 对持证人进行委员会认为适当的察看,并就持证人的实践施加委员会所指明的条件。

如委员会撤销或吊销针灸师执照,在委员会认为持证人遵守委员会最终纪律处分令中规定的所有条款和条件,并且持证人有能力安全地和道德地从事针灸和相关技术实践之前,不得恢复执照。一旦持证人书面要求恢复执照后,委员会应进行审查,以确定是否应重新颁发执照。

第 六 节

A. 持证专业人员的违禁行为: 如任何申请执照续期的申请人就法案或本条例所涵盖的任何行动或程序向委员会提供虚假信息或作出虚假陈述,将受到纪律处分,包括拒绝、撤销或吊销执照。在做出吊销或撤销持证人执照的最终命令或对持证人施加其他制裁之前,委员会将以书面形式向持证人送达投诉及听证通知。持证人应享有听证权利,而委员会有责任证明投诉中所控事实及违反法律行为。

下列作为或不作为可视为委员会在通知及听证会后采取纪律处分或拒绝执照申请的理由:

（1）专业能力不足: 不具备或者不能应用专业知识,或不能运用针灸师通常使用的技能和治疗手段,并适当考虑所在地区的情况。

（2）未能遵循适当的器械灭菌程序: 未能使用无菌器械或未按美国国家针灸师资格考试委员会（NCCA）发布的《针灸师洁针技术手册》的现行版本,遵照适当的器械灭菌程序,包括使用生物监测仪和保存灭菌周期和设备保养的准确记录。本规定不适用于针刺针,在任何情况下针灸针不得重复使用或消毒后用于多名患者。

(3)未能遵循洁针技术:未能按照美国国家针灸师资格考试委员会(NCCA)发布的《针灸师洁针技术手册》的现行版本中定义的洁针技术。

(4)虚假报告:故意以针灸师身份在实践过程中作出虚假报告或记录,或提交虚假陈述以收取未提供的服务的费用。

(5)州外纪律处分:任何作为或不作为导致针灸师或针灸执照申请人在其他州、准州或国家受到针灸执照委员会或纪律部门或法院的纪律处分。

(6)通过贿赂、欺诈、欺骗手段获得执照:通过虚假陈述或者提供执照申请相关的虚假信息,获得或者试图获得或者续期针灸及其相关技术执照或者临时针灸执照。如针灸师或申请人试图向委员会成员支付现金或提供任何有价值的东西,作为颁发执照的回报,即构成受贿罪。

(7)谎报:以他人名义进行广告宣传、实践或企图实践。

(8)虚假广告:以任何具有误导性、欺骗性或不实的方式进行招标或宣传。针灸师自称为医生或医师也构成虚假广告。

(9)教育欺诈:在针灸和相关技术的教育计划中实施欺诈、欺骗、重大过失或不当行为。

(10)未能保存记录:未能保留反映患者治疗过程的书面记录。记录须保存不少于五年,并须由委员会审查。

(11)未能向患者提供记录:未能按要求向患者或委托人提供由持证人持有或保管,且由患者或委托人准备的和支付的文件副本。

(12)违反保密条款:未征得患者或者委托人事先同意,透露以专业身份获得的个人身份事实、数据或者信息,法律授权或要求的除外。

(13)委托给不具资格的人员:

a. 在针灸师知情或应当知情的情况下,将专业职责委托给不具备履行该职责的教育水平、经验或执照或证书的资格的人员;或

b. 未能对只能在针灸师监督下执业的临时持证人或学生进行适当监督。

(14)为了与患者发生性行为的目的,在医患关系中施加影响:为了与患者发生性行为的目的,在医患关系中施加影响。

(15)不适合执业:继续执业及为患者提供治疗,当持证人:

a. 因疏忽、习惯或其他相关原因而精神不健全或不能胜任的;或

b. 习惯性地放纵或沉迷于成瘾性药物、毒品及酗酒。

(16)保险欺诈:在提交与患者的健康或福利相关的保险表格、文件或信息时故意欺诈或欺骗,或故意允许雇员提交与健康或福利相关的虚假的保险表格、文件或信息。

(17)故意违反:故意或多次违反法案或本条例任何规定,或委员会的任何合法命令。

(18)张贴执照:经委员会批准的针灸师,须在其诊所或执业地点的显著位置张贴其执照;如未能张贴执照,可视为违反职业道德的行为。

（19）公共健康和卫生：

a. 未能在针灸服务中使用一次性消毒针灸针的。

b. 在针灸实践中使用针灸钉的。

c. 未能在处理针灸针前以及治疗不同患者之前用肥皂、水或其他消毒剂洗手的。

d. 在针灸实践中，重复使用针灸针的。

（20）第 17－3－102 条中所列罪行：对第 17－3－102 条中所列罪行已认罪或不抗辩或已被裁定有罪。

（21）不称职和违反职业道德的行为：上述违反职业道德的行为的规定不排除委员会认为构成不称职或违反职业道德的行为的作为和不作为的情形。

B. 紧急措施

（1）如委员会发现公众健康、安全或福利急需采取紧急措施，并将该裁断纳入其命令内，委员会可立即吊销、限制或约束执照。第五条 B.4 的通知要求不适用，且不得解释为在最早可行的时间内阻止听证会进行。

（2）紧急令：

紧急裁决令必须包含一项调查结果，即公众健康、安全和福利迫切需要委员会采取紧急行动。书面命令必须包括通知委员会诉讼程序计划完成的日期。

书面通知：

书面紧急裁决令将立即送交需要遵守该命令的人。将采用下列一种或多种程序：

a. 专人递送。

b. 挂号邮件，要求回执，寄往委员会存档的最后地址。

c. 普通邮件寄往委员会存档中的最后地址。

d. 传真。如果要求遵守紧急令的人提出书面要求，要求委员会紧急令必须以传真方式发出，并提供了传真号码，则传真可以作为唯一的送达方法。

e. 口头通知。除非该书面紧急令在发出当日以专人递送方式送达，否则委员会须尽快以电话方式联络须遵守该命令的人。

f. 电子邮件发送到最后已知的电子邮件地址，并要求立即确认收到。

（3）除非法律另有规定，否则委员会必须在依据本规则 B.(1) 项采取紧急行动后十日内，启动正式的暂停或吊销程序。

C. 自愿放弃执照

持证人可提出放弃其执照，以代替正式纪律处分程序，但须经委员会接受其放弃执照，从而代替正式纪律处分程序。

D. 吊销后恢复

（1）吊销执照的命令可规定任何希望恢复执照的人，向委员会提交一份要求恢复执照的核实呈请。

（2）呈请恢复必须列明以下事项：

a. 申请人已充分且及时遵守本条第五节 B.5(e) 规定的关于被批准的专业人员职责要求。

b. 在执照吊销期间,禁止申请人从事该职业。

c. 申请人的执照费正在或已向委员会缴交。

d. 申请人已充分遵守作为恢复的条件而施加的要求。

（3）任何故意做出对事实的虚假陈述,均可构成拒绝或撤销恢复的理由。

（4）如未能遵循本规则的规定,则不得考虑恢复。

（5）除非阿肯色州针灸及相关技术委员会以多数票通过恢复,否则均不得恢复。

E. 重新申请吊销或放弃的执照

（1）任何已被吊销执照或已放弃执照的人,除非向委员会提出申请,否则不予颁发执照。在吊销或交回执照至少两年后,才能重新申请执照。

（2）申请人须承担举证责任,证明其在吊销或放弃执照后已恢复,且可从事该执照所授权的行为而不会对公众健康、安全和福利造成不必要的危险,并证明其在其他方面有资格根据第 17－102－101 条及其后各条颁发执照。

（3）委员会可对执照施加任何适当条件或限制,以保障公众健康、安全及福利。

（4）委员会可规定要求重新获得执照的人参加执照考试。

北卡罗来纳州

北卡罗来纳州针灸法[①]

第 90－450 条　目的

本节旨在通过建立有序的针灸执照制度,促进北卡罗来纳州民众的健康、安全和福祉,并为制定执照颁发要求提供有效的方法。

第 90－451 条　定义

下列定义适用于本节:

(1) 针灸。针灸系指由传统和现代中医理念发展而来的一种保健形式,采用针灸诊断、治疗及辅助疗法和诊断技术,旨在促进、维持和恢复健康并预防疾病。

(2) 委员会。系指针灸许可委员会。

(3) 针灸实践。系指在针灸诊断基础上,在人体特定部位实施针刺或灸法为主的治疗方法。针灸范围内的辅助疗法包括按摩、器械治疗、温针治疗、电针治疗、电磁治疗以及草药、膳食指南和治疗性运动。

第 90－452 条　禁止无执照从事针灸实践

(a) 违法行为。根据本节规定,无执照从事针灸实践属违法行为。在未持有本款要求的执照情况下,宣传或以其他方式表示自己有资格或被授权从事针灸实践属违法行为,构成一级轻罪。

(b) 豁免。本条不适用于以下人群:

(1) 根据本章第 1 节获得针灸执照的医师。

(2) 在执业针灸师直接监管下从事针灸实践的学生,其实践为委员会批准的针灸学习课程内容。

(3) 根据第 90 章第 8 节获发执照的整脊疗法医师。

第 90－453 条　针灸执照委员会

(a) 成员。针灸执照委员会由九名成员组成,其中三名由州长任命,六名由大会任命。

---

① 根据《北卡罗来纳州制定法》注释版第 90 章第 30 节"针灸服务"译出。

大会任命的六名成员应获得在本州从事针灸实践的执照,且不得根据本章第 1 节成为执业医师。在委员会选举期间,这六名成员无须持有执照,但须符合《北卡罗来纳州制定法》(G.S.)90 - 455(a)(4)、(5)规定的要求。州长任命的三名成员中,一名应为非卫生保健专业人员;一名应为根据本章第 1 条获得执照的医师,且应顺利完成美国医学针灸学会推荐的二百学时的医学针灸课程,获得美国医学会第一类学分;一名应在本州取得针灸执照。在大会任命的六名成员中,三名应根据众议院议长推荐任命,另外三名应由参议院临时议长推荐任命。大会必须按照《北卡罗来纳州制定法》(G.S.)120 - 121 的规定任命成员。

成员应听从任命机构的指示。职位空缺应由原任命机构填补,任期应为未届满期限。大会任命成员的空缺应按照《北卡罗来纳州制定法》(G.S.)120 - 122 的规定填补。

(b)任期。州长最初任命的成员均应于 1994 年 6 月 30 日结束任期。大会根据众议院议长推荐任命的成员,一名应于 1995 年 6 月 30 日结束任期,另一名应于 1996 年 6 月 30 日结束任期。大会根据参议院临时议长推荐任命的成员,一名应于 1995 年 6 月 30 日结束任期,另一名应于 1996 年 6 月 30 日结束任期。初次任命的成员任期结束后,后续所有成员的任期自 7 月 1 日始,为期三年。委员会成员最多连任两届。

(c)会议。委员会每年应在新成员任命后四十五日内至少召开一次会议。在新成员任命后的每年度委员会首次会议上,成员应选出一名委员会主席和一名年度秘书。委员会主席最多连任五届。委员会应在其他时间召开会议以履行其职责。委员会成员的多数构成处理事务的法定人数。

(d)薪酬。委员会成员有权按照《北卡罗来纳州制定法》(G.S.)93B - 5 的规定获得旅费报销和生活津贴。

第 90 - 454 条 委员会的权力与责任

委员会可:

(1)根据其通过的规则拒发、颁发、吊销及撤销针灸执照,并可收取费用、调查违反本节规定的行为,也可以其他方式执行本节规定。

(2)赞助或授权其他单位提供针灸继续教育课程,并批准用于续期执照的继续教育要求。

(3)制定本州针灸学校的课程要求,收取学费以及批准建立针灸学校。课程要求至少应与针灸与东方医学行业协会核心课程标准同等严格。

(4)起诉违反(G.S.)90 - 452 规定的行为。未经授权从事针灸实践,即便无人员受伤,法院也可发布禁令。

(5)采用印章对委员会的正式文件进行验证。

(6)聘用及厘定执行委员会职能所需人员及专业顾问(包括法律顾问)的薪酬,以及为委员会运作而购买、租赁、出租、出售或以其他方式处置个人资产及不动产。

(7)根据需要从本节收取费用所产生的收入和利息中支出款项,以执行本节的规定。

(8)根据《北卡罗来纳州制定法》(G.S.)第 150B 章的规定,制定本节实施细则。

(9)制定实践规范,自 1995 年 7 月 1 日起生效。实践规范应适用于一般和专业领域的实践。委员会应定期审查实践规范,并要求持证者确定使用的规范、护理计划以及根据护理计划使用的治疗方式。

第 90‑455 条　执照资格;续期;非执业、吊销、到期或失效执照

(a)初始执照。要取得针灸执照,申请者必须满足以下要求:

(1)按照委员会要求提交一份完整的申请。

(2)缴纳委员会要求的费用。

(3)提交证明,证实已经顺利完成委员会管理或批准的执照考试。

(4)提供符合下列教育、培训标准或者经验证明之一的书面证明:

a. 顺利完成针灸学院三年研究生课程或委员会批准的培训课程。

b. 在本州申请执照之前,在另一州或其许可条件达到或超过本州条件的另一州的机构连续获得针灸执照至少十年,且在申请执照期间没有受过或即将受任何纪律处分。申请人在提交申请时须证明在申请执照前的十年中,每年至少平均完成《北卡罗来纳州制定法》(G.S.)中的二十项继续教育,即关于针灸或医疗保健的相关研究。

(5)提交证明,证实已经顺利完成针灸和东方医学委员会提供的洁针技术课程。

(6)具有良好品德。

(7)目前没有或从未参与过任何根据《北卡罗来纳州制定法》(G.S.)90‑456 规定构成纪律处分的实践行为。

(8)提交一份由申请人签署的表格,证明申请人有意完全遵守委员会通过的道德标准。

(b)执照续期。针灸执业执照每两年更新一次。在提交所有续期所需的声明、文件和费用后,申请人的执照应在不超过一百二十日的期限内保持信誉良好。在此期间,委员会应开会审查续期申请并采取行动。申请人续期执照须:

(1)按照委员会要求提交一份完整的申请。

(2)缴纳委员会要求的费用。

(3)按照委员会的要求,在每个续期内提交证明,证实已经接受四十个学时获委员会认可的继续教育课程。

(c)非执业执照。持证针灸师在本州内未积极从事针灸实践,且不愿对执照进行续期,可向委员会请示将执照列入非执业状态。自列入非执业状态之日起,执照可保持八年的非执业状态。在申请人证明已修毕四十学时获委员会认可的继续教育课程,并已缴付所有费用后,委员会确定申请人未从事任何违反《北卡罗来纳州制定法》(G.S.)90‑456 纪律规定的活动,且在非执业状态期间未从事任何违禁活动,委员会可重新激活执照。

(d)吊销执照。吊销执照应符合本条规定的续期要求,并可按本条规定续期。在未取消吊销状态前,此续期不授权持证针灸师参与任何执业活动或其他任何违反暂时吊销命令或判决的行为或活动。若要恢复因违纪而吊销的执照状态,持证人应缴纳续期费和滞纳金。

(e)到期执照。因未能根据本条(b)款续期而到期的执照,可在到期后两年内续期。续期日期为委员会批准续期的日期。为续期到期执照,申请人应:

(1)按照委员会的要求提交一份完整的续期申请。

（2）提交完成所有继续教育课程要求的证明。

（3）支付累计的续期费用，以及执照到期费用。

（f）失效执照。因执照到期后两年内未续期或者列入非执业状态后八年内未恢复使用而失效的，视为失效执照。失效执照不可续期、激活或恢复。执照失效者可根据本条（a）款申请新执照。

第90－456条 禁止的活动

执业针灸师或申请者有以下情况的，委员会可拒绝颁发、吊销或撤销执照，要求其接受补救教育或发出谴责信：

（1）从事虚假或欺诈行为，证明其不能胜任针灸实践，包括下列任何活动：

a. 在申请执照或委员会调查相关事项中存在谎报行为。

b. 试图提前收费。

c. 虚假广告，包括承诺针灸可以治愈疾病。

d. 主动向转诊患者的人分摊或同意分摊针灸服务费。

（2）有下列不能正确控制针灸实践行为之一的：

a. 协助无证人士从事针灸实践。

b. 在针灸师知情或应当知情的情况下，将专业职责委托给不具备资格的人员。

c. 对于与针灸师一同参与针灸实践工作的无执照人员，未能进行适当的管理。

（3）未能以适当方式保存下列任何一项记录的：

a. 未能保留描述每位患者治疗过程的书面记录。

b. 拒绝向患者提供由患者准备或支付的病历。

c. 未经同意泄露患者个人身份信息，法律另有规定的除外。

（4）未能对患者进行适当的护理，包括以下任何一种情形：

a. 在没有为连续护理做出合理安排的情况下放弃或忽视患者。

b. 在针灸师与患者的关系中，通过性挑逗、提出性行为要求或将此类行为作为一种治疗条件来施加或试图施加不当影响。

（5）表现出习惯性滥用药物或患有精神障碍，以致妨碍提供有效治疗的能力。

（6）被判有罪或认罪，或对任何证明其不适合从事针灸实践的罪行不予抗辩。

（7）由于疏忽而在执业过程中未能以专业认可的技术水平从事针灸实践。

（8）故意违反本节或委员会的任何规定。

（9）在另一司法管辖区，因任何原因而被拒绝颁发、吊销或撤销执照，且相关行为在本州也应受到同样处理。

第90－457条 费用

委员会可确定费用标准，但不得超过以下金额：

（1）申请和考试费：一百美元。

（2）执照颁发费：五百美元。

（3）执照续期费：三百美元。

（4）执照续期滞纳金：二百美元。

（5）执照复本费：二十五美元。

（6）代理资格证复本费：五十美元。

（7）执业针灸师标签费：一百五十美元。

（8）退还支票费：四十美元。

（9）执照验证费：四十美元。

（10）更名费：二十五美元。

（11）继续教育课程审批费：五十美元。

（12）继续教育课程提供者审批费：二百美元。

（13）首次入学申请费：一千美元。

（14）学校续期批准费：七百五十美元。

（15）非执业执照续期费：五十美元,每延长两年,到期付款一次。

第90-457.1条　继续教育

（a）执照续期申请人应在续期日前的两个日历年内完成要求的继续教育课程。

（b）委员会应对针灸执业范围内的特定科目设置最短学时以及任何与保健服务和与针灸实践有关科目的最长学时。除正式组织的课程外,委员会可以批准事先获委员会审批的课程,如非认证项目的个人培训和教学诊断与治疗。

（c）为本节之目的,一个继续教育课程单位应为一个面授学时或五十分钟。

（d）委员会可选择审核任何已申报及宣誓遵守继续教育规定的持证人记录。对任何持证人的审核不得超过每两年一次。

（e）若未能遵守继续教育要求,则应当禁止续期执照,并在续期结束时使其执照成为到期状态。

（f）因服兵役、家庭紧急情况或长期患病等不可预见事件,持证人可向委员会申请延长完成继续教育要求的时间。委员会可酌情延长执照有效期,最长不超过一个有效期。委员会应不迟于执照续期日前30日收到申请。申请人应证明申请是一份完整及准确的声明,并应包括以下内容:

（1）持证人未能完成继续教育要求的原因。

（2）持证人已修毕的继续教育课程及学时一览表。

（3）持证人对完成继续教育要求的规划。

第90-458条　头衔的使用及执照的展示

"执业针灸师"或"针灸师"的头衔只能由根据本节获得针灸执照的人使用。根据本节取得执照并非授权其自称为医生或医师。每名获准执业的针灸师,应将执照展示在其执业地点的显著位置。

第90-459条　第三方补偿

本节的任何内容均不得解释为要求直接的第三方补偿根据本节获得执照的人员。

第90-460条—第90-469条　保留

北卡罗来纳州针灸行政法①

第0100节 执 照

第01.0101条 执照申请和执业要求

为《北卡罗来纳州制定法》(G.S.)第90-455条之目的,申请针灸执照的申请人应满足下列要求的第(1)~(6)款及(8)款,或满足第(1)~(5)款及(7)和(8)款:

(1) 提交一份完整的申请。

(2) 按照本节0103条规则缴费。

(3) 确保文凭、成绩单、执照或证书、考试成绩或申请所需的其他文件的正式副本由发证单位或其继受机构或指定的国家机构直接转交给委员会。文件应加盖官方或政府公章或附有书面证明。

(4) 申请人若在2004年6月30日或之前已参加国家针灸与东方医学认证委员会(NCCAOM)认证考试,应提交NCCAOM或其继受机构出示的关于其已通过针灸笔试和穴位定位考试的证明。若申请人于2004年6月30日之后参加针灸执照考试,则须提交通过NCCAOM认定的"东方医学基础""针灸""生物医学"和"穴位"四门课程的证明。

(5) 提交通过针灸与东方医学行业协会(CCAOM)或其继受机构提供并认定的洁针技术课程的证明。

(6) 提交满足下列教育要求的证明文件:

(a) 在美国接受过培训的申请人。所有在美国接受过培训的申请人均应自针灸及东方医学教育审核委员会(ACAOM)或其继受机构认可的或获得候选资格的三年制研究生针灸学院毕业。

(b) 在外国接受过培训的申请人。所有在外国接受培训的申请人均应自符合ACAOM课程要求的研究生针灸学院毕业。学院还应获得以下任意一方的批准:

(i) 外国政府教育部。

(ii) 外国政府卫生部。

(iii) 与美国政府负责教育认证的部门相当的政府机构;或

(iv) 外国私营认证机构,其认可程序和标准与ACAOM的认可程序和标准基本同等,并得到与美国政府负责教育认证的部门基本同等的外国政府机构的认可。该教育机构应符合ACAOM的课程要求。

(c) 为证明在美国接受过培训的申请人符合规定要求,应提交如下文件:

(i) 申请人根据教育项目或从政府机构获得证书或文凭,负责该教育项目的机构或该政府机构应将申请人成绩单的正式副本直接用密封信封寄送至委员会。

---

① 根据《北卡罗来纳州行政法典》第21卷第1章"针灸许可委员会"译出。

（ⅱ）负责教育项目的机构或政府机构提交成绩单后,应核实申请人是否顺利完成针灸及东方医学教育审核委员会(ACAOM)学术和临床教育要求,并完成指定的课程和每门学科的学时。

（d）为证明在外国接受过培训的申请人符合规定要求,应提交如下文件:

（ⅰ）申请人根据教育项目或从政府机构获得证书或文凭,负责该教育计划的机构或该政府机构应将申请人成绩单的正式副本直接用密封信封寄送至委员会。

（ⅱ）负责教育项目的机构或政府机构提交成绩单后,应核实申请人是否顺利完成临床教育要求,并完成指定的课程和每门学科的学习时间。

（ⅲ）申请人应自费对所提交的全部文件进行翻译,提交一份准确的英文译文。翻译文件应附有翻译人员的书面证明,证明其精通文件源语及英语,且该译文准确完整地翻译出原文件。每份翻译文件亦须附有申请人的宣誓书,证明该翻译文件是原文件准确完整的译本。每份宣誓书都应在公证人面前签署;且

（ⅳ）在外国接受培训的申请人应自费提交外国学历评估服务处评估的成绩单,据此确定申请人所学课程是否与针灸及东方医学院校委员会所要求的三年制研究生针灸学院的课程相当。主要包括对于符合 ACCAOM 课程要求的科目进行对照分析,此类课程要求在NCCAOM 对针灸笔试与穴位确认考试进行认证时有效。申请人可以向国家认证评估服务协会(NACES)或美国大学注册办公室和招生办公室(AACRAO)的现任成员提出申请。

（7）执业要求:

（a）申请人应满足《北卡罗来纳州制定法》(G.S.)第90-455条的要求。

（b）《北卡罗来纳州制定法》(G.S.)第90章第30节所称纪律处分,是指谴责、吊销或撤销,但不包括警告信、警告或告诫;且

（8）提交一份说明申请人纪律表现的执照记录,以反映其任何谴责、吊销或撤销状态。该记录应由申请人获发针灸执照的各州委员会直接送至北卡罗来纳州针灸许可委员。

第 01.0102 条 《北卡罗来纳州制定法》(G.S.)90-455

执照申请人如寻求豁免本节第0101条的规定,应:

（1）在 1994 年 12 月 31 日前提交一份完整的申请,且

（2）按照本节第0103条的规定缴纳不可退还的费用,且

（3）提供自 1993 年 1 月 1 日起在北卡罗来纳州居住的证明,且

（4）完成以下任意一项:

（a）提交经发证机构认证的文件副本,包括由委员会批准的针灸学院的毕业证明(经批准的针灸学院是指提供至少两个学年的培训,并经所在州或国家认证或批准的针灸学院),或

（b）提交顺利完成洁针技术(CNT)课程的证明,并取得本条第(4)(b)(ⅰ)及(ⅱ)款所述不少于十五学分的成绩,以符合委员会批准的培训计划要求。

（ⅰ）提交在国家针灸师认证委员会考试中得分不低于70%的成绩证明:十五学分;或

（ⅱ）培训:累积十五学分[本条第(4)(b)(ⅱ)(A)及(B)款两类均不低于五学分]。

（A）教育:

（Ⅰ）规划记录完成委员会批准的正式培训计划,每完成一百学时:一学分。正式培训

计划是由其所在州或国家认证或批准的针灸学院。

（Ⅱ）学徒制。在针灸师的监督下进行学徒训练（经针灸师证实），每完成一百五十学时：一学分。

（B）经验：申请人必须在本条第（4）（ii）（B）（Ⅰ）及（Ⅱ）款的任何组合中，累积最少五学分。针灸必须至少占申请人执业过程的90%。若戒烟及减肥疗法占申请人执业过程的40%以上，则该等疗法并不足以符合经验要求。

（Ⅰ）在申请执照前的最近三年内，对不少于一百名不同患者进行不少于二千学时的治疗：五学分。

（Ⅱ）在申请执照前的最近三年内，对不少于一百名不同患者进行不少于四千学时的治疗：十学分。

（5）将所有材料，包括仅可以手写或打印的申请表，提交至北卡罗来纳州针灸许可委员会，北卡罗来纳州阿什维尔市，邮政信箱25171号，邮编28803（North Carolina Acupuncture Licensing Board, P.O.Box 25171, Asheville, NC 28803）。

第 01.0103 条　费用

应当缴纳以下费用：

序　号	缴 纳 项 目	金　额
（1）	申请费（不可退还）	一百美元
（2）	初始两年期执照	五百美元
（3）	两年期执照续期	三百美元
（4）	执照续期滞纳金（附加）	二百美元
（5）	非执业执照续期费（两年续期一次）	五十美元
（6）	执照复本费	二十五美元
（7）	代理资格证复本费	五十美元
（8）	邮寄标签费	一百五十美元
（9）	退还支票费	四十美元
（10）	北卡罗来纳州执照核实费	二十五美元
（11）	更名费	五美元
（12）	继续教育单项课程审批费	五十美元
（13）	继续教育课程提供者审批费	五十美元
（14）	首次入学申请费	一千美元
（15）	两年一次制学校续期批准	五百美元

第 01.0104 条　定义

除《北卡罗来纳州制定法》(G.S.)第 90－451 条所载定义外,下列定义适用于本章:

(1)"执业针灸师"或"针灸师"是北卡罗来纳州针灸许可委员会根据北卡罗来纳州一般法规第 90 章第 30 条授予的头衔。根据(G.S.)第 90－458 条规定,只有在获得"博士"或"博士学位"头衔的情况下,执业针灸师或针灸师才可自称北卡罗来纳州的医生(doctor)。

(2)"针灸辅助疗法"包括《北卡罗来纳州制定法》(G.S.)第 90－451(3)款中列出的辅助疗法。该疗法还包括用于刺激穴位和经络的以下任何方法:拔罐,热法,磁疗和刮痧技术。

(3)"针灸诊断技术"包括但不限于望、听、闻、问、触诊、脉诊、舌诊、腹诊、面诊、五行对应、良导络、赤谷、电针。

(4)"针灸针"与联邦法规第 21 章第 880.5580 条同义,在此通过引用并入,包括后续修正案和版本,可在 https://www.gpo.gov/fdsys/pkg/CFR－2016－title21－vol8/pdf/CFR－2016－title21－vol8－sec880－5580.pdf 免费查阅。"针灸针"包括实心毫针、皮内针、梅花针、揿针和三棱针。

(5)"膳食指南"包括但不限于营养咨询以及食品和补充剂的推荐。

(6)"电刺激"包括但不限于使用经皮电刺激神经疗法、压电电刺激、耳镜治疗和耳穴治疗装置,和Ⅲa 类 5 毫瓦激光装置来治疗或诊断能量失衡。所有激光产品应当符合作为联邦法规第 21 章第 1040.10 条和 1040.11 条规定的性能标准,包括后续修正案和版本,可在 https://www.gpo.gov/fdsys/pkg/CFR－2012－title21－vol8/pdf/CFR－2012－title21－vol8－part1040.pdf 免费查阅。

(7)"中草药"包括但不限于酊剂、专利药物、汤剂、药粉、稀释中草药、冻干中草药、药膏、膏药、药油和搽剂。

(8)"按摩和手法技术"包括但不限于穴位按压、指压按摩、推拿、气血治疗和医疗气功。

(9)"治疗性运动"包括但不限于气功、道家养生功、导引、太极拳、八卦和冥想练习。

(10)"热疗法"包括但不限于艾灸、冷热包敷和激光针灸。激光针灸应按照联邦法规第 21 章第 890.5500 条及后续修正案和版本进行使用,可在 https://www.gpo.gov/fdsys/pkg/CFR－2017－title21－vol8/pdf/CFR－2017－title21－vol8－sec890－5500.pdf 免费查阅。

第 01.0105 条　通过执照互惠获得执照资格

申请北卡罗来纳州针灸执业执照的申请人应:

(1)提交一份完整的申请。

(2)按照本节第 0103 条规则缴费。

(3)已直接向北卡罗来纳州针灸许可委员会提交与该委员会签订互惠许可协议的另一司法管辖区许可委员会的正式信函,证明申请人目前已获得执照并在该管辖区内信誉良好。

第 01.0106 条　姓名或地址更改

凡根据本条获发执照的,如其姓名或地址有任何变更,应在更改后六十个日历日内以书面形式告知委员会。

第 01.0107 条　委员会邮寄地址

所有材料应邮寄至以下地址:

北卡罗来纳州针灸许可委员会

北卡罗来纳州罗利市邮政信箱 10686 号

邮编 27605

第 0200 节 执 照 续 期

第 01.0201 条 执照续期

执照续期的程序及要求如下:

(1)两年续期一次。持证人必须在初次获得执照后第二年的 7 月 1 日续期执照,此后每两年在 7 月 1 日前进行续期。

(2)继续教育。继续教育持证人若要续期,委员会应按照准备的表格核实该申请人是否已完成本章第 0301 条规定所需的继续教育标准。续期表格应包括以下信息:

(a)持证人的身份信息和联系信息。

(b)完成委员会规定的继续教育要求的信息。

(c)有关执照续期及适用情况的声明。

(d)继续教育课程的信息,包括已修课程的数量和每门已修课程的完成数量。

(3)费用。持证人必须缴纳本章第 0103 条规定的续期费。

(4)吊销执照。被吊销执照的持证人在被吊销执照期间,必须符合《北卡罗来纳州制定法》(G.S.)第 90-455(b)款规定的续期条件,否则根据《北卡罗来纳州制定法》(G.S.)第 90-457.1(e)款的规定,执照将到期。

(5)到期执照。若到期执照持有人未收到执照到期通知,并不会免除其满足继续教育要求的责任,即若执照有效,则须满足继续教育要求。这些继续教育学时不适用于后续续期的要求。根据《北卡罗来纳州制定法》(G.S.)第 90-455(e)款,续期执照必须提交经批准的申请材料,提交继续教育完成证明,缴纳因执照到期而产生的滞纳金和所需的续期费。根据《北卡罗来纳州制定法》(G.S.)第 90-455(c)款的规定,在执照到期后两年未续期,或根据《北卡罗来纳州制定法》(G.S.)第 90-455(f)款的规定,如执照列入非执业状态八年内未重新激活,将视为已失效。

第 01.0202 条 取得非执业执照的程序;激活执照

(a)申请执照非执业状态的程序和要求如下:

(1)非执业执照的书面申请。未从事针灸实践的执业针灸师可向委员会提交书面申请,要求将其执照列入非执业状态。

(2)非执业执照有效期为八年,逾期为无效执照。

(b)激活执照的程序和要求如下:

(1)在委员会提供的表格上提交激活执照的申请。

(2)申请人如符合《北卡罗来纳州制定法》(G.S.)第 90-455(c)款所列关于激活执照的要求,应向委员会提交一份经签署的声明,证明其在执照非执业状态期间未参与《北卡罗来纳州制定法》(G.S.)第 90-456 款所列任何违禁活动。

(3)为作出该决定,委员会可以依照本法第 0710 条撤销及吊销执照的规定举行听证。

（4）申请人应向委员会表明，依照《北卡罗来纳州制定法》（G.S.）第90-455款，申请人已于申请前两年内完成四十学时的继续教育课程。

（c）费用：申请人应在委员会通知后，每两年支付一次非执业执照的延期费用。

（d）若申请人已缴付所有费用，完成继续教育课程要求且未从事任何构成违反《北卡罗来纳州制定法》（G.S.）第90-456款规定的纪律基础的禁止活动，委员会应激活其执照。

第0300节 继续教育

第01.0301条 继续教育的标准

（a）除非另有说明，本条所称的一个继续教育课程单位应为一个面授学时或五十分钟。

（b）所有申请人应每两年完成四十个继续教育课程单位。详情如下：

（1）二十五个继续教育课程单位应该与针灸实践有关。在这二十五个继续教育课程单位中，其中十五个应包括针灸针的使用和在人体上施灸的课程内容。剩下十个可以是辅助疗法相关课程内容，包括按摩、器械治疗、热疗、电针和电磁治疗，以及草药的推荐、膳食指南和治疗性运动。

（2）其余十五个继续教育课程单位可以由下列任何组合组成：

（A）十五个与本规则第（b）（1）项所载任何内容有关的继续教育课程。

（B）本条第（e）款所述的医院或机构进行针灸或中医研究的继续教育课程，不超过十门。

（C）在本条第（c）（2）项所述的正式组织课程中教授中医的继续教育课程，不超过十门。

（D）本条第（g）款规定的在同行评审期刊上发表文章的继续教育课程，不超过十门；或

（E）用于获得或维持心肺复苏术认证的两门课程。

（c）为完成继续教育课程单位而修的所有课程应满足以下要求：

（1）经下列一个或多个组织或其继受机构的批准：

（A）针灸及东方医学教育审核委员会（ACAOM）认可或候选的针灸学校。

（B）国家针灸与东方医学认证委员会。

（C）针灸研究协会。

（D）国家针灸戒毒协会。

（E）美国医学针灸学会（AAMA）。

（F）北卡罗来纳州针灸许可委员会（NCALB）。

（2）是正式组织。正式组织的课程应符合下列要求：

（A）课程主办者保存四年的出席记录。本记录应在委员会要求时提供。

（B）教授课程的讲师应持有所涉及领域的执业证书，或具有教授指定课程的资格，根据其所受教育、培训和实践经验，委员会可决定允许其进行针刺技术操作的演示。

（C）该课程应载明课程目标、教学大纲或课程内容描述，并附有课程大纲。

（D）由每位学员通过讲师提供的评价表对所修课程进行评价；且

（E）每门课程结束后，课程提供方应向每名学员颁发结业证书，其中应包括：

（i）课程名称。

（ii）学员姓名。

（iii）全体讲师姓名。

（iv）提供方名称。

（v）课程时间和地点。

（vi）继续教育完成学时。

（d）申请人可通过完成由本规则（c）款第（1）项规定的组织批准的在线课程，获得最长二十八学时的继续教育课程。

（e）在获批医院或教育机构从事针灸或中医研究的申请人可在每个续期内取得十个继续教育课程单位。为获得继续教育课程的研究项目只能提交一次。为了获得研究批准的继续教育课程，必须将以下内容提交委员会审查和批准：

（1）机构审查委员会（IRB）的批准。

（2）研究摘要。

（3）参与研究人员的姓名和证书。

（f）在针灸及东方医学教育审核委员会（ACAOM）认可的教育机构或北卡罗来纳州针灸许可委员会（NCALB）认可的继续教育课程中进行针灸教育教学，每次续期最多可获得十个继续教育课程单位。每三学时（不超过三十学时）可获得一个教育课程学分。所有继续教育课程教学应在开始前得到委员会批准。为获批准，持证人应提交以下信息：

（1）课程名称。

（2）课程内容或课程大纲摘要。

（3）课程地点。

（4）课程时间。

（5）教授时长。

（6）将提供给学生的课程评估副本。

（7）课程费用和退款政策。

（g）在同行评审的针灸或中医期刊上发表文章可以获得十个继续教育课程，委员会应考虑的期刊示例包括：

（1）《中医杂志》。

（2）《美洲中医药杂志》。

（3）《世界中医药杂志》。

（h）任何指定的继续教育课程单位只可用于满足一次续期的需求。

（i）每位持证人应将所有参与的继续教育项目记录保留四年，以此表明：

（1）课程或项目名称。

（2）学员姓名。

（3）全体讲师姓名。

（4）提供方名称。

（5）课程时间和地点。

（6）继续教育完成学时。

（j）依照《北卡罗来纳州制定法》（G.S.）第 90－457.1（b）款规定,委员会可审核任何持证人的记录,以确保符合本细则的继续教育要求。任何持证人每两年接受一次审核。

（k）所有预先批准的申请必须于开课前六十日递交。

（l）依照《北卡罗来纳州制定法》（G.S.）第 90－457.1（f）款,持证人可向委员会申请延长时间。

第 0400 节　执业范围和程序

第 01.0401 条　执业范围

以下是北卡罗来纳州针灸师的执业范围:

（1）执业针灸师应在经国家针灸与东方医学院校认可委员会认可的学院或候选学院提供的培训范围内开展执业。

（2）执业针灸师应在其培训范围内执业。患者的诊断和治疗参数包括"五行""八纲""阴阳理论""经络理论""脏腑理论""六经"和"卫气营血"。

第 01.0402 条　针灸程序

针灸实践应遵循以下程序:

（1）执业环境:

（a）治疗应在提供隐私和保密的环境中进行。

（b）若在公共环境的社区针灸诊所中从事针灸实践,则应在患者首次治疗前获得并保留每位患者签署的放弃在私密场所治疗权利的同意书。

（c）每一间针灸诊所应始终保持清洁,并应设有无障碍洗手间。

（d）应满足所有经修订或替换的适用的职业安全与健康标准（OSHA）,包括血源性病原体相关标准,此类标准可在 https://www.gpo.gov/fdsys/pkg/CFR－2017－title29－vol6/pdf/CFR－2017－title29－vol6－sec1910－1030.pdf 免费查阅。

（e）所有针灸实践和记录的保存应符合所有与医疗记录保密性有关的州和联邦法律法规,包括经修订或替换的 HIPAA 法案制定的安全和隐私法规,包括联邦法规第 45 章第 160 节,可在 https://www.gpo.gov/fdsys/pkg/CFR－2017－title45－vol1/pdf/CFR－2017－title45－vol1－part160.pdf 免费查阅。包括第 164 节 A 和 E 分节,可分别在 https://www.gpo.gov/fdsys/pkg/CFR－2017－title45－vol1/pdf/CFR－2017－title45－vol1－part164－subpartA.pdf 和 https://www.gpo.gov/fdsys/pkg/CFR－2017－title45－vol1/pdf/CFR－2017－title45－vol1－part164－subpartE.pdf 免费查阅。

（2）持证人在治疗前应从患者处获得包括以下信息的书面或口头形式的病史:

（a）信息应包括当前和过去患过的疾病、治疗史、住院史、当前使用的药物和药物过敏史。

（b）包括使用烟草、酒精、咖啡因和娱乐性药物的社会史。

（c）应列出现有执业医师的名字。

（d）应概述目前的诉求以及已经尝试和正在进行的疗法。

（e）应确定是否怀孕或体内是否存在生物医学装置,如人工关节或心脏起搏器。

（3）费用。治疗前应提供有关费用的信息。

（4）承诺。对于能否治疗成功,不给予任何明示或暗示的承诺。应提供合理的治疗时间和通常的治疗结果。

（5）诊断:

（a）诊断应采用本章第0104(2)款所列的与东方医学传统有关以及在针灸及东方医学教育审核委员会(ACAOM)教育计划范围内的方法。

（b）每次就诊时应记录所有使用的针灸诊断技术。

（6）治疗。每次就诊时应记录治疗的具体内容。治疗应符合在针灸培训计划中获得的亚洲和生物医学知识。

（7）医疗记录。每次患者就诊和沟通的日期记录应保存七年。在共享任何患者信息之前,应获得公布病历的授权。在得到授权后,应将医疗记录发放给患者。《北卡罗来纳州制定法》(G.S.)第90-411款规定了卫生保健提供者可以就医疗记录副本收取的费用数额。持证人向患者收取病历费用时,应遵循《北卡罗来纳州制定法》(G.S.)第90-411款所写的或随后修订的规定。

（8）治疗无效:

（a）若对患者的治疗无效,则应考虑其他治疗方式或转诊给其他卫生保健专业人员。

（b）对于持续性、不明原因的疼痛,或持续治疗过程中任何情况都无法解释的恶化病症,应进行转诊或咨询。在选择转诊时,应优先考虑曾就诊过的执业医师。

（c）应当始终尊重患者的要求,提供关于其他治疗形式的信息或转诊至另一名卫生保健专业人员的请求。

第0500节　针灸学校和学院

第01.0501条　在北卡罗来纳州建立针灸学校的资格

（a）为本条之目的,"针灸项目"系指由学术机构持续提供的针灸培训。

（b）除了满足《北卡罗来纳州制定法》(G.S.)第90-454(3)款的要求,为获批针灸学院,所设机构必须符合下列标准:

（1）提交一份完整的申请。

（2）按照本章第0103条规则缴费。

（3）提供至少三个学年、六个学期、九个季度或二十七个月针灸课程,时长至少为一千八百学时,其中至少包括九百学时的教学及理论培训以及六百五十学时的督导临床实习。六百五十学时的临床培训至少包括四百学时的实操治疗。

（4）开课一年内,在国家针灸和东方医学院校认证委员会取得候选资格,并在多年的执业中维持资格。

（5）提供成绩单(作为学生成绩记录的一部分),包括以下内容:姓名、地址、出生日期、课程名称、所获成绩、每门课程的学时数。

（6）只有当学生顺利完成针灸教育培训,参加所有必修课程并达到培训要求后,才能授予文凭。

第0700节　行政程序

第01.0701条　对委员会拒绝颁发执照决定的行政复议

当北卡罗来纳州针灸许可委员会确定申请人未能满足其申请资格而拒发执照时,应立即通知申请人其决定,并说明申请人在何方面未能满足要求。若申请人在收到委员会的决定后六十日内向委员会秘书所在地北卡罗来纳州加纳市阿弗斯波罗路 1418 号(邮编 27529)(1418 Aversboro Rd.,Garner,NC 27529)提交或邮寄复议,应为该申请人举办有争议案件听证会,并阐明该要求的原因。委员会应在收到此类请求后二十日内通知申请人公开听证会的时间和地点,并应在六十日内举行听证会。申请人须承担提请委员会进行执照资格审查的责任。听证会后,委员会须决定申请人是否有权获发执照。

第01.0702条　提交投诉

(a)总则。任何有理由相信执业针灸师违反针灸法律的人都可以向北卡罗来纳州针灸许可委员会提交投诉。投诉应向北卡罗来纳州针灸许可委员会秘书提交,地址为北卡罗来纳州加纳市阿弗斯波罗路 1418 号(1418 Aversboro Rd.,Garner,NC 27529),邮编 27529。

(b)投诉形式。投诉可以是正式或非正式,但必须以书面形式提出:

(1)非正式投诉。委员会应将任何违反针灸管理法律且对投诉人最有利的书面函件,视为非正式投诉。

(2)正式投诉。投诉人应在秘书提供的表格上以书面形式正式宣誓提出投诉。投诉书应写明被指控违反的法规则,并简要陈述构成违法的作为和不作为,包括所述作为或不作为发生的日期。

(c)秘书对投诉的回应。秘书应审查任何投诉,以确定是否存在有重大或轻微违规。若秘书确定所指控的违规行为是轻微的,应设法与投诉人和被投诉的针灸师进行非正式沟通以解决投诉。若秘书确定所指控的违规行为是重大的,且投诉人尚未提出正式起诉,应协助投诉人提出正式起诉。

第01.0703条　合理根据的确定

(a)总则。北卡罗来纳州针灸许可委员会应当对正式投诉进行调查。委员会应举行听证会,以确定是否有合理根据相信被指控针灸师违反有关针灸法律。

(b)听证会通知。秘书应至少在合理根据听证会开始前十五日,以挂号邮件通知被投诉的针灸师。

(c)召开合理根据听证会。合理根据听证会应是非正式的。秘书可酌情制定为便于审查证据所必需的程序。委员会可以在合理根据听证会上审议证据,若在有争议案件的听证会上提出证据,则这些证据不予受理。

(d)委员会采取的行动。在审查合理根据听证会上所提出证据后,委员会可在正式投诉中处理每项指控,详情如下:

(1)若无合理根据,认为已经发生违反《北卡罗来纳州制定法》(G.S.)第 90 – 456 款的行为,则可以驳回指控。

(2)若答辩人承认该项指控,可以指示其停止违反《北卡罗来纳州制定法》(G.S.)第

90 - 456 款的行为。

（3）若指控被驳回并找到合理根据，或指控已被承认，但其严重性足以实施适当的惩罚性制裁，则申诉人应将控诉提交委员会，由其依照《北卡罗来纳州制定法》（G.S.）150B 章第3A 条酌情决定。

第 01.0704 条　非正式程序

（a）除根据《北卡罗来纳州制定法》（G.S.）第 90 - 456 款举行正式听证会外，委员会还可采取非正式程序，以非正式方式解决争端事项。获得委员会颁发执照或其他授权从事针灸实践的人士可被邀请参加委员会的非正式会议，讨论委员会认为适当的事项。不得对此类程序进行公开记录，也不得宣誓作证。以非正式方式出席委员会会议的人士讨论的事项，可在其后举行的正式听证会（若举行）中当作对该人不利的证据。

（b）此类非正式会议结果是，委员会可以建议该人采取某些行动，可以为其提供机会，签署将成为公开记录的同意令，也可以就该人提起有争议的案件，或者可以就每一案件采取委员会认为适合的其他行动。

（c）非正式会议不作出席要求，被邀请者可自行决定是否出席。应邀参加非正式会议的人可以聘请律师出席此类会议。

第 01.0705 条　举行正式听证会

（a）根据《北卡罗来纳州制定法》（G.S.）第 90 - 456 款，北卡罗来纳州针灸许可委员会可给予执业针灸师或申请人纪律处分。

（b）在收到任何有能力提供信息作为行动依据的人的书面请求和证实信息后，北卡罗来纳州针灸许可委员会应进行充分调查，以确定是否存在合理原因以采取纪律处分。

（c）该人士有机会在下次委员会会议上举行听证。

第 01.0706 条　延期审理

任何被传唤出席有争议案件听证会的人士，均可通过向委员会执行秘书提交申请以寻求延期审理，只要延期审理的原因已知且合理，就可以提出具体的延期审理动议。由于个人或家庭疾病、死亡或天灾等原因，应准予延期。延期的动议应由委员会主席及执行秘书作出裁决，如无委员会主席，则由秘书及执行秘书作出裁决。

第 01.0707 条　因个人偏见而取消资格

任何被传唤出席有争议案件听证会的人士，均可基于个人偏见或其他理由，质疑任何一名委员是否适合及胜任听证有关该名人士的证据，并权衡此类证据。应以动议的方式陈述质疑，并附有宣誓书，具体说明质疑的理由，并应在收到信后十四日内向委员会执行秘书提出。本条所载的任何规定，均不得阻止被传唤出席有争议案件听证会的人士就委员会成员对该宗案件的了解情况及个人偏见，向其进行个人询问。

第 01.0708 条　保留作将来编纂之用

第 01.0709 条　吊销执照的程序

（a）若北卡罗来纳州针灸许可委员会确定存在根据《北卡罗来纳州制定法》（G.S.）第90 - 456 款给予纪律处分的合理原因，则委员会应准备书面指控并确定应采取的行动。

（b）委员会应向该人提供书面指控的副本，并通知该人，除非该人在收到通知后的六十日内依照《北卡罗来纳州制定法》(G.S.)150B 章第 3A 条提起行政诉讼,否则委员会将采取确定的行动。通知将以挂号邮件寄出,要求回执。

(c) 若该人提起行政诉讼,北卡罗来纳州针灸许可委员会应推迟对该事项的最终行动,直至诉讼完成。若该人未在收到通知后六十日内提起行政诉讼,北卡罗来纳州针灸许可委员会可在下次会议上实施确定的行动。

(d) 北卡罗来纳州针灸许可委员会可以恢复吊销或撤销的执照,也可以在申请和证明符合委员会要求后授予新的执照。

第 01.0710 条　撤销或吊销执照前的听证

在委员会撤销、限制或吊销其颁发的任何执照之前,应向持证人发出书面通知,说明对其提出的指控、控告或投诉的一般性质。本通知可由委员会指定的一名或多名委员会成员组成的委员会拟备,并述明该持证人将有机会在该通知所述的时间和地点或此后委员会指定的时间和地点就该指控或投诉进行听证。委员会应在自该持证人送达该通知之日起不少于三十日内举行听证,在听证期间,持证人可亲自出席听证会及通过律师代为出席,也可讯问证人并为其自身提交证据。

第 01.0711 条　申请变更规则的规定

任何人士如欲申请通过、修订或废除规则,应向委员会提交下列资料:

(1) 拟议规则的草案或规则的修正案。

(2) 提案理由。

(3) 现有规则的效果。

(4) 支撑该提案的数据。

(5) 对所涉领域现有做法的影响,包括成本。

(6) 最有可能受影响的人的姓名及地址。

(7) 呈请人的姓名和地址。北卡罗来纳州针灸许可委员会应就驳回申请或启动规则制定程序作出决定。

佛 罗 里 达 州

佛罗里达州针灸法[①]

第 **457.01** 条　在 **1955** 年《佛罗里达州制定法》中重新编号为 **485.011**

详见 F.S.A. § 485.011。

第 **457.011** 条　根据 **1976** 年《佛罗里达州制定法》第 **76 – 168** 章第 **3** 条；**1979** 年《佛罗里达州制定法》第 **79 – 165** 章第 **1** 条废止

第 **457.02** 条　在 **1955** 年《佛罗里达州制定法》中重新编号为 **485.021**

详见 F.S.A. § 485.021。

第 **457.021** 条　根据 **1976** 年《佛罗里达州制定法》第 **76 – 168** 章第 **3** 条；**1979** 年《佛罗里达州制定法》第 **79 – 165** 章第 **1** 条废止

第 **457.03** 条　在 **1955** 年《佛罗里达州制定法》中重新编号为 **485.031**

详见 F.S.A. § 485.031。

第 **457.031** 条　根据 **1976** 年《佛罗里达州制定法》第 **76 – 168** 章第 **3** 条；**1979** 年《佛罗里达州制定法》第 **79 – 165** 章第 **1** 条废止

第 **457.04** 条　在 **1955** 年《佛罗里达州制定法》中重新编号为 **485.041**

现见于佛罗里达州制定法注释版第 485.041 条

第 **457.041** 条　根据 **1976** 年《佛罗里达州制定法》第 **76 – 168** 章第 **3** 条；**1979** 年《佛罗里达州制定法》第 **79 – 165** 章第 **1** 条废止

第 **457.05** 条　在 **1955** 年《佛罗里达州制定法》中重新编号为 **485.051**

现见于《佛罗里达州制定法》注释版第 485.051 条

第 **457.051** 条　根据 **1976** 年《佛罗里达州制定法》第 **76 – 168** 章第 **3** 条；**1979** 年《佛罗里达州制定法》第 **79 – 165** 章第 **1** 条废止

第 **457.06** 条　在 **1955** 年《佛罗里达州制定法》中重新编号为 **485.061**

详见 F.S.A. § 485.061。

---

① 　根据《佛罗里达州制定法》注释版第 32 卷第 457 章"针灸"译出。

第 457.061 条　根据 1976 年《佛罗里达州制定法》第 76－168 章第 3 条;1979 年《佛罗里达州制定法》第 79－165 章第 1 条废止

第 457.07 条　在 1955 年《佛罗里达州制定法》中重新编号为 485.071

现见于《佛罗里达州制定法》注释版第 485.071 条

第 457.071 条　根据 1976 年《佛罗里达州制定法》第 76－168 章第 3 条;1979 年《佛罗里达州制定法》第 79－165 章第 1 条废止

第 457.08 条　在 1955 年《佛罗里达州制定法》中重新编号为 485.081

现见于《佛罗里达州制定法》注释版第 485.081 条

第 457.081 条　根据 1976 年《佛罗里达州制定法》第 76－168 章第 3 条;1979 年《佛罗里达州制定法》第 79－165 章第 1 条废止

第 457.09 条　在 1955 年《佛罗里达州制定法》中重新编号为 485.091

现见于《佛罗里达州制定法》注释版第 485.091 条

第 457.091 条　根据 1976 年《佛罗里达州制定法》第 76－168 章第 3 条;1979 年《佛罗里达州制定法》第 79－165 章第 1 条废止

第 457.10 条　根据 1976 年《佛罗里达州制定法》第 76－168 章第 3 条;1979 年《佛罗里达州制定法》第 79－165 章第 1 条废止

第 457.101 条　立法声明

为了保护公民的健康、安全和福利,立法机关基于公共健康利益的考虑管理本州的针灸实践,使这种医疗技术能够为所需之人使用。

第 457.102 条　定义

下列定义适用于本章:

（1）"针灸"系指基于中国传统医学理念和现代东方医学技术,采用针灸诊断、治疗及辅助疗法和诊断技术,旨在促进、维持和恢复健康并预防疾病的一种初级保健形式。针灸应包括但不限于在人体特定部位插针、施灸,以及使用电针、气功、东方按摩、草药疗法、膳食指南和其他辅助疗法,以上根据委员会规则进行定义。

（2）"针灸师"系指按本章规定获得执照,作为初级卫生保健提供者从事针灸实践的人。

（3）"委员会"系指针灸委员会。

（4）"执照"系指部门对从事针灸实践的人员出具的授权文件。

（5）"部门"系指卫生部门。

（6）"东方医学"系指使用针灸、电针、气功、东方按摩、草药疗法、膳食指南和其他辅助疗法。

（7）"处方权"系指针灸和东方医学实践中针具和器械、限制用器械和处方用器械的处方、管理和使用。

第 457.103 条　针灸委员会;成员资格;任命和任期

（1）针灸委员会在部门内设立,由七名成员组成,由州长任命,并经参议院批准。委员会的五名成员必须是佛罗里达州执业针灸师。两名成员必须为非专业人员,即当前和过去均不是针灸师或任何密切相关职业的专业人员。委员会成员的任期为四年,或未届满期限的剩余任期。

（2）第456章有关委员会的所有条文均适用。

第457.104条　规则制定权

委员会有权根据《佛罗里达州制定法》第120.536（1）款和120.54条通过规则，以实施本章赋予其职责的规定。

第457.105条　执照资格和费用

（1）任何人在本州从事针灸实践均属违法行为，除非此人已获得委员会颁发的执照、正在接受委员会批准的研究课程或本章另有豁免。

（2）任何人如向部门提出申请，且满足以下条件的，可获发针灸执照：

（a）年满二十一岁，具有良好品德，并且有能力用英语沟通，这种能力可通过国家英语笔试证明，如果以外语进行笔试，则还应通过国家认可的英语水平考试。

（b）从经认证的高等院校完成六十学分认证，作为报名获授权的三年针灸和东方医学课程学习的前提，并已完成三年针灸和东方医学课程的学习，且于2001年7月31日起，完成四年针灸和东方医学课程的学习，课程符合委员会所规定的标准，这些标准包括但不限于顺利完成西方解剖学、生理学、病理学、生物医学术语、急救、心肺复苏（CPR）等专业课程。但是，任何在1997年8月1日之前报名参加了获授权的针灸课程学习的，必须完成两年课程的学习，并达到委员会规定的标准，包括但不限于顺利完成西方解剖学、生理学和病理学的专业课程。

（c）已经顺利完成了委员会批准的国家认证程序，在考试要求与本州基本同等或更严格的州持有有效执照，或通过部门的考试，该考试旨在测试申请人的针灸和东方医学实践的能力和知识。应任何申请人的要求，在考试中应使用穴位的东方术语。该考试应包括现代、传统针灸和东方医学所需知识和技能的实践考试，包括诊疗技术和操作方法。

（d）支付委员会规则所规定的费用，但不得超过以下金额：

1. 考试费：五百美元，加上每个申请人的实际支出，用于购买委员会批准的国家机构的书面和实践考试。

2. 申请费：三百美元。

3. 复试费：五百美元，加上每个申请人的实际支出，用于购买委员会批准的国家机构的书面和实践考试。

4. 两年一次的初始执照费：如果在两年期的前半期获得执照，则支付四百美元；如果在两年期的后半期获得，则支付二百美元。

第457.107条　执照续期；继续教育

（1）部门在收到执照续期申请后，须按委员会规则规定的费用续期，费用不超过五百美元。

（2）部门应制定规则，建立两年一次的执照续期程序。

（3）委员会须在规则中规定每两年不超过三十学时继续教育的要求，作为执照续期的条件。凡有助于提高、拓展或加强与针灸实践有关的专业技能和知识的教育计划，无论是非营利性或营利实体组织的，均有资格获得批准。继续专业教育的要求必须是针灸或东方医学科目,包括但不限于解剖学、生物科学、辅助疗法、卫生和消毒、急救方案和疾病学。委员会可以为每个继续教育提供者设定不超过一百美元的费用。持证人应当在其记录中保存完成继续专业教育要求的证书。经批准,所有国家和州的针灸和东方医学机构、学校均可根据本款提供继续专业教育。

第 457.108 条　非执业状态;到期;重新激活执照

(1) 经向部门申请,非执业执照可根据本条重新激活。委员会应在规则中规定继续教育要求,作为重新激活执照的条件。执照处于非执业状态期间,继续教育要求不得超过十个学时。此外,还必须在执照列为非执业状态之日完成续期所需的学时。

(2) 委员会必须制定有关非执业状态的申请程序、非执业执照续期及重新激活执照的规则。委员会应根据规则规定非执业状态的申请费、续期费、逾期费和重新激活执照的费用。这些费用不得超过委员会为执业执照规定的两年一次的续期费用。

(3) 部门不得重新激活执照,除非非执业执照或逾期执照的持证人已支付任何适用的两年续期费或逾期费,或两者都支付,并支付了重新激活费。

第 457.108.5 条　感染控制

在 1986 年 11 月 1 日之前,委员会须制定有关预防感染、安全处置任何可能的传染性物质及其他保护公众健康、安全和福利相关要求的规则。从 1997 年 10 月 1 日开始,所有用在患者身上的针灸针都必须是无菌的、一次性的,而且每根针只能使用一次。

第 457.109 条　纪律处分;理由;委员会的行动

(1) 根据《佛罗里达州制定法》456.072(2)的规定,以下行为构成不予颁发执照或给予纪律处分的理由:

(a) 企图通过贿赂、欺诈性的不实陈述或部门的差错来获得或续期针灸执照。

(b) 针灸执照被其他州、准州或国家的发证机构撤销、吊销或采取其他行动,包括不予颁发针灸执照。

(c) 在任何司法管辖区被判有罪,无论判决如何,而该罪行与针灸实践或实践能力有直接关系。为本章之目的,任何不抗辩答辩应视为定罪。

(d) 发布虚假、欺骗性的或误导性的广告或发布声称针灸能治疗任何疾病的广告。

(e) 以他人名义进行广告宣传、执业或者企图执业。

(f) 持证人明知任何人有违反本章或部门规则的行为而未向部门通报。但是,持证人明知他人由于疾病,或使用酒精、毒品、麻醉剂、化学品或任何其他类型的物质,或由于精神、身体病症而无法在保证患者安全的情况下采取合理手段为患者提供针灸服务,可以向第456.076 条中所述的残障从业者计划的顾问报告,而无须向部门报告。

(g) 帮助、协助、促使、雇用或建议任何无证人士违反本章或部门规则从事针灸实践。

(h) 没有履行任何法定或法律义务的执业针灸师。

(i) 制作或提交持证人明知是虚假的报告,故意或大意地未按照州或联邦法律的要求提交报告或记录,故意妨碍或阻碍提交报告或诱导他人故意妨碍或阻碍提交报告。此类报告或记录应仅包括以执业针灸师身份签署的报告或记录。

(j) 在患者针灸师关系中施加影响,以使患者发生性行为。应推定患者无法自由、充分和知情地同意与其针灸师发生性行为。

（k）在针灸实践中作出欺骗性、不真实或欺诈性的陈述，或在针灸实践中使用不符合社会普遍治疗标准的方案或技巧。

（l）通过欺诈、恐吓、不当影响或实施一系列过分或无理的行为，亲自或通过代理人招揽患者，直接或隐晦地要求接受治疗者立即口头回应任何要求。

（m）没有保存证明患者治疗过程的书面医疗记录。

（n）对患者施加影响，为持证人或第三方的经济利益而剥削患者。

（o）由于疾病，或使用酒精、毒品、麻醉剂、化学品或任何其他类型的物质，或由于精神、身体病症而无法在保证患者安全的情况下采取合理手段为患者提供针灸服务。在执行本项规定期间，经州卫生局局长或其指定人员发现，由于上述的原因，有理由认为持证人无法担任针灸师，部门有权发出命令，强迫持证人接受部门指定医生的精神、体格检查。如果持证人拒绝服从该命令，要求此类检查的命令可向持证人所在地巡回法院申请强制执行。被申请执行的持证人不得在任何公开法庭记录或文件中以名字缩写命名，并且该程序不向公众开放。部门有权采用《佛罗里达州制定法》第51.011条规定的简易程序。因本款受影响的针灸师应在合理的时间间隔内向患者证明他或她能够以合理的手段，在保证患者安全的情况下恢复并胜任针灸工作。本项规定的任何程序中，程序记录或部门命令均不得在任何其他程序中被用来反对针灸师。

（p）出现严重的医疗事故或反复出现医疗事故，或未能达到一个合理谨慎的针灸师认为在类似的条件和情况下可接受的护理、技术和治疗水平。

（q）超出法律允许的范围从事针灸实践或提出从事针灸实践，或接受和履行持证人明知或应当知道他或她不能胜任的专业职责。

（r）在持证人明知或应当知道该人员在培训、经验或执照方面没有资格履行专业职责时，将该等职责委派给该人员。

（s）违反委员会曾在纪律听证会中发出的合法命令，或不遵守部门依法发出的传票。

（t）与他人串谋，或单独实施企图胁迫、恐吓或阻止另一持证人合法宣传其服务的行为。

（u）在教学过程中有欺诈、欺骗、重大过失、不称职或不当行为。

（v）不遵守州、县、市有关公共卫生和传染病防治的规定或报告要求的。

（w）不遵守委员会关于健康和安全的任何规则，包括但不限于针具和器械的消毒以及处理可能具有传染性的物质。

（x）违反本章或第456章的任何规定或据此通过的任何规则的。

（2）对于任何被裁定违反本条第（1）款的任何规定的执照申请人或持证人，或被裁定违反《佛罗里达州制定法》第456.072（1）条的任何规定的执照申请人或持证人，委员会可发出命令不予颁发执照或实施第456.072（2）条所列任何罚款。

（3）在委员会确信针灸师已遵守最终命令中规定的所有条款和条件，并且能够安全地从事针灸实践之前，部门不得恢复针灸师的执照，或向其认为不合格的人员颁发执照。

第457.11条　根据法律1976，c.76‐168，§3；法律1979，c79‐165，§1废止

第457.111条　根据法律1986，c.86‐265，§12，eff.Oct.1，1986废止

第 457.116 条　被禁止的行为；处罚

（1）任何人不得：

（a）从事针灸实践，除非该人根据《佛罗里达州制定法》第 457.101～457.118 条获得执照。

（b）在其姓名或营业地点使用包含"针灸""针灸师""认证针灸师""执业针灸师""东方医生"等字样的任何服务名称或描述；"L.Ac""R.Ac""A.P."或"D.O.M."；或任何其他表明或暗示他或她从事针灸实践的词、字母、缩写或标记，除非他或她持有根据第 457.101～457.118 条颁发的有效执照。

（c）将他人的执照作为自己的执照出示。

（d）故意向委员会或其成员提供虚假或伪造的证据。

（e）使用或企图使用已被吊销、撤销或处于非执业或逾期状态的执照。

（f）雇用任何没有根据《佛罗里达州制定法》第 457.101～457.118 条获得执照的人从事针灸实践。

（g）隐瞒与违反《佛罗里达州制定法》第 457.101～457.118 条有关的信息。

（2）违反本节规定，构成二级轻罪，依照《佛罗里达州制定法》第 775.082 条、第 775.083 条的规定处罚。

第 457.118 条　本章对其他卫生保健实践的影响

本章不得解释为扩大或限制根据《佛罗里达州制定法》第 458 章、第 459 章、第 460 章、第 461 章、第 466 章、第 474 章或第 486 章获得执照的任何卫生保健专业人员的执业范围，因为该执业范围是由法规界定的。

第 457.119 条　根据法律 1986, c.86‑265, §12, eff.Oct.1,1986 废止

第 457.12 条　根据法律 1976, c.76‑168, §3；法律 1979, c 79‑165, §1 废止

第 457.13 条　根据法律 1976, c.76‑168, §3；法律 1979, c 79‑165, §1 废止

第 457.14 条　根据法律 1976, c.76‑168, §3；法律 1979, c 79‑165, §1 废止

第 457.15 条　根据法律 1976, c.76‑168, §3；法律 1978, c.78‑323, §4；法律 1979, c. 79‑165, §1 废止

第 457.16 条　根据法律 1976, c.76‑168, §3；法律 1979, c 79‑165, §1 废止

佛罗里达州针灸行政法[①]

第 64B1‑1 节　组　　织

第 64B1‑1.003 条　其他与委员会有关事务

为《佛罗里达州制定法》第 456.011 条第（4）款规定的委员会成员薪酬之目的，"其他与委员会有关事务"定义包括：

---

① 根据《佛罗里达州行政法典》第 64 卷第 64B1 编"针灸委员会"译出。

（1）委员会议。

（2）委员会各工作委员会会议。

（3）委员会成员应部门或委员会的要求与部门工作人员或部门承办商举行的会议。参会成员无论是否收到参会通知，将在委员会办公室存档。

（4）可能展开的小组会议。

（5）所有委员会授权并参与或受邀参加的专业协会会议，包括但不限于所有委员会参与的国家协会会议，以及经委员会授权，参加涉及教育、管理或专业审查的国家或行业协会或组织的会议，委员会对其拥有法定权力。

（6）召开计划采取颁发执照或纪律处分且持续时间超过四小时的会议；或者在紧急情况下召开的会议。

第64B1－1.0035条　可免责缺席事由

（1）委员会成员患病或受伤。

（2）委员会成员直系亲属患病、受伤或死亡。

（3）履行陪审员义务。

（4）在州或联邦服兵役。

第64B1－1.008条　公众意见

针灸委员会邀请并鼓励所有公众人士就委员会或工作委员会的事项和提议发表意见和建议。发表意见或建议应遵循以下规定：

（1）公众人士将有机会在正式出席的委员会会议上，在提出议程项目后发表意见和建议。

（2）公众人士发表意见时间应当限制在五分钟以内。该段时间不包括发表者回答委员会成员、工作人员或委员会顾问问题所用的时间。如果时间允许，委员会主席可以延长发表意见时间。

（3）公众人士如有兴趣就委员会审议的某项提议或事项进行聆讯，应书面通知委员会工作人员。书面通知内容应当指明其为个人或机构，表明支持、反对或中立，并确定将代表团队或五人或五人以上的团体或派别发言。在董事会露面的任何个人或机构如果不希望被识别，可以使用假名。

第64B1－2节　费　　用

第64B1－2.001条　费用

（1）初始申请费为二百美元。

（2）初始执照费为二百美元。

（3）执业执照的两年续期费为二百七十五美元。

（4）非执业执照的两年续期费为一百五十美元。

（5）非执业状态的申请费为二百美元。

（6）停用执照的申请费为五十美元。

（7）停用状态的费用为五十美元。

（8）除续费外,任何时间更改状态的费用为二百美元。

（9）重新激活执照的费用为二百七十五美元。

（10）逾期费为二百美元。

（11）继续教育提供者的初始注册费为一百美元。

（12）继续教育提供者两年续期费为一百美元。

（13）证书或执照副本费为二十五美元。

第64B1‑2.0015 条废除

第64B1‑2.004 条废除

第64B1‑2.005 条废除

第64B1‑2.006 条废除

第64B1‑2.009 条废除

第64B1‑2.0095 条废除

第64B1‑2.010 条废除

第64B1‑2.011 条废除

第64B1‑2.012 条废除

第64B1‑2.014 条废除

64B1‑2.015 条　公开记录认证费

委员会应当收取二十五美元公开记录认证费。

第64B1‑2.016 条废除

第64B1‑2.018 条废除

第64B1‑3节　定义;针灸师考试

第64B1‑3.001 条　定义

（1）针灸系指基于中医理念,采用针灸诊断、治疗及辅助治疗和诊断技术,旨在促进、维持和恢复健康并预防疾病的初级保健形式。针灸应包括但不限于在人体特定部位实施针刺或灸法。

（2）针灸应包括但不限于:

（a）耳、手、鼻、面、足和/或头皮穴位的针灸治疗。

（b）用下列任何一种方法刺激穴位及经络:

1. 针刺、艾灸、拔火罐、热疗法、磁石、刮痧和腧穴。

2. 手动刺激包括穴位按摩(指用不刺穿皮肤的器械进行刺激)、按摩、针压法、反射疗法、指压按摩和推拿。

3. 电刺激包括电针疗法,经皮和经皮神经电刺激。

4. 根据食品和药物管理局规章条例在内的相关联邦法律,激光生物刺激在首次使用前不少于十四日,针灸委员会须收到关于拟使用激光生物刺激的书面通知,并提供符合联邦要求的证明。

（3）针灸诊断技术应当包括但不限于运用望诊、听诊、嗅诊、问诊、触诊;观察脉搏、舌头、面相;利用五行对应、良导络、赤谷、德国电针、克里安影像和热影像技术。

（4）针灸针应为实心丝状器械,包括但不限于皮肤针、梅花针、压针、三棱针和一次性采血针。禁止使用其他任何针头。

（5）辅助疗法应当包括但不限于:

（a）营养咨询、推荐符合食品和药物管理局标签要求的非处方药,作为促进健康的膳食补充剂。

（b）推荐呼吸技巧和治疗性运动。

（c）生活方式和压力咨询。

（d）推荐所有经食品和药物管理局和美国顺势疗法药典委员会批准的顺势疗法制剂。

（e）草药学。

第64B1－3.003 条废除

第64B1－3.004 条　针灸考试

国家针灸与东方医学认证委员会（NCCAOM）考试是获委员会批准的,由东方医学基础模块、穴位针灸模块、生物医学模块和中草药模块组成的考试。

第64B1－3.008 条废除

第64B1－3.009 条　通过国家认证背书的执照

根据《佛罗里达州制定法》第457.105 条（2）（c）款,针灸委员会将通过背书方式认证下列申请人的执照:

（1）提供 NCCAOM 东方医学有效认证的证明。

（2）满足《佛罗里达州制定法》第457.105 条（2）（a）款和（d）款的要求。

（3）满足《佛罗里达州行政法》64B1－4.001（4）、（5）和（6）中规定的要求。

第64B1－3.010 条　通过其他州执照背书的方式颁发执照

根据《佛罗里达州制定法》第457.105 条（2）（c）款,针灸委员会为下列申请人颁发执照:

（1）提交在其他州获得有效执照的证明,该州在申请人首次获得执照时的执照要求须与本州基本同等,或更加严格。申请人必须通过请求他州发证机构,向委员会提供一份声明,说明截止日期时申请人执照当前状态,他州执照的有效期以及为申请人颁发执照时他州有效的执照颁发依据,包括他州的法律法规和考试要求。

（2）符合《佛罗里达州制定法》第457.105 条（2）（a）和（d）款的要求。

（3）达到《佛罗里达州行政法》64B1－4.001（4）、（5）和（6）款的最低要求。

第64B1－4 节　考试和执照的资格

第64B1－4.001 条　针灸培训课程的要求

申请人必须证明其已符合下列最低要求,方可获准参加执照考试或有资格通过背书方式获得执照。

（1）申请人在1997 年8 月1 日之前没有入学,并于2001 年7 月31 日以后结业的,必须完成与针灸及东方医学教育审核委员会（ACAOM）的东方医学硕士水平课程相当的核心课程,并接受不少于两千七百学时的监督指导。

（2）申请者在 1997 年 8 月 1 日之前没有入学，并于 2001 年 7 月 31 日以前结业的，在完成三年的针灸和东方医学课程以前，必须完成六十个经认证的专科学校的学分，并接受不少于二千〇二十五学时的监督指导。

（3）申请人在 1997 年 8 月 1 日以前入学的，必须完成不少于九百学时的传统东方针灸的监督指导和不少于六百学时监督下的临床经验。所有符合本规定的申请人必须在 1998 年 2 月 1 日前开始上课。

（4）所有申请人必须完成六十学时注射疗法学习，包括：

（a）针灸注射疗法的历史和发展。

（b）鉴别诊断。

（c）定义、概念和病理生理学。

（d）草药、顺势疗法和营养注射剂的性质、功能、归经和禁忌。

（e）针灸注射疗法适应证以及适合治疗此类疾病的注射药物。

（f）确定适当的治疗穴位，包括触诊。

（g）解剖学和推荐区域综述。

（h）普遍预防措施，包括血源性病原体和有害生物废料的管理。

（i）注射程序，包括准备注射剂、禁忌证和注意事项。

（j）对一名或多名患者的十学时临床实践。

（k）所需的管理技术和设备。

如果提交的官方成绩单上没有记录六十学时的注射疗法学习，则必须提交获委员会批准的提供者出具的证书，以证明完成了学习。

（5）所有申请人必须完成十五学时普遍预防措施的监督指导和二十学时《佛罗里达州制定法》法律法规的监督指导，包括《佛罗里达州制定法》第 456 章和 457 章以及本章规则。如果提交的给官方成绩单上没有记录这两项学习内容，必须提交获委员会批准的提供者出具的证书，以证明完成了学习。

（6）申请人必须完成八学时课程或同等课程，包括在针灸和东方医学实践中安全有效地使用实验室检查和影像学检查结果。如果提交的官方成绩单上没有记录八学时课程，必须提供获委员会批准的提供者出具的证书，以证明完成了课程。

第 64B1‑4.0011 条　申请执照所需文件

正式填写申请应当将针灸许可申请表提交卫生部（DH‑MQA1116,2020 年 6 月），该表格作为委员会申请，在此引用和合并，并在网站（http://www.flrules.org/Gateway/reference.asp?No=Ref‑12187 或 http://floridaacupuncture.gov/resources/）上查阅。填妥申请表后，请附上适当的费用和证明文件，并提交至申请须知上所列明的地址。

第 64B1‑4.0012 条　执照的英语能力要求

（1）申请者用英语以外的任何一种语言通过国家笔试，均必须具备英语交流能力，在美国教育考试服务中心管理的国家英语水平考试（以下简称"托福"，TOEFL）或者英语口语考试（以下简称"TSE"）中取得及格分数。用于本条时，托福考试的及格分数定为：笔考总分不低于五百分；机考总分不低于一百七十三分；网络考试总分不低于六十一分。TSE 考试的及格分数定为不低于五十分。申请人须自行申请托福考试或 TSE 考试,并于申请执照前向考试服务中心取得其官方成绩报告。申请人应当在提交申请时一并提交官方成绩报告副本。

（2）申请人通过考试申请执照,并在申请中表明希望以英语以外的任何语言参加佛罗里达州的国家笔试的,应当在他们的申请中提交一份官方成绩报告表明已经通过托福考试或者 TSE 考试。

第 64B1－4.0015 条　监督指导的定义

为《佛罗里达州行政法》第 64B1－4.001 条之目的,委员会对"监督指导"的定义如下:

（1）"监督指导"系指对学生进行有计划、有监督的指导,在此过程中学生能够亲自动手治疗针灸患者。

（2）在前二百个学时的监督指导中,学生应当观察导师诊断和治疗患者。

（3）在第二个二百学时的监督指导中,学生必须接受导师的直接监督。"直接监督"系指导师与学生在同一间教室进行的所有实际操作的监督。

（4）在接下来的监督指导时间里,学生必须接受导师直接或间接的监督。"间接监督"系指导师亲自在场,以便在学生需要时立即出现在学生身边。

（5）在接下来的监督指导时间里,学生必须诊断和治疗至少三十个不同的患者。

（6）申请人在 2001 年 7 月 31 日以后入学的,在监督指导期间,学生必须在患者诊疗过程中观察并使用实验室检查和影像学检查结果。

第 64B1－4.004 条　草药疗法

"草药疗法"系指草药疗法、植物疗法的使用、处方、建议和管理,包括植物药、动物药和/或矿物药,以及所有促进、维持、恢复健康并预防疾病的顺势疗法制剂。

第 64B1－4.005 条　东方按摩

东方按摩涵盖中国传统和现代东方医学手法,包括用手工和机械方式刺激穴位、经络、阿是穴;各种东方经络顺势疗法,包括穴位按压、推拉、刮痧疗法、腹部按摩、牛痧、灵气疗法、足底按摩、指压按摩、推拿、牵引和对抗牵引、震动和其他神经肌肉、身体和物理疗法技术等针灸和东方医学技术以促进、维持、恢复健康并预防疾病。

第 64B1－4.006 条　气功

气功系指中国的能量培育术,通过姿势、动作、功法、呼吸、冥想、观想、意念等来调动或净化气,以促进、维持、恢复健康并预防疾病。

第 64B1－4.007 条　电针

电针系指在使用针头或不使用针头的情况下,通过运用经皮电神经和组织刺激;和/或使用微电流、低电压、高电压、干扰电流、化电流和针刺治疗仪刺激穴位、经络和阿是穴。

第 64B1－4.008 条　辅助疗法

辅助治疗应包括针灸刺激穴位、阿是穴、耳穴、经络、微系统等;使用空气、芳香疗法、颜色、冷冻疗法、电灸术、顺势疗法、热疗、离子注入（ion pumping cords）、虹膜学、克里安影像术、激光针灸、生活方式咨询、磁石疗法、石蜡、光子刺激、推荐呼吸技巧、治疗性运动和日常活动、声音（包括音叉疗法）、牵引、水、热疗以及《佛罗里达州行政法》第 64B1－4－010 条规定归为中医理念和现代东方医学技术的其他辅助疗法和诊断技术。

第64B1‑4.009条　膳食指南

膳食指南应当包括针灸和东方医学中使用的营养咨询,以及促进、维持、恢复健康和预防疾病的营养补充的管理、处方和/或建议。

第64B1‑4.010条　传统中医理念,现代东方医学技术

传统中医理念和现代东方医学技术,应包括针灸诊断和治疗,预防和纠正痼疾、疾病、损伤、疼痛、毒瘾、其他疾病、身体功能失调;调节气的流通;平衡患者精力和功能;促进、维持、恢复健康;用于疼痛治疗和姑息治疗;针刺麻醉;运用下列方式预防疾病:刺激穴位、阿是穴、耳穴、经络和微系统,包括使用赤谷;过敏消除技术;呼吸;冷冻;五色;感应;拔火罐;膳食指南;电;电针刺激;经皮电活动(EDS);功法;八纲;五行;卫气营血;腹部按摩;热疗;草药疗法;包括植物药、动物药和/或矿物药;红外线和其他形式的光;询问病史;经络;听诊;艾灸;脱敏;望诊;东方按摩‑手工和机械方法;触诊;相面术;微点放血疗法;脉搏;气;血和津液;良导络;三焦;六经;嗅;舌;太极拳;气功;五轮八廓;阴阳;脏腑;印度草药按摩、中国、日本、韩国、蒙古、越南等东亚针灸和东方医学理念和治疗技术、法国针灸、德国针灸包括电针和诊断,以及使用实验室检查和影像学检查结果。

第64B1‑4.011条　诊断技术

协助针灸诊断、确诊和监测针灸治疗方案或决定将患者转诊至其他卫生保健提供者的诊断技术包括:传统中医理念和现代东方医学技术;推荐家庭诊断筛查;体格检查;使用实验室检查结果;使用影像学成像;报告或试验结果;头发、唾液和尿液的诊室筛查;肌肉反应测试;触诊;反射;活动范围;感官测试;温度记录;激痛点;生命体征;急救;保健和卫生设施。

第64B1‑4.012条　穴位注射疗法

2002年3月1日起生效的辅助疗法包括穴位注射疗法,系指通过皮下注射针将中草药、顺势疗法和其他无菌形式的营养补充剂注入穴位,而非静脉注射疗法,用于促进、维持和恢复健康;疼痛治疗和姑息治疗;针刺麻醉和预防疾病。

第64B1‑6节　继续教育

第64B1‑6.002条　定义

(1)"批准"系指佛罗里达州针灸委员会批准。

(2)"委员会"系指佛罗里达州针灸委员会。

(3)"继续教育委员会"系指委员会下设的继续教育委员会。

(4)"联系人"系指负责提交提供者批准申请、确保遵守规则,保存完整的参与者名册并了解提供者课程的人员。

(5)"函授课程"系指通过邮件提供的获批课程,其中规定的课程由参与者完成,并由提供者对其表现进行评估,并对学员完成课程的满意或不满意程度进行评级。

(6)"学时"系指不少于五十分钟,且不多于六十分钟的上课时间。半个学时意味着不少于二十五分钟,且不多于三十分钟的课程时间。

(7)"部门"系指卫生部门。

（8）"参与者"系指参加提供者提供的课程以完成该课程既定目标的针灸师。

（9）"课程"系指基于既定目标处理特定内容的有计划教育经历。

（10）"提供者"系指指导继续教育课程的个人、组织或机构。

第 64B1－6.005 条　继续教育学分核准标准

（1）继续教育课程必须有助于提高、扩展或增强持证人的针灸和东方医学实践相关的知识和技能。课程内容应当包括针灸的历史和理论、针灸诊断和治疗技术、辅助疗法技术、针灸师-患者沟通和职业道德等。所有继续教育课程都必须经过委员会的评估和批准，以确定继续教育课程是否符合委员会制定的标准。委员会对每项课程所授予学分的学时数有最终决定权。

（2）提供继续教育学分的各项课程必须由满足以下条件的人员讲授：至少拥有经认可的学院或大学或佛罗里达州许可的高等教育机构的学士学位，且主修该科目；或从针灸学校毕业，或已经完成了与该州要求相当的辅导课程，且该课程获得州发证机构、全国认可的针灸/东方医学协会或基本同等的评审机构批准，并且拥有三年针灸执业经验；在过去的两年内，在专业会议、专业团体或任何针灸学校就申请批准的课程讲授过至少三次，或已完成课程主修科目的专门培训，并在主修科目方面有至少两年的实践经验。

（3）为了满足继续教育的要求，持证人提交的继续教育课程必须符合委员会制定的标准。

（4）对于主要致力于针灸服务的行政或商业管理方面的课程将不给予学分。

（5）持证人首次续期执照时，为获得 HIV/AIDS 课程的学分，该课程不得少于三学时，且必须涉及《佛罗里达州制定法》第 456.033 条指定的领域。委员会接受卫生部提出或实施的 HIV/AIDS 的课程方案，以及其他卫生专业管理委员会批准的方案。

（6）生物医学相关的继续教育课程应提供与该课程临床相关的课程内容，同时提高、扩展或增强持证人在生物医学方面的技能和知识。

第 64B1－6.006 条　对继续教育提供者的要求

每位提供者应当：

（1）通过 OE Broker.com 注册，并直接向 CE Broker 支付适当的提供者注册费。提供者注册费不可退还，应在每个两年期内发生以下事件时（以最早日期为准）支付：

（a）提供者提交新课程或多项课程供委员会批准时。

（b）提供者提供《佛罗里达州制定法》第 457 章中的继续教育课程时，持证人可通过该课程获得执照续期学分。

（2）确保提供者提供的继续教育课程符合规则。

（3）在每次课程展示后，保留一份完整的、按字母顺序排列的、清晰易读的参加者名册，保存期为三年。

（4）保存一份有参与者签名的签到表和签名离开表。

（5）为每位学员提供证书，证明学员已顺利完成课程。该证书在课程完成后颁发，并应当包含提供者的名称、课程名称、课程日期、地点和学时数。

（6）如本规则所述的标准维持有任何重大变更，应当通知委员会。

（7）确保每个人获得同一课程的学分不超过一次。

（8）经批准课程的讲师出现任何变更，都应当通知委员会，并证明新讲师符合《佛罗里达州行政法》64B1－6.005 条（2）款所规定的标准。

（9）指定一个负责并且了解每个课程的联系人。联系人应当将课程中任何重大变更或标准维持的失误通知委员会。

（10）新讲师应当符合《佛罗里达州行政法》64B1－6.005 条（2）款所规定的标准。在函授继续教育课程中，每个提供者有责任从每个持证人处获得一份签字声明，声明参与者确实阅读了材料，进行了实践并亲自参加了考试。

（11）如果交付方式需要技术或其他专长，应有足够的人员协助处理行政事务，且应有足够人员具备在内容领域之外的能力。

（12）提供者应当保存个人要约的记录以供检查，记录应当包括科目、目标、教员资格、评核机制、学时和参加者名单。

第 64B1－6.008 条　课程批准程序

（1）为了获得委员会批准的两年制针灸执照的一个或多个课程的继续教育学分，提供者应当上交 DOH/AP006 表格申请批准，《继续教育课程批准》现作为参考编入本文件，生效日期至 2004 年 7 月 26 日，《继续教育课程批准》复印件可向委员会领取，并上交委员会办公室审批。

（2）下列课程中，符合本条规定的可以获得委员会批准：

（a）由国家或州针灸和/或东方医学组织主办的学习课程。

（b）由认证的针灸和/或东方医学学校主办的学习课程。

（3）委员会保留旁听和/或监督任一提供者所开课程的权力及权限。如果提供者散布任何与继续教育课程有关的虚假或误导性信息，或未能遵守委员会的规则，委员会将拒绝批准提供者提供的个别课程。

（4）如获批准，提供者可在宣传单或其他广告中标明该课程"已获得佛罗里达州针灸委员会批准，可提供继续教育学分"。

第 64B1－6.009 条　继续教育学分的教学时间

（1）经批准提供继续教育学分的课程任教老师，每学时可申请三学时继续教育学分，每两年不得超过九学时。

（2）学校任教老师的继续教育学分不能仅仅作为常规教学任务的学分。

第 64B1－6.010 条废除

第 64B1－7 节　执 照 续 期

第 64B1－7.001 条　废除

第 64B1－7.0015 条　继续教育要求

（1）作为执照两年一次续期的条件，每个持证人每两年至少应当完成三十学时的继续教育，满足《佛罗里达州制定法》第 457.107 条和《佛罗里达州行政法》规则第 64B1－6.005 条的要求，其中应当包括：

（a）按照《佛罗里达州行政法》第 64B1－6.005 条规定，生物医学课程的继续教育学分需达到不少于五学时的要求。

(b) 按照《佛罗里达州制定法》第 456.003 条(2)款和《佛罗里达州行政法》第 64B1－6.005 条(5)款的规定,HIV/AIDS 课程的继续教育学分需达到三学时的要求。

(c) 按照《佛罗里达州制定法》第 456.013 条(7)款的规定,预防医疗错误课程的继续教育学分需达到 2 学时的要求。

(d) 在《佛罗里达州制定法》第 456 和 457 章以及本委员会颁布的规则有二学时的继续教育学分。各持证人可通过出席另一持证人受到纪律处分完整的委员会会议,或者在标准护理纪律案件中作为合理根据小组成员,提供专家意见而不给予赔偿,来满足此要求。

(2) 在首次颁发执照后的第一次续期时,持证人免于遵守《佛罗里达州行政法》第 64B1－7.0015 条的继续教育要求,但因医疗过错而强制要求的继续教育学时数和三学时的 HIV/AIDS 课程除外。

(3) 学时不得追溯或累积。所有学分必须在申请后的两年内获得。

第 64B1－7.002 条　非执业执照的重新激活要求

(1) 非执业执照应当按照《佛罗里达州行政法》第 64B1－2.001 条(9)款中规定支付重新激活费,并证明被持证人完成了《佛罗里达州行政法》规则第 64B－7.0015 条中规定的继续教育要求后,非执业执照将重新激活。

(2) 但持证人的执照连续处于非执业状态超过两个两年周期,且过去四年中有两年没有在另一司法管辖区执业的,应当要求其出席委员会会议,并培养足够的医疗实践能力和技能,以保护公众健康、安全和福利。在这种情况出现时,持证人应当:

(a) 表明符合上述第(1)项的规定。

(b) 说明在执照处于非执业状态期间,任何在本州或任何其他司法管辖区从事的针灸实践相关活动,以及确定在任何司法管辖区没有渎职或受到纪律处分。

(c) 证明符合《佛罗里达州制定法》第 456.048 条和《佛罗里达州行政法》第 64B－12.001 条的财务责任要求。

(d) 证明符合《佛罗里达州制定法》第 456.033 条和《佛罗里达州行政法》第 64B1－7.0015 条。

(3) 对于下列持证人,卫生部不得重新激活执照:

(a) 在本地或任何其他司法管辖区犯下的任何行为或罪行,将构成《佛罗里达州制定法》第 457.109 条规定的惩罚执照持有人。

(b) 未能遵守《佛罗里达州制定法》第 456.048 条和《佛罗里达州行政法》第 64B1－12.001 条规定的财务责任要求。

(c) 未能遵守《佛罗里达州制定法》第 456.033 条和《佛罗里达州行政法》第 64B1－7.0015 条的规定。

第 64B1－7.0025 条　重新激活停用执照

持证人可以根据以下要求重新激活停用状态的执照:

(1) 支付重新激活费。在持证人处于停用状态的两年执照周期内,该费用与本规则规定的处于执业状态的持证人的续期费用相同。

（2）对于持证人的执照处于停用状态的两年期,证明符合《佛罗里达州行政法》第64B1‑7.0015 条的继续教育要求。

第64B1‑7.004 条　通知机构持证人的邮寄地址和执业地点

（1）各持证人有义务向卫生部提供关于其当前通信地址和执业地点的书面通知。为本规则之目的,"执业地点"系指持证人从事针灸实践的主要场所的地址。

（2）任何持证人的当前通信地址和执业地点如有更改,应在更改后十日内向卫生部提供书面通知。持证人的书面通知应发送到下列地址:针灸委员会,佛罗里达州塔拉哈西市,C‑06 片区,落羽松街道 4052 号,邮编 32399‑3256。可以接收发送到 MQA.Acupuncture@flhealth.gov 的电子通知,并有责任确保卫生部收到了电子通知。

第64B1‑8节　感　染　控　制

第64B1‑8.001 条　定义

（1）针系指用于针灸实践的实心丝状器械,包括但不限于:皮肤针、梅花针、压针、三棱针和一次性柳叶刀。根据《佛罗里达州制定法》第 457.1085 条,所有用于患者的针灸针必须是无菌和用后即丢弃的,而且每根针只能使用一次。

（2）灭菌:杀死进入组织的所有微生物,包括所有细菌孢子。灭菌是将清洁后的物品通过高压蒸汽灭菌或干热灭菌完成的。

第64B1‑8.002 条　监测灭菌和感染控制

（1）针灸针以外的器械,当器械穿透组织或接触血液时,应当按照高压灭菌器生产厂家的说明,用适当的高压灭菌方法完成灭菌。

（2）（a）灭菌指示剂应用于每次高压灭菌以监测灭菌过程。

（b）贴片必须标明暴露于蒸汽和高于 250 华氏度。

（3）所有灭菌后的物品都必须以保持无菌的方式储存和处理。

（4）使用高压灭菌技术的每个针灸诊所应张贴灭菌流程,并应保存所有高压灭菌器工作的文件。

（5）针灸师有责任确保负责按照本规则执行灭菌程序的人员得到充分的培训。

（6）灭菌所用的流程和设备必须定期进行有效性检验。压力下的蒸汽(如高压灭菌器)必须通过适当的生物监测来验证其有效性,至少每四十小时(二千四百分钟)使用一次或至少每三十日一次,任选为准。

第64B1‑8.003 条　诊室卫生

针灸诊室应当保持安全卫生。

第64B1‑8.004 条　生物医学废物的处置

生物医学废物必须按照 2015 年 12 月 2 日生效的《佛罗里达州行政法》第 64E‑16 章的规定进行管理,该章在此参考编印,可从 http://www.flrules.org/Gateway/reference.asp?No=Ref‑10517 获取。

第64B1‑8.005 条　感染控制培训

在开始临床培训以前,经批准的学习和辅导课程都应提供关于洁针技术和普遍预防措施的培训,以防止血源性病原体和其他传染病的传播,包括 HIV/AIDS、肝炎、葡萄球菌和结核病。

第 64B1‑8.006 条　实验室检查及影像学检查结果教育

在教学和临床培训期间,且作为继续教育的一部分,针灸委员会要求学习有关在针灸和东方医学实践中安全和有益地使用实验室检查和影像学检查结果的课程。

第 64B1‑9 节　纪　　律

第 64B1‑9.001 条　纪律规定

(1) 当委员会发现任何人触犯《佛罗里达州制定法》第 456.072(1)条或 457.109(1)条中规定的任何行为时,应发布最终命令,按照以下纪律规定的建议实施适当的处罚。以下确定违纪的语言只是描述性的。在确定所引用的行为时,必须参考所引用的每条法定条款的全文。

(a) 试图通过贿赂、欺诈性的谎报,或通过卫生部或委员会的失误来获得或续期针灸执照。

[《佛罗里达州制定法》第 457.109(1)(a)款,第 456.072(1)(h)款]

1. 通过卫生部或针灸委员会的失误

现场注册	最　低　处　罚	最　高　处　罚
首次违纪	关注函,或法律法规继续教育	一千美元罚款
随后违纪	法律法规继续教育	一千美元罚款
远程医疗注册者		
首次违纪	吊销执照并提供整改方案	撤销执照
再次违纪	撤销执照	

2. 通过贿赂或欺诈性的谎报

现场注册	最　低　处　罚	最　高　处　罚
首次违纪	谴责和一万美元罚款	一万美元罚款和撤销执照
随后违纪	谴责和一万美元罚款	一万美元罚款和撤销执照
远程医疗注册者		
首次违纪	撤销执照	
再次违纪	撤销执照	

（b）针灸执照被其他州、地区或国家发证机构撤销、吊销或采取其他行动,包括拒绝颁发针灸执照。

[《佛罗里达州制定法》第457.109(1)(b)款,第456.072(1)(f)款]

现场注册	最 低 处 罚	最 高 处 罚
首次违纪	关注函	吊销执照和/或罚款和/或继续教育
随后违纪	五百美元罚款和吊销执照和/或继续教育	撤销执照
远程医疗注册者		
首次违纪	关注函	吊销执照并提供整改方案
再次违纪	吊销执照1年并提供整改方案	撤销执照

（c）在任何司法管辖区,无论判决如何,因与针灸实践或针灸服务能力有关的行为被定罪或被判有罪,或对该犯罪进行不争辩答辩。

[《佛罗里达州制定法》第457.109(1)(c)款,第456.072(1)(c)款]

现场注册	最 低 处 罚	最 高 处 罚
首次违纪	关注函	吊销执照和/或罚款和/或继续教育
随后违纪	吊销执照和/或罚款和/或继续教育	撤销执照
远程医疗注册者		
首次违纪	吊销执照并提供整改方案	撤销执照
再次违纪	吊销执照1至2年	撤销执照

（d）发布虚假的、欺骗性的或误导人的广告或发布声称针灸能治疗任何疾病的广告。

[《佛罗里达州制定法》第457.109(1)(d)款]

现场注册	最 低 处 罚	最 高 处 罚
首次违纪	关注函	一千美元罚款
随后违纪	吊销执照和/或罚款和/或继续教育	撤销执照
远程医疗注册者		
首次违纪	关注函	谴责
再次违纪	吊销执照并提供整改方案	撤销执照

（e）以他人名义做广告、执业或试图执业。

[《佛罗里达州制定法》第457.109（1）（e）款]

现场注册	最　低　处　罚	最　高　处　罚
首次违纪	关注函	一千美元罚款
随后违纪	吊销执照和/或罚款和/或继续教育	撤销执照
远程医疗注册者		
首次违纪	关注函	谴责
再次违纪	吊销执照并提供整改方案	撤销执照

（f）未向卫生部报告持证人所知道的任何违反本章或卫生部或针灸委员会规则的人。

[《佛罗里达州制定法》第457.109（1）（f）款，第456.072（1）（i）款]

现场注册	最　低　处　罚	最　高　处　罚
首次违纪	关注函	五百美元罚款
随后违纪	吊销执照和/或罚款和/或继续教育	撤销执照
远程医疗注册者		
首次违纪	关注函	谴责
再次违纪	吊销执照并提供整改方案	撤销执照

（g）帮助、协助、唆使、雇用或建议任何无证人士从事针灸实践，违反《佛罗里达州制定法》第457章或第456章，或卫生部或针灸委员会的规定。

[《佛罗里达州制定法》第457.109（1）（g）款，第456.072（1）（j）款]

现场注册	最　低　处　罚	最　高　处　罚
首次违纪	谴责和五百美元罚款和继续教育	五千美元罚款和/或吊销执照
随后违纪	五千美元罚款和/或吊销执照	撤销执照
远程医疗注册者		
首次违纪	谴责	撤销执照
再次违纪	吊销执照并提供整改方案	撤销执照

（h）没有履行任何法定或法律义务的针灸师。

［《佛罗里达州制定法》第 457.109（1）（h）款，第 456.072（1）（k）款］

现场注册	最 低 处 罚	最 高 处 罚
首次违纪	关注函和五百美元罚款	吊销执照和一千美元罚款
随后违纪	吊销执照和一千美元罚款	撤销执照
远程医疗注册者		
首次违纪	谴责	吊销执照并提供整改方案
再次违纪	吊销执照并提供整改方案	撤销执照

（i）以执业针灸师的身份签署或提交报告，持证人明知是虚假的，但故意或疏忽未提交州或联邦法律要求的报告或记录、故意阻止或妨碍提交或诱导他人实施该行为。

［《佛罗里达州制定法》第 457.109（1）（i）款，第 456.072（1）（l）款］

现场注册	最 低 处 罚	最 高 处 罚
首次违纪	关注函和五百美元罚款	五千美元罚款和/或吊销执照
随后违纪	五千美元罚款和继续教育	撤销执照
远程医疗注册者		
首次违纪	谴责	撤销执照
再次违纪	吊销执照并提供整改方案	撤销执照

（j）在患者-针灸师的关系中施加影响，目的是使患者发生性行为，或试图使患者参与性活动。

［《佛罗里达州制定法》第 457.109（1）（j）款，第 456.072（1）（v）款］

现场注册	最 低 处 罚	最 高 处 罚
首次违纪	谴责和五百美元罚款	一万美元罚款,吊销执照和/或撤销执照
随后违纪	五千美元罚款和吊销执照	撤销执照
远程医疗注册者		
首次违纪	吊销执照并提供整改方案	撤销执照
再次违纪	撤销执照	

（k）在针灸服务中或与针灸服务有关的情况下作出误导、欺骗性、不真实或欺诈性的陈述，或在针灸实践中使用技巧或计划，而该技巧或计划未能符合社会普遍采用的治疗标准。

［《佛罗里达州制定法》第 457.109（1）（k）款］

现场注册	最 低 处 罚	最 高 处 罚
首次违纪	谴责和一万美元罚款	一万美元罚款和撤销执照
随后违纪	谴责和一万美元罚款	一万美元罚款和撤销执照
远程医疗注册者		
首次违纪	关注函	谴责
再次违纪	吊销执照并提供整改方案	撤销执照

（1）通过欺诈、恐吓、不当影响或某种形式的过分干涉或无理取闹的手段，亲自或通过代理人招揽患者。

［《佛罗里达州制定法》第 457.109（1）（1）款，第 456.072（1）（y）款］

现场注册	最 低 处 罚	最 高 处 罚
首次违纪	谴责和一万美元罚款	一万美元罚款，吊销执照和/或撤销执照
随后违纪	谴责和一万美元罚款	一万美元罚款，吊销执照和/或撤销执照
远程医疗注册者		
首次违纪	谴责	吊销执照并提供整改方案
再次违纪	谴责	撤销执照

（m）未保存符合针灸护理标准的书面病历的。

［《佛罗里达州制定法》第 457.109（1）（m）款］

现场注册	最 低 处 罚	最 高 处 罚
首次违纪	关注函和文件编制继续教育	谴责和一千美元罚款
随后违纪	谴责和一千美元罚款	察看期和/或吊销执照
远程医疗注册者		
首次违纪	谴责	吊销执照并提供整改方案
再次违纪	吊销执照并提供整改方案	撤销执照

（n）对患者施加影响,利用患者为持证人或第三方谋取经济利益。

[《佛罗里达州制定法》第 457.109（1）（n）款,第 456.072（1）（n）款]

现场注册	最　低　处　罚	最　高　处　罚
首次违纪	谴责和一千美元罚款	吊销执照和/或一万美元罚款
随后违纪	两千美元罚款和吊销执照	撤销执照
远程医疗注册者		
首次违纪	谴责	吊销执照并提供整改方案
再次违纪	谴责	撤销执照

（o）因疾病、酒精、毒品、麻醉品、化学品或任何其他物质,或由于任何精神或身体病症,无法在保证患者安全的情况下采取合理手段为患者提供针灸服务。

[《佛罗里达州制定法》第 457.109（1）（o）款,第 456.072（1）（z）款]

现场注册	最　低　处　罚	最　高　处　罚
首次违纪	吊销执照直至持证人能够向委员会证明其有能力以合理的技巧和安全性执业	撤销执照
随后违纪	吊销执照直至持证人能够向委员会证明其有能力以合理的技巧和安全性执业	撤销执照
远程医疗注册者		
首次违纪	吊销执照并提供整改方案	撤销执照
再次违纪	吊销执照并提供整改方案	撤销执照

（p）严重或多次发生医疗事故,或未能以合理审慎的针灸师认可的在类似条件和情况下可接受的技巧和治疗水平进行针灸。

[《佛罗里达州制定法》第 457.109（1）（p）款]

现场注册	最　低　处　罚	最　高　处　罚
首次违纪	关注函和继续教育	一千美元罚款,吊销执照和继续教育
随后违纪	察看期或吊销执照和/或五千美元罚款	撤销执照
远程医疗注册者		
首次违纪	谴责	吊销执照并提供整改方案
再次违纪	吊销执照并提供整改方案	撤销执照

（q）在法律允许的范围以外从事针灸实践或提出从事针灸实践，或接受和履行持证人知道或应当知道他或她不能胜任的专业职责。

［《佛罗里达州制定法》第457.109（1）（q）款，第456.072（1）（o）款］

现场注册	最　低　处　罚	最　高　处　罚
首次违纪	关注函和继续教育	一千美元罚款，吊销执照和继续教育
随后违纪	察看期或吊销执照和/或两千美元罚款	撤销执照
远程医疗注册者		
首次违纪	谴责	吊销执照并提供整改方案
再次违纪	吊销执照并提供整改方案	撤销执照

（r）当持证人向他人委派或承包专业职责时，知道或有理由知道该人在培训、经验或执照方面没有资格履行相关职责。

［《佛罗里达州制定法》第457.109（1）（r）款，第456.072（1）（p）款］

现场注册	最　低　处　罚	最　高　处　罚
首次违纪	关注函和继续教育	一千美元罚款，吊销执照和继续教育
随后违纪	察看期或吊销执照和/或两千美元罚款	撤销执照
远程医疗注册者		
首次违纪	谴责	吊销执照并提供整改方案
再次违纪	吊销执照并提供整改方案	撤销执照

（s）违反《佛罗里达州制定法》第457或456章的任何条文、针灸委员会或卫生部的规则或针灸委员会的合法命令，或未能遵守依法发出的卫生部传票。

［《佛罗里达州制定法》第457.109（1）（s）款，第456.072（1）（q）款］

现场注册	最　低　处　罚	最　高　处　罚
首次违纪	关注函和五百美元罚款	吊销执照
随后违纪	五百美元罚款和吊销执照	撤销执照
远程医疗注册者		
首次违纪	谴责	撤销执照
再次违纪	吊销执照并提供整改方案	撤销执照

（t）与他人串谋实施意图胁迫、恐吓或阻止另一持证人合法宣传其服务的行为。

[《佛罗里达州制定法》第457.109（1）（t）款]

现场注册	最　低　处　罚	最　高　处　罚
首次违纪	关注函	一千美元罚款
随后违纪	一千美元罚款和吊销执照	撤销执照
远程医疗注册者		
首次违纪	关注函	谴责
再次违纪	吊销执照并提供整改方案	撤销执照

（u）在某一课程中存在欺诈、欺骗或重大过失、不称职或不当行为。

1. 重大过失、不称职或不当行为：

[《佛罗里达州制定法》第457.109（1）（u）款]

现场注册	最　低　处　罚	最　高　处　罚
首次违纪	谴责和两千美元罚款	一万美元罚款和察看期或吊销执照
随后违纪	吊销执照和两千美元罚款	一万美元罚款和撤销执照
远程医疗注册者		
首次违纪	吊销执照并提供整改方案	撤销执照
再次违纪	撤销执照	

2. 欺诈或欺骗：

现场注册	最　低　处　罚	最　高　处　罚
首次违纪	谴责和一万美元罚款	一万美元罚款和撤销执照
随后违纪	谴责和一万美元罚款	一万美元罚款和撤销执照
远程医疗注册者		
首次违纪	吊销执照并提供整改方案	撤销执照
再次违纪	吊销执照	撤销执照

（v）未遵守州、县、市有关公共卫生和传染病控制的规定或报告要求的。

[《佛罗里达州制定法》第457.109（1）（v）款]

现场注册	最 低 处 罚	最 高 处 罚
首次违纪	谴责和五百美元罚款和继续教育	谴责和一千美元罚款和继续教育
随后违纪	谴责和一千美元罚款和继续教育	谴责和五千美元罚款和继续教育
远程医疗注册者		
首次违纪	谴责	吊销执照并提供整改方案
再次违纪	吊销执照并提供整改方案	撤销执照

（w）未遵守麻管局有关健康和安全的任何规则,包括但不限于针头和设备的消毒以及可能具有传染性的材料的处置。

[《佛罗里达州制定法》第457.072(1)(w)款,第456.072(1)(b)款]

现场注册	最 低 处 罚	最 高 处 罚
首次违纪	谴责和五百美元罚款和继续教育	谴责和一千美元罚款和继续教育
随后违纪	谴责和一千美元罚款和继续教育	谴责和五千美元罚款和继续教育
远程医疗注册者		
首次违纪	谴责	吊销执照并提供整改方案
再次违纪	吊销执照并提供整改方案	撤销执照

（x）未遵守继续教育要求,包括 HIV/AIDS 教育的要求。

[《佛罗里达州制定法》第457.109(1)(x)款,第456.072(1)(b)(e)款]

现场注册	最 低 处 罚	最 高 处 罚
首次违纪	吊销执照直至完成继续教育	一千美元罚款和吊销执照直至完成继续教育
随后违纪	吊销执照直至完成继续教育	撤销执照
远程医疗注册者		
首次违纪	关注函	谴责
再次违纪	吊销执照并提供整改方案	吊销执照并提供整改方案

（y）因故意向部门提交虚假的报告或投诉书,诽谤另一持证人,而在民事诉讼中被裁定须负法律责任。

[《佛罗里达州制定法》第456.072(1)(g)款]

现场注册	最 低 处 罚	最 高 处 罚
首次违纪	谴责和五百美元罚款	吊销执照和一千美元罚款
随后违纪	吊销执照和两千美元罚款	撤销执照
远程医疗注册者		
首次违纪	谴责	吊销执照
再次违纪	吊销执照	撤销执照

（z）不正当地干涉法律授权的调查或检查，或任何纪律处分程序。

[《佛罗里达州制定法》第456.072（1）（r）款]

现场注册	最 低 处 罚	最 高 处 罚
首次违纪	关注函	一千美元罚款和/或吊销执照
随后违纪	两千美元罚款和吊销执照	撤销执照
远程医疗注册者		
首次违纪	关注函	谴责
再次违纪	吊销执照并提供整改方案	吊销执照并提供整改方案

（aa）持证人在任何司法管辖区被判有罪或判有罪后三十日内，未以书面向委员会报告，或就任何罪行（不论裁决如何）放弃答辩。

[《佛罗里达州制定法》第456.072（1）（x）款]

现场注册	最 低 处 罚	最 高 处 罚
首次违纪	关注函	两千美元罚款和继续教育
随后违纪	谴责和五百美元罚款	两千美元罚款和继续教育
远程医疗注册者		
首次违纪	关注函	谴责
再次违纪	吊销执照并提供整改方案	撤销执照

（bb）利用由执法人员或根据《佛罗里达州制定法》第316.066条所作的意外报告所提供的涉及机动车事故相关人士的资料，或利用源于此类报告的其他信息，例如报纸或其他新闻出版物的信息，或通过电台、电视广播发布的信息，旨在招揽事故当事人。

[《佛罗里达州制定法》第456.072(1)(y)款]

现场注册	最 低 处 罚	最 高 处 罚
首次违纪	谴责和五百美元罚款	吊销执照
随后违纪	谴责和一千美元罚款	撤销执照
远程医疗注册者		
首次违纪	吊销执照并提供整改方案	吊销执照并提供整改方案
再次违纪	吊销执照并提供整改方案	撤销执照

(cc)根据18U.S.C规则下第669条,第285~287条,第371条,第1001条,第1035条,第1341条,第1343条,第1347条,第1349条,或者第1518条,或42U.S.C规则第1320a-7b条有关医疗补助项目,任何被判犯有任何轻罪或重罪,或进行有罪答辩或放弃答辩的,不论判决如何。

[《佛罗里达州制定法》第456.072(1)(ii)款]

现场注册	最 低 处 罚	最 高 处 罚
首次违纪	谴责和一万美元罚款	撤销执照
随后违纪	谴责和一万美元罚款	撤销执照
远程医疗注册者		
首次违纪	撤销执照	
再次违纪	撤销执照	

(dd)未按照最后的命令、判决、规定或和解,将因医疗补助项目多付的款项汇给州政府。

[《佛罗里达州制定法》第456.072(1)(hh)款]

现场注册	最 低 处 罚	最 高 处 罚
首次违纪	吊销执照	撤销执照
随后违纪	吊销执照	撤销执照
远程医疗注册者		
首次违纪	吊销执照并提供整改方案	吊销执照并提供整改方案
再次违纪	吊销执照并提供整改方案	撤销执照

（ee）根据《佛罗里达州制定法》第409.913条的规定,任何其他州医疗补助计划或联邦医疗保险项目从州医疗补助项目中被终止,除非该从业者被终止的资格已经恢复。

[《佛罗里达州制定法》第456.072(1)(jj)款]

现场注册	最 低 处 罚	最 高 处 罚
首次违纪	吊销执照直至履行	撤销执照
随后违纪	吊销执照直至履行	撤销执照
远程医疗注册者		
首次违纪	吊销执照并提供整改方案	撤销执照
再次违纪	吊销执照并提供整改方案	撤销执照

（ff）在任何司法管辖范围内与医疗欺诈有关的任何轻罪或重罪,或进行有罪答辩或放弃答辩,不论判决如何。

[《佛罗里达州制定法》第456.072(1)(kk)款]

现场注册	最 低 处 罚	最 高 处 罚
首次违纪	撤销执照	撤销执照
远程医疗注册者		
首次违纪	撤销执照	
再次违纪	撤销执照	

（gg）故意不遵守《佛罗里达州制定法》第627.64194或641.513条,且频率较高,表明其为一般商业行为。

[《佛罗里达州制定法》第456.072(1)(ll)款]

现场注册	最 低 处 罚	最 高 处 罚
首次违纪	一万美元罚款	一万美元罚款和/或吊销执照或撤销执照
随后违纪	一万美元罚款	一万美元罚款和撤销执照
远程医疗注册者		
首次违纪	撤销执照	
再次违纪	撤销执照	

（hh）未能遵守，未能顺利完成，或被终止执业医师治疗项目。

[《佛罗里达州制定法》第456.072（1）（oo）款]

现场注册	最 低 处 罚	最 高 处 罚
首次违纪	谴责和一千美元罚款	四千美元罚款和吊销执照
随后违纪	五千美元罚款和察看期	一万美元罚款和撤销执照
远程医疗注册者		
首次违纪	吊销执照并提供整改方案	撤销执照
再次违纪	吊销执照并提供整改方案	撤销执照

（ii）根据F.S.第760.27条的规定，在不知道某人有残疾，或与残疾有关的对特定情感支持动物的需求的情形下，提供信息（含书面文件）表明某人有残疾或支持某人对情感支持动物的需求。

[《佛罗里达州制定法》第456.072（1）（pp）款]

现场注册	最 低 处 罚	最 高 处 罚
首次违纪	谴责和一千美元罚款	吊销执照和四千美元罚款
随后违纪	吊销执照和八千美元罚款	撤销执照
远程医疗注册者		
首次违纪	吊销执照并提供整改方案	撤销执照
再次违纪	吊销执照并提供整改方案	撤销执照

（jj）除了法律另有规定以外，未能遵守《佛罗里达州制定法》第1014.06条规定的父母知情同意的要求。

[《佛罗里达州制定法》第456.072（1）（rr）款]

现场注册	最 低 处 罚	最 高 处 罚
首次违纪	谴责和一千美元罚款	谴责和两千美元罚款
随后违纪	吊销执照和两千五百美元罚款	撤销执照
远程医疗注册者		
首次违纪	谴责	吊销执照并提供整改方案
再次违纪	吊销执照并提供整改方案	撤销执照

（kk）被判有罪的、进行有罪答辩或放弃答辩的，不管判决与否，或犯下或企图、教唆或共谋犯下违反《佛罗里达州制定法》第456.074（5）条所列任何犯罪，或者在另一个管辖区内犯下类似罪行。

［《佛罗里达州制定法》第456.072（1）（ss）款］

现场注册	最 低 处 罚	最 高 处 罚
首次违纪	撤销执照	NA
随后违纪	NA	NA
远程医疗注册者		
首次违纪	撤销执照	NA
再次违纪	NA	NA

（2）针灸委员会可考虑下列因素而采取纪律处分，并采取除上述建议以外的纪律处分：

（a）对公众的危险。

（b）重复犯罪的次数，但持证人目前正被处罚的已判决的犯罪除外。

（c）自违反日期起的时间长度。

（d）对持证人提出的投诉数目。

（e）持证人针灸实践的时间长度。

（f）对患者实际身体或其他方面损伤。

（g）刑罚的威慑作用。

（h）罚款对持证人生计的影响。

（i）对康复所做的努力。

（j）持证人对违规行为的实际了解。

（k）持证人试图纠正或停止违法行为，或拒绝纠正或停止违法行为。

（l）在另一州与纪律或拒绝颁发证书或执照有关的任何行动，包括有罪或无罪的认定、适用的标准、施加的惩罚和已履行的惩罚。

（3）违法行为及处罚范围。根据第120.57（1）和（2）条给予申请人和持证人纪律处分时，委员会应根据纪律规定行事，并在与违法行为相应的范围内处以罚款。以上任何一种处罚都可以包括继续教育。对申请人来说，任何违反以上规定的行为，均足以构成拒绝颁发执照的理由。除罚款外，委员会须追讨有关个案的调查及检控费用。此外，如审裁处裁定与违例行为有关的金钱利益或私利，则审裁处须要求退还向患者或代表患者向第三者收取的费用。

（4）上述第（1）到（4）款的规定不得解释为《佛罗里达州制定法》第457.116条或者第450.072条所述的禁止民事诉讼和刑事诉讼的规定，以及上述第（1）至（4）款的规定不得解释为限制针灸委员会根据第120.57条第（4）款与被告订立有约束力的规定的能力。

（5）远程保健指南。

（a）对州外注册的远程保健服务提供者的纪律处分范围，按严重程度从小到大依次为：关注函、谴责、吊销营业和撤销执照。

（b）吊销执照可以是一段确定的期限，也可以附带由委员会制定的纠正行动计划。

（c）只有经委员会批准，才可提前终止一定期限的暂停营业。在存在整改计划的情况下，可在遵守整改计划或由委员会决定的其他情况下终止吊销执照。

（d）"整改计划"必须与吊销执照同时进行，并必须包括委员会设置的复原条款，以便委员会能够妥善处理违反法纪的行为。为了满足整改计划，注册人必须向委员会提供完成所有条款的证明。整改计划可以在吊销执照一定时间后实施。本规定不应被解释为限制委员会施加一段吊销执照期限的能力，也不意味着整改计划需要附加条件。

第 64B1－9.002 条　传票

（1）定义。下列定义适用于本规则：

（a）"传票"系指符合《佛罗里达州制定法》第 456.077 条规定要求的文书，并送达被执行人以评估本规则规定的罚款金额。

（b）"主体"系指持证人、申请人、个人、合伙企业、公司或其他被指控违反本规则规定的实体。

（2）为了取代《佛罗里达州制定法》第 456.073 条规定的纪律处分程序，本部门特此授权在投诉提交后 6 个月内向当事人发出传票（传票的基础）以处理这里指定的任何违规行为。

（3）委员会特此指出下列违规行为为违规引证行为，应处以五百美元的罚款：

（a）违反《佛罗里达州制定法》第 457.109 条（1）（d）或（e）项。

（b）违反《佛罗里达州行政法》第 64B1－10.002 条规定。

（c）未能以适当继续教育学分续期执照的。

第 64B1－9.003 条　违规行为通知

（1）定义。

（a）"违规行为通知"系指部门向持证人发出的通知，作为对轻微违反委员会规则的第一反应，不伴随罚款或其他纪律处罚。

（b）"轻微违反"系指违反委员会规则，但不造成对某人的经济或身体伤害，或对公共健康、安全和福利产生不利影响，或造成损害的重大威胁。

（2）委员会指定以下为轻微违规，如果第一次违规时未提供持证人当前邮寄地址和执业地点的书面通知，则可能会发出违规行为通知，违反《佛罗里达州行政法》第 64B1－7.004 条规则。

第 64B1－9.004 条　合理根据确定

（1）对于是否有合理根据相信发生了违反《佛罗里达州制定法》第 456 章或第 457 章或根据该章颁布的规则的情况，应由委员会合理根据陪审团以多数票决定。

（2）合理根据陪审团应由根据《佛罗里达州制定法》第 456.073 条授权的成员组成，并可包括一名任期不得超过一年的前委员会成员，除非由委员会主席重新任命。

（3）合理根据陪审团应由委员会主席选定。

（4）合理根据陪审团应在委员会主席或委员会行政主管要求的时间召开会议。

（5）陪审员的审裁官应由委员会主席选定。

第 64B1－9.006 条　调解

（1）"调解"系指该部门委任调解员的程序，以鼓励和协助解决充足合法的投诉。这是一种非正式的、非对抗性的程序，目的是帮助当事人或申诉人和申诉对象达成双方都能接受的协议。

（2）委员会认为调解是一种可以接受的解决争端的方法，因为第一次被指控违反了在广告中没有明显地指明持证人的名字，违反了《佛罗里达州行政法》规则第 64B1－9.007 条。

第 64B1－9.007 条　广告

（1）根据《佛罗里达州制定法》第 457 章授权或认证的人的广告，只要所传播的信息没有任何虚假、欺骗性或误导性，只要所传播的信息没有声称针灸治疗任何疾病是有用的，都是允许的。任何广告如符合以下条件均应被视为虚假的，欺骗性的，或具有误导性。

（a）包含谎报事实。

（b）只披露部分相关事实。

（c）对有益的辅助造成错误或不合理的期望。

（d）包含任何声明或申诉，而提出申诉的人无意履行该声明或申诉。

（e）包含任何其他误导或欺骗的陈述、声明或主张。

（f）未能在广告中明显指明持证人的姓名。

（2）本委员会规则中所使用的"广告"系指任何口头或书面的，向公众传播的话语，旨在直接或间接地推广专业服务，或提议提供专业服务，或诱使公众成员承担与该等专业服务相关的任何义务。

（3）任何根据《佛罗里达州制定法》第 457 章获得许可或认证的人使用以下缩写或术语，不得被视为虚假、欺骗或误导：

（a）L.Ac.。

（b）R.Ac.。

（c）A.P.。

（d）D.O.M.。

（e）执业针灸师（L.Ac.）。

（f）注册针灸师（R.Ac.）。

（g）针灸医生（A.P.）。

（h）东方医学医生（D.O.M.）。

（4）任何通过代理或推荐服务做广告的持证人应对该等广告的内容负责，并应确保该等广告符合本规则和《佛罗里达州制定法》第 457 章。

第 64B1－10 节　针灸医疗记录

第 64B1－10.001 条　医疗记录的内容和保留

（1）针灸师必须保留书面医疗记录，证明每个患者的治疗过程是合理的。这些记录必须包括每位患者至少以下内容：

（a）患者病史。

（b）针灸诊断征象。

（c）每次就诊时使用的穴位或治疗程序。

（d）针灸师的建议。

（e）患者病程记录。

（f）适当和医疗必要时提供实验室检查结果。

（g）适当和医疗必要时提供影像学篇、报告或测试结果。

（2）所有医疗记录必须由针灸师保存五年，自最后一次记录的日期起算。

第 64B1－10.002 条　针灸师死亡、终止执业或搬迁的医疗记录；保留；时间限制

（1）已故针灸师的遗嘱执行人、管理人、个人代表或遗嘱对其执照情况按照《佛罗里达州制定法》第 457 章，应当保留与已死亡针灸师有关的患者的现有病历自针灸师的死亡日期后至少两年。

（2）在针灸师死亡之日起一个月内，其遗嘱执行人、管理人、个人代表或遗属应在该针灸师所在县发行量最大的报纸上发表，向已故针灸师的患者发出通知，写明患者或其适当组成的代表可以从某一地点获得针灸师的医疗记录。

（3）针灸师的死亡之日起二十四个月的时间内，或者此后，遗嘱执行人、管理员、个人代表，或其遗属应当连续四星期，在其针灸办公室所在县发行量最大的报纸上，每周出版一次、连续四周向已故针灸师的患者发出通知，指明该针灸师的医疗记录将于公布的第四个星期的最后一日起计一个月或之后销毁。

（4）根据《佛罗里达州制定法》第 457 章，获发执照的针灸师在终止执业或搬迁而不再向其患者提供服务时，须确保其患者的医疗记录在终止执业或搬迁后至少保留两年。

（5）依照《佛罗里达州制定法》第 457 章，被许可的针灸师如果终止执业或迁址，不再为其患者提供针灸服务，并且没有将其执业转移到其他针灸医生或医生，应当向美国针灸师或医生提供此类终止或搬迁的书面通知，邮寄给所有在终止或迁址前六十日内接受治疗并需要积极、持续治疗的患者，通知应告知患者，在某一地点，患者或其代表可以获得针灸师的医疗记录。该通知须告知患者针灸师的医疗记录可由患者或其正式组成的代表从特定地点的特定人士处获得。

（6）在其他情况下，针灸师在执业或搬迁的终止日期之前至少六十日之前，理应在针灸师办公室所在县发行量最大的报纸上每周出版一次、连续四周向该针灸师的患者发出通知，表明该针灸师的医疗记录可以在某一地点由患者或他们的正式组成代表获得。

（7）在针灸师终止执业或搬迁结束时两年后，针灸师理应在针灸师办公室所在县发行量最大的报纸上每周出版一次、连续四周向该针灸师的患者发出通知，表明该针灸师的医疗记录将于公布的第四个星期的最后一日起计一个月或之后销毁。

第64B1-12节 经济责任

第64B1-12.001条 经济责任

作为获得执照或执照续期的先决条件,每一位针灸师都必须维持医疗事故保险或提供此处规定的财务责任证明:

(1)根据《佛罗里达州制定法》第624.09条定义,从626.914条(2)款规定的盈余线保险人,从第627.942条规定的风险自留组,从第627.351条(4)款规定的联合承保协会,或通过第627.357条规定的自我保险计划,从一个授权保险公司获取和维护专业责任保险金额不少于一万美元索赔,最低的年度总额不少于三万美元。

(2)根据《佛罗里达州制定法》第675章,获取并维持设立的未到期的、不可撤销的信用证,每次索赔金额不低于一万美元,最低可获得信贷总额不少于三万美元。经出示表明责任并判定由针灸师承担责任和损害赔偿的最终判决,或者经出示由协议各方签署的和解协议,如果该终局的判决或和解是由针灸师提供或不能提供针灸师服务引起的索赔导致,则该信用证应支付给作为受益人的针灸师。该信用证不可转出或转让。该信用证应由根据佛罗里达州法律组织并存在的银行或储蓄协会,或根据美国法律组织的银行或储蓄协会签发,其主要营业地点在该州或在该州法律或美国法律授权下接受存款的分支机构。

(3)获得并维持每宗金额不低于一万美元的履约保证,且由在该州有营业执照并被Best's评级为A+的公司出具履约保证,每年至少不低于三万美元。

(4)经向针灸委员会提出申请后,下列持证人可免于符合本条的规定:

(a)专门作为联邦政府或佛罗里达州或其机构或分部的官员、雇员或代理人执业的针灸师。佛罗里达州的代理人、其机构或分支机构是指符合资格投保任何根据《佛罗里达州制定法》第768.28条(14)款规定授权的自我保险或保险计划的人,或根据《佛罗里达州制定法》第110.501条(1)款规定的志愿者。

(b)根据《佛罗里达州制定法》第457章,其执照已处于非执业状态,且不在本州执业的任何人。申请重新激活执照的任何人必须证明该持证人持有长尾保险,为1993年10月1日或之后发生的事件提供责任保险;或本州的初始许可日期(以较晚者为准)和事故发生在执照失效日期之前;或者该类持证人必须提交一份宣誓书,说明在申请重新启动时,该持证人不存在不满意的医疗事故判决或和解。

(c)任何根据《佛罗里达州制定法》第457章获得执照或认证的人,其只在认证学校从事与教学工作相关的工作时,该人员可以从事针灸实践,这种服务是附带的,是与学校教学职位相关的职责的必要部分。

(d)任何根据《佛罗里达州制定法》第457章持有有效执照但不在本州执业的人。如果这类人在本州开始或恢复执业,他(她)必须通知相关委员会。

(e)任何能向针灸委员会证明他(她)在佛罗里达州没有医疗事故的人。

肯 塔 基 州

肯塔基州针灸法[①]

第 311.671 条　《肯塔基州修订版制定法》第 311.671 条至 311.686 条的适用范围

为了保护公众的生命、健康和安全,任何人以针灸师身份从事针灸实践或提出从事针灸实践,都应根据《肯塔基州修订版制定法》第 311.671 条至第 311.686 条的规定获得执照。任何未根据《肯塔基州修订版制定法》第 311.671 条至第 311.686 条规定获得执照的人,继续从事针灸执业实践,或使用任何头衔、标志、卡片或装置来表明他或她是针灸师,都属违法行为。《肯塔基州修订版制定法》第 311.671 条至第 311.686 条中所列规定并非旨在限制、排除或以其他方式干扰在肯塔基、联邦机构或委员会相应机构注册、许可的卫生保健提供者的实践行为,该等卫生保健提供者的实践行为和培训可能包含与执业针灸师的实践行为性质相同的要素。

第 311.672 条　第 311.671 条至 311.686 条涉及的定义

在《肯塔基州修订版制定法》第 311.671 条至第 311.686 条中,除了上下文另有明确规定外,下列词汇与短语应当做如下界定:

(1)"针灸师"系指经委员会许可的针灸执业人员。

(2)"委员会"系指州医疗许可委员会。

(3)"咨询委员会"系指州医疗许可委员会下设的针灸咨询委员会。

(4)"执照"系指州医疗许可委员会颁发执照许可其从事针灸实践。

(5)"针灸实践"系指在伴有或不伴有电刺激或热刺激的情况下,在人体表面的某些穴位或经络上插入针灸针,以改变体内能量流动的方法,包括穴位按压、拔罐、艾灸或皮肤摩擦(推拿)。但针灸实践不应包括激光针灸、整骨疗法、整脊疗法、物理治疗或手术。

法律研究委员会(LRC)提示

法律研究委员会提示(7 - 12 - 06):2006 年《肯塔基州法案》第 249 章第 2 节第 3 款载

[①]　根据《肯塔基州修订版制定法》第 26 卷第 311 章"理疗师、整骨师、足病诊疗师及相关医疗执业者"译出。

明:"理事会"系指在州医疗许可委员会下设的针灸咨询理事会。2006 年《肯塔基州法案》第 249 章第三节创设了针灸咨询委员会,而非前者。在编纂法典的过程中,州制定法的修订者根据《肯塔基州修订版制定法》7.136(1)(h)将"理事会"改为"委员会"。

第 311.673 条　管理制度;针灸咨询委员会;成员;会议;职责

(1) 委员会应当根据《肯塔基州修订版制定法》第 13A 章颁布有关针灸师的执照与管理的行政法规(包括针灸师的临时执照)。针灸法规包括继续教育要求和收费表。

(2) 委员会应设立一个由八名成员组成的针灸咨询委员会,就委员会收到的与针灸师相关的事项进行审查并向委员会提出建议,包括但不限于:

(a) 针灸执照认证申请书。

(b) 执照续期的相关规定。

(c) 费用。

(d) 针灸从业者适用的实践标准。

(e) 继续教育规定。

(f) 咨询委员会的轮岗。

(g) 应委员会其他机构的要求,给予纪律处分。

(h) 颁布和修订行政规章。

(3) 委员会负责任命针灸咨询委员会的成员,任期为四年,且可以以轮岗的方式获得连任。此外,咨询委员会应当由下列人员构成:

(a) 一名州医疗许可委员会成员。

(b) 两名经州医疗许可委员会颁发执照的医师,且其执业范围包含针灸。

(c) 一名与针灸行业无关联或无经济利益的公众成员。

(d) 四名由州医疗许可委员会颁发执照的针灸从业者。

(4) 咨询委员会的主席和秘书长应当由该委员会成员每年以多数票的形式选举产生。主席应当负责主持定期召开的会议,且每个日历年不少于两次。应主席的要求或至少三名咨询委员会成员提出的书面要求,可以在每个日历年举行额外会议。秘书长应将咨询委员会的会议记录存档。咨询委员会的五名成员构成处理事务的法定人数。

(5) 咨询委员会成员应按照国家对公务员差旅费报销的政策,对因出席委员会会议产生的支出进行报销。

(6) 如收到其他成员的请求或查证某成员有出席委员会会议次数较少、玩忽职守或渎职的情况,委员会有权解除任何成员的职务。

第 311.674 条　针灸师执照颁发;执业申请的批准与驳回;续期;互惠原则

(1) 为获得委员会颁发的针灸执照,申请人应当:

(a) 提交经州医疗许可委员会批准的申请,妥善填写相关内容,并缴纳所需费用。

(b) 具有良好品德和声誉,符合《肯塔基州修订版制定法》第 335B 章的要求。

(c) 在国家针灸与东方医学认证委员会(NCCAOM)组织的针灸考试中取得及格分数。

(d) 已完成经针灸及东方医学教育审核委员会(ACAOM)批准的一千八百学时的培训

课程,其中包括三百学时的临床培训。

所有申请人员在首次申领针灸师执照前,必须满足本款项下全部规定,包括完成(d)款所规定的培训课程。

(2)在另一州合法从事针灸实践且目前在该州信誉良好的针灸师,若该州执行的标准与本州标准基本同等,可经其执业所在州认可,为其颁发执照。

(3)州医疗许可委员会可以要求申请人提供一切合理的资料以及委员会为做出知情决定所必需的其他额外资料。申请人须签署任何必要的弃权书或免责声明,以便委员会可以从间接渠道获得必要的信息。若申请人已完成全部所需的申请事项,且委员会已收到申请人和间接渠道提供的全部补充信息,则申请程序完成。

(4)针灸执照应当在满足下列要求的情况下每两年续期一次:

(a)申请人已在规定的时间内提交委员会批准的续期申请,已填写所有必要内容,并已缴纳所需费用。

(b)申请人具有良好品德和声誉。

(5)在收到申请人完整的申请后,委员会须在一百二十日内以书面的方式将批复结果通知各申请人。

(6)尽管本条就颁发执照有任何规定,在通知申请人其批复结果并为其提供合理的陈述机会后,委员会若发现申请人违反本条任何规定或在其他方面有不适合从事针灸实践的情形,可在不事先举行听证会的情况下拒绝向申请人颁发执照。若委员会驳回申请,应当将驳回的理由通知申请人。申请人也可根据《肯塔基州修订版制定法》第311.593条的规定就其申请被驳回的事项提出申诉。

法律研究委员会(LRC)提示

法律研究委员会提示(7-12-06):为了进一步明确《肯塔基州修订版制定法》7.136(1)(c)的权力,州制定法的修订者进一步拆分了2006年《肯塔基州法案》第249章第四节第一款。

第311.675条 临时针灸执照;临时执照的注销通知

(1)若州医疗许可委员会行政主管根据申请书中已核实的信息认为,根据《肯塔基州修订版制定法》第311.671条至第311.686条,申请针灸执照的申请人具有相应资格,则行政主管可代表委员会向申请人颁发一张临时执照。自颁发执照之日起,临时执照持有人可从事最多六个月的针灸实践。行政主管可以在未召开听证会的情况下根据充分的理由与许可委员会进行适当磋商,随时取消该临时执照。在收到该委员会指示或申请被委员会驳回的情况下,行政主管应当立即注销其颁发的临时执照。此外,临时执照不得续期。

(2)行政主管应当将临时执照持有人所提出的申请提交给委员会。如委员会向临时执照持有人颁发正式执照,则申请人因临时执照支付的费用同样适用于正式执照。

(3)若行政主管注销某临时执照,应当立即以挂号邮件的方式通知该临时执照持有人,地址应当以持有人向委员会提交的文件中最后一次更新的地址为准。临时执照应当在注销通知以挂号邮件的形式发出之日起三日后终止,并不再有效。

第311.676条　称号的使用和执照展示;禁止行为;处罚

(1)在其投放的全部广告、发表的专业文献和与其执业有关的账单中,针灸从业者可在其姓名之后附加"执业针灸师"或"L.Ac."。

(2)由州医疗许可委员会颁发的执照必须在持证针灸师营业处所的显著位置进行展示。

(3)未经《肯塔基州修订版制定法》第311.671条至第311.686条认证的人员不得使用任何意在表明或暗示其在从事针灸执业活动的术语、词汇、缩略词、字母或标志。

(4)任何违反本条规定的行为均构成一类轻罪。

第311.677条　《肯塔基州修订版制定法》第311.671至311.686条不适用的人员与活动

《肯塔基州修订版制定法》第311.671条第311.671条至第311.686条,所载规定不适用于:

(1)根据《肯塔基州修订版制定法》任何其他条款获得执照、许可或已经注册的人员。但这些人员可以提供与规范其职业实践和职业道德的法律相一致的服务。

(2)参加经州医疗许可委员会批准的针灸教育机构进修的实习生或学员(若此人被指定为针灸实习生或受训学生,并且其活动在监督下进行且构成受监督学习计划的一部分)。

(3)在经州医疗许可委员会批准的机构或委员会批准的研讨会或辅导机构中从事教学工作且具有其他州颁发的合法执业资格的客座针灸师。本款所称"职责"系指课堂教学和相关技术演示。但不包括向患者提供服务以收取费用的行为;或

(4)作为联邦政府雇员、以个人身份从事相关活动、提供相关服务或使用相关职称的行为。

第311.678条　需要向患者披露的信息;知情同意

针灸师应当以符合本州规定且通行的方式取得每位患者的知情同意,并且至少应当在患者首次就诊之前或就诊期间以书面的形式披露下列信息:

(1)针灸师的资质,包括其教育程度、证明材料,以及针灸执业在本州的定义和范围。

(2)可能出现的治疗效果,包括疼痛、挫伤、感染、晕针或其他可能出现的副作用。

第311.679条　报告与记录保存要求

(1)针灸师应当遵守本州和本州各市指定的所有针对医疗服务人员的相关公共卫生报告要求。

(2)针灸师应按照符合本州规定和通行的职业标准为每位接受治疗的患者保留一份记录,该记录至少应该包括:

(a)针灸师根据《肯塔基州修订版制定法》第311.678条的规定向患者披露信息的签字副本。

(b)针灸师就患者的病史和当前的身体状况进行医患沟通的证据。

(c)针灸师进行传统针灸检查的证据。

(d)治疗记录,包括所治疗的穴位。

(e)针灸师对治疗的评价和指示。

第 311.680 条　患者访谈与医疗急救的书面处理方案;危重患者的治疗;行政规章

(1)所有执业针灸师应当制定一份符合委员会行政条例要求的书面处理方案,以方便为患者问诊、紧急转院或转诊到适当医疗机构或具有相应执业范围的其他卫生保健从业者处。书面处理方案除了应提交至州医疗许可委员会,还应在针灸师的执业地点保留一份。此外,该方案还应根据监管要求进行更新。

(2)在就患者的病史进行医患沟通时,若患者透露其曾患有本条第(3)款所列的某种严重疾病或症状,则针灸师在提供针灸治疗之前须确认该患者目前已得到医师的诊疗并向其主治医师就其病情进行咨询。若患者拒绝提供病史或拒绝透露下列任何一种情形,则针灸师不得向其提供针灸治疗。

(3)本条所称的"严重疾病或病症"是指:

(a)高血压和心脏病。

(b)急性严重腹痛。

(c)未诊断的神经病变。

(d)在不到三个月的时间内出现不明原因的体重减少或增加,且幅度超过百分之十五的。

(e)疑似骨折或脱臼。

(f)疑似全身性感染。

(g)严重失血性疾病。

(h)无既往病史的急性呼吸窘迫。

(i)妊娠。

(j)糖尿病。

(k)癌症。

第 311.681 条　执照续期;宽限期;终止、吊销、撤销和恢复

(1)已获得执照成为针灸师的人员应每两年将其证书续期一次,且应向委员会缴纳其规定的续期费。该项费用应在证书到期当年的 6 月 1 日或之前缴纳。自 6 月 1 日起六十日内未能按期续期的执照将到期。

(2)州医疗许可委员会应根据针灸师最后登记的地址向其发出续期通知。通知中应包含续期申请和续期费用等事项。执业针灸师不能以未能收到通知为由要求免于缴纳滞纳金。

(3)证书到期当年的 6 月 1 日后的六十日为宽限期,其间针灸师可以继续执业。针灸师在缴纳委员会行政条例中规定的续期费和滞纳金之后,允许续期执照。

(4)在宽限期结束后未能续期的执照将失效。此后该针灸师不再有资格在本州从事针灸实践。在缴纳续期费和委员会在行政条例中规定的恢复费用之后,持有失效执照的人员可以申请恢复执照。若该申请在其执照失效后的五年内提出,则申请人无须参加恢复执照考试。

(5)被吊销且未续期的执照将到期并失效。被吊销的执照续期后,在执照吊销期间或委员会决定恢复其执照之前,该执业针灸师依然不得从事针灸实践。

（6）被撤销的执照将失效且不得续期。若针灸师欲恢复其被撤销的执照，则须根据本条第（1）和（4）款的规定缴纳续期费和恢复费。

（7）如某人执照失效后五年内未申请恢复，则不得申请续期、恢复或补发该执照。如欲获得新执照，则应根据《肯塔基州修订版制定法》第 311.674 条的规定重新申请。

第 311.682 条　继续教育要求

（1）按照州医疗许可委员会的行政规章，持证人须每两年参加一次不超过三十学时的继续教育，作为其执照续期的条件。继续教育可以选择与针灸相关的专业技能和知识提升、拓展或提高的项目，由非营利机构或营利机构提供的均可。此外，继续教育必须涉及针灸或东方医学相关科目，包括但不限于解剖学、生物科学、辅助疗法、卫生与消毒、急救方案和疾病。

（2）委员会有权为各继续教育主办机构确定相关费用。

（3）执业针灸师须保留完成继续教育的证明记录，以证明其符合本条规定。

（4）国家和州级针灸和东方医学机构和学校均可根据本条的规定为相关人员提供继续教育。

法律研究委员会(LRC)提示

法律研究委员会提示（7‑12‑06）：为进一步明确并执行《肯塔基州修订版制定法》7.136（1）（c）的规定，州制定法的修订者将 2006 年《肯塔基州法案》第 249 章第十二节拆分为多款。

第 311.683 条　申请执照转为非执业状态；重新激活为执业状态

（1）根据《肯塔基州修订版制定法》第 311.674 条和第 311.675 条获得执照者，在提交申请并缴纳执照非执业状态费用之后，可以申请将其执照转为非执业状态。

（2）向州医疗许可委员会提交申请可激活非执业执照。若执照已处于非执业状态超过五年，持证人须重新申请执照并需符合《肯塔基州修订版制定法》第 311.674 条及第 311.675 条的所有认证要求。申请认证要求应包括：

（a）持证人已缴纳非执业状态费用的证据。

（b）缴纳首次申请执照所需费用。

第 311.684 条　撤销执照；书面警告；其他处罚程序

（1）州医疗许可委员会有权：

（a）撤销执照。

（b）吊销执照，期限不超过五年。

（c）驳回执照申请。

（d）拒绝续期执照。

（e）对执照施加无限期限制。

（f）对单项违法行为和/或因诉讼产生的费用处以最高两千美元的罚款。

（g）将某人转为察看状态，期限不超过五年。

（h）对针灸师发出警告。

（i）在证明针灸师存在下列行为后，实施上述处罚中的任意组合：

1. 故意做出或出示，或唆使他人做出或出示与执照申请有关的具有虚假性、欺诈性或伪造性的声明、文书、证书、文凭或其他文件。

2. 进行与执业资格认证考上有关的欺诈、伪造、欺骗行为，协助或唆使他人做出上述行为，或与他人串谋或共谋。

3. 根据肯塔基州或美国法律，认罪或不抗辩，或被肯塔基州境内或境外的任何法院判定犯有重罪或即将成为重罪的行为。

4. 认罪或不抗辩，或因以不诚实为基本及必要因素被肯塔基州境内或境外的任何法院判有轻罪，包括但不限于盗窃、挪用公款、虚假宣誓、伪证、欺诈或谎报。

5. 对酒精、毒品或任何非法药物上瘾，或滥用上述药物。

6. 因出现身体或心理障碍或其他疾病而导致其继续从事针灸执业活动的行为会对患者、公众或其他医护人员产生危险。

7. 在与针灸相关的任何文件中故意或使他人作出、协助或唆使他人作出虚假陈述。

8. 帮助、协助或教唆他人非法行医或从事针灸实践。

9. 故意违反保密通信规定。

10. 以违反职业道德、不称职或重大/长期过失的方式提供针灸服务。

11. 被任何医疗机构或专业协会因违反职业道德、不称职或违反本条任何规定而免职、吊销执照、开除或列入察看状态。

12. 违反与针灸实践相关的法律或行政规章的相关规定。

13. 违反委员会发出的最终命令或议定命令中规定的任何条款。

14. 未能完成继续教育所需的学时数。

（2）所有针对针灸师的纪律处分程序均应根据《肯塔基州修订版制定法》第311.591条、第311.592条、第311.593条、第311.599条、第13B章以及第311节中载明的相关行政条例进行。

（3）（a）在做出下列判决时，委员会可向执业针灸师发出书面警告：

1. 该针灸师被指控的违法行为并不严重。

2. 调查后提交给委员会的证据（包括针灸师根据委员会依法提供的机会而做出的答复）清楚地表明其被指控的违法行为属实。

（b）书面警告的副本应保存在该执业针灸师的永久档案中。

（c）针灸师有权在收到警告后的三十日内做出答复，该答复也应存入其永久执照档案中。

（d）执业针灸师可在收到警告后的三十日内向委员会提出请求，要求召开听证会。

（e）委员会在收到关于举行听证会的请求后，应暂缓执行书面警告相关的操作，并根据《肯塔基州修订版制定法》第13B章的规定准备听证会事宜。

（4）在调查或举行听证会的过程中，委员会可随时发出议定命令，或让针灸师作出保证，表示其会自愿服从委员会的裁决。

（5）经受害方同意，委员会可以采用调解的方式处理针灸师的违纪事宜。委员会可委任任意一名或多名委员会成员或工作人员负责处理调解事宜。

（6）委员会有权重新审议、修改或撤销其作出的违纪处分。

法律研究委员会(LRC)提示

法律研究委员会提示(7-12-06)：为了进一步明确并执行《肯塔基州修订版制定法》7.136(1)(c)的规定，州制定法的修订者将2006年《肯塔基州法案》第249章第十四节一款拆分为多款。

第 311.685 条　实施违纪处分前举行听证会；举行听证会和上诉的权利；申请补发被撤销的执照；察看期；不受司法审查约束的委员会决议

（1）在根据《肯塔基州修订版制定法》第 311.671 条至第 311.686 条的规定吊销或撤销某执业针灸师的执照、将其转入察看状态、对其执业行为进行监管、作出行政罚款、发出书面警告或采取上述组合处罚措施之前，委员会应当根据《肯塔基州修订版制定法》第 13B 章的规定召开听证会。

（2）在根据《肯塔基州修订版制定法》第 311.671 条至第 311.686 条的规定驳回针灸师提出的申请或发出书面警告后，委员会可应受害方的请求，根据《肯塔基州修订版制定法》第 13B 章的规定召开听证会。

（3）除旨在驳回执照的首次申请或续期请求的最终命令或根据《肯塔基州修订版制定法》第 13B 章第 125(3)款的规定发出的最终命令外，委员会发出的有关针灸执照的其他最终命令均应在通知送达持证人后三十日内生效（除非另有约定）。但若委员会调查小组基于充分、合理的理由认为患者或公众的健康、福祉和安全会因通知的延迟生效而受到威胁的话，委员会可命令该通知立即生效。

（4）若委员会对任何针灸师发出最终命令，拒绝其首次申请执照或对执照进行续期，或给予持证人纪律处分，则该针灸师可根据《肯塔基州修订版制定法》第 13B 章的规定向该委员会办公所在地的巡回法院提出呈请，要求对该项命令进行司法审查。但委员会调查小组就恢复被撤销执照的申请而做出的决议并非最终命令，因此不受司法审查的约束。

（5）法院不得在未向委员会提供陈述机会的情况下对其发出禁令救济。

（6）被撤销执照的针灸师可在撤销令生效之日起五年后，向委员会提交重新申请执照的呈请，从而再次获得在肯塔基州从事针灸实践的资格。

（7）法院不得强制要求委员会颁发新执照，委员会就拒绝重新颁发执照的决议也不受司法审查的约束。在根据本条第(6)款规定提出呈请后，除非原持证人能够向委员会证明其品德良好，身体和心理健康，具备恢复行医的条件，且不会对患者或公众造成不必要的风险或危险，否则不予颁发新的执照。

（8）若委员会决定在本条所述的情况下向被撤销执照的人员重新颁发执照，则须为新获发执照的人员设置二到五年的察看期，具体时长由委员会确定。若上述人员在察看期内出现任何违法行为，则其执照自动撤销。

第311.686条 吊销、限制执照的紧急命令—投诉/控告与听证—听证的程序规则—最终命令发布后紧急命令作废

（1）当根据《肯塔基州修订版制定法》第311.591条成立的调查小组有合理根据相信针灸师已违反《肯塔基州修订版制定法》第311.550(19)款下界定的命令条款，或者已违反纪律条款，或者针灸师的行为对患者和公众健康和福祉构成危险时，为保证患者和公众的安全，调查小组可根据《肯塔基州修订版制定法》第13B章第125条的规定发布紧急命令，吊销该针灸师的执照，或对其执照进行限制。

（2）为据《肯塔基州修订版制定法》第311.592条就依本条而发布的紧急命令举行的听证会之目的，紧急命令涉及的事实调查结果应构成可反驳推定，即存在构成对患者或公众健康、福祉或安全构成直接危险的、违反法律的实质性证据。为本条所称听证会之目的，委员会应就根据传闻对针灸师作出的投诉/控告进行受理，且传闻可作为委员会调查结果的依据。

（3）除非申诉理由成立，否则不得发出本条项下第（1）款所述的紧急命令。调查小组应在听证会举行前提出申诉，否则紧急命令无效。

（4）在按照申诉程序向被申诉针灸师送达《肯塔基州修订版制定法》第311.550(20)款中定义的最终命令后，不得继续执行吊销或限制其执照的紧急命令。就紧急命令提出的申诉不得妨碍委员会对相关申诉进行处理。

路易斯安那州

路易斯安那州针灸法[①]

第 1356 条　定义

下列定义适用于本节：

（1）"针灸"系指为达到诱导麻醉、减轻疼痛、治疗人体疾病、机体失调或功能失调或就此而言的治疗或预防效果之目的，并基于人体器官相关穴位或穴位组合的生理相互关系理论，通过机械、热或电刺激，在预先确定的穴位或穴位组合进行针刺，或对该穴位采用热刺激或电刺激的治疗方式。

（2）"针灸戒毒"缩写为"acu detox"，系指在耳朵上的多个穴位插入针灸针进行治疗。

（3）"针灸戒毒专家"，即 A.D.S，系指经认证可以进行针灸戒毒的个人。

（4）"委员会"系指路易斯安那州医学委员会。

（5）"执业针灸师"系指除医师以外的经委员会认证并按照 R.S.第三十七章 1358 条的规定从事针灸实践的个人。

（6）"NADA"系指国家针灸戒毒协会。

（7）"医师"系指在路易斯安那州持有医师执照的个人。

（8）"针灸医师"系指经委员会认证并按照 R.S.第三十七章 1357 条的规定从事针灸实践的医师。

（9）自 2016 年，废止。第 550 号法令第 2 条。

第 1357 条　针灸医师

委员会应向已在路易斯安那州获得医师执照，并顺利完成以下任何一项的医师颁发针灸医师执照：

（1）在委员会规定的学校或诊所接受为期六个月的针灸培训。

（2）完成三百学时的针灸继续医学教育，该教育由美国医学会指定为一类继续医学教育学时。

[①]　根据《路易斯安那州制定法》注释版第 37 卷第 15 章第 4 节"针灸服务"译出。

第 1357.1 条　针灸戒毒实践；认证；规定颁布；突发公共卫生事件

A. 委员会应向符合以下条件的个人颁发执照：在获得委员会许可于该州执业的医师或针灸师的一般监督下工作，且顺利完成以下事项：

（1）由 NADA 注册培训师进行的 NADA 培训。

（2）具有 NADA 出具的资质证书。

（3）向委员会登记注册。

B. 根据本条的规定，委员会应与其中西医结合医学委员会合作，颁布必要的规章制度，以规范州内针灸戒毒专家认证和针灸戒毒实践。此类规章制度应包括但不限于以下内容：

（1）关于收费的规定。

（2）关于拒绝、吊销、撤销或在执业范围之外从事违反职业道德的行为的规定。

（3）关于对针灸戒毒专家进行一般监督的规定。

C. 在公共卫生紧急事件期间且路易斯安那州卫生部认为需要继续提供紧急服务的时段内，应允许其他州的经 NADA 认证的针灸戒毒专家，根据委员会制定的规章制度，在路易斯安那州执业。

第 1358 条　执业针灸师

该委员会应当向满足以下两种情况的个人颁发执照：

（1）国家针灸与东方医学认证委员会（NCCAOM）中表现积极。

（2）顺利通过 NCCAOM 资格考试，包括生物医学考试。

第 1359 条　向立法机构提交年度报告

委员会应每年向立法机构报告本州针灸实践的状况。

第 1360 条　路易斯安那州医学委员会的权力和职责

除在 R.S.第三十七章 1270 条中规定的权力和职责外，路易斯安那州医学委员会可以实施以下任何一项行为：

（1）根据《行政诉讼法》，通过、修订和执行《行政诉讼案》认为必要的规则和规章，以确保辨明申请人能力、保护公众利益及实施本节条款。

（2）批准执业申请人的执照，拒绝、吊销或撤销任何超出执业范围或从事违反职业道德行为的持证人的执照，或将其列入察看期。

（3）就要求拒绝、吊销、撤销或拒绝续期执照的指控举行听证会。

（4）根据 R.S.第三十七章 1281 条的规定，为实施本节条款而收取费用。

（5）设立针灸咨询委员会，提供委员会认为在实施本节条款时必要的协助。

路易斯安那州针灸行政法[①]

第一节　总　　则

2101　适用范围

本章规则适用于路易斯安那州针灸医师、执业针灸师以及针灸戒毒专家的认证。

2103　定义

用于本章和第 51 章时，下列术语应具有规定的含义。

针灸实践法案或法案——R.S. 第 37 卷 1356‑1360 条及其修订或补充版本。

针灸：为达到诱导麻醉、减轻疼痛、治疗人体疾病、机体失调或功能失调或就此而言的治疗或预防效果之目的，并基于人体器官相关穴位或穴位组合的生理相互关系理论，通过机械、热或电刺激，在预先确定的穴位或穴位组合进行针刺，或对该穴位采用热刺激或电刺激的治疗方式。

针灸戒毒：根据国家针灸戒毒协会的技术规程，将针灸针插入耳朵上的多个穴位进行治疗。针灸戒毒疗法构成针灸实践的一个子类别。

针灸戒毒专家（ADS）：持有由委员会正式颁发的现行执照的个人，可在医师或执业针灸师的监督下从事针灸戒毒疗法。

申请人：向委员会申请认证为路易斯安那州的针灸医师、执业针灸师或针灸戒毒专家的个人。

申请：为获得在路易斯安那州从事针灸或针灸戒毒疗法实践的执照，按照委员会规定格式向委员会提交并由委员会接收的申请，该申请还包括所有按委员会格式要求的信息、执照、文件及其他材料。

委员会：路易斯安那州医学考试委员会。

执照：委员会对个人现行证书的正式认可，由委员会正式颁发，证明委员会依法对该个人的认证。

一般监督：用于本章和第 51 章时，应指对本规则第 5106.B 条规定的针灸戒毒专家所提供服务进行负责任的监督。

良好品德：用于申请人时，意味着：

a. 申请人（如属医师）在向委员会提出申请之前或期间，根据 R.S. 第 37 卷 1285 的规定，未因任何作为、不作为、情况或情形导致医疗执照被拒绝颁发、吊销或撤销。

b. 申请人（如属针灸医师、执业针灸师或针灸戒毒专家）在向委员会提出申请之前或期间，不存在任何根据本规定第 5113 条可导致执照被吊销或撤销的作为、不作为、情况或情形。

[①]　根据《路易斯安那州行政法典》第 46 卷第 45 编第 2 篇第 21 章"针灸师和针灸排毒专家"译出。

c. 申请人在申请之前或在申请相关流程期间,没有在知情或不知情的情况下,就某一重要事实向委员会作出任何虚假或误导性陈述,或遗漏对申请具有重要意义的任何事实或事项;或

d. 申请人在达到或获得本章要求的认证资格时,未作出任何陈述或未能作出陈述,或有任何虚假、欺骗、欺诈或误导性的作为或不作为。

执业针灸师(LAc):除持有现行执照的医师外,在本州从事针灸实践的持有由州针灸委员会正式颁发执照的个人。

NADA:国家针灸戒毒协会。

针灸医师:持有委员会正式颁发的执照、可以从事针灸实践的医师。

主要执业地点:医师、执业针灸师或针灸戒毒专家花费大部分时间使用委员会颁发的执照或认证行使执业权限的地点。

拟任督导执业针灸师:已向委员会提交申请获批为针灸导师的执业针灸师。

拟任督导医师:已向委员会提交申请获批为督导医师的医师。

督导执业针灸师:根据本章在委员会注册的执业针灸师,对针灸戒毒专家实施监督工作。

督导医师:根据本章在委员会注册的医师,负责监督针灸戒毒专家。

普遍预防措施:由美国疾病控制中心(CDC)制定的一套预防措施,旨在于提供急救或卫生保健时防止人类免疫缺陷病毒(HIV)、乙型肝炎病毒(HBV)和其他血源性病原体的传播。在普遍的预防措施下,所有患者的血液和某些体液都视为可能感染 HIV、HBV 和其他血源性病原体。

本章任何地方使用的阳性名词也应视为包括阴性名词。

第二节　针灸医师的认证

2105　本节适用范围

本节条款规定了在路易斯安那州获得针灸医师执照所需的资格和程序。

2107　针灸医师的认证资格

A. 要获得针灸医师认证的资格,申请人应当:

1. 是一名医生,持有委员会正式颁发的在路易斯安那州不受限制的现行医师执照。

2. 具有第 2103.A 条所定义的良好品德。

3. 已顺利完成:

a. 在委员会根据本章第 2118－2121 条确定的学校或诊所接受不少于六个月的针灸培训;或

b. 不少于三百学时的针灸继续医学教育,该教育被美国医学会指定为一类继续医学教育学时。

B. 申请人应承担向委员会证明其任职条件和资格的责任。除非申请人按照委员会规定的方式提供证据证明该资格,并获得委员认可,否则不得视申请人为符合此类任职条件。

2109　针灸医师的申请程序

A. 针灸医师的认证申请应当符合委员会规定的格式。

B. 本章规定的认证申请应包括：

1. 以委员会认可的形式证明申请人具备本章规定的资格。

2. 委员会可能要求的其他信息和文件，以证明认证资格。

C. 采用英语以外语言提交的文件，应附有由申请人以外的翻译人员核证的英文译本。翻译人员应证明该译本的准确性，并遵循伪证相关的法律条款。

D. 委员会可以拒绝考虑任何细节不完整的申请，包括提交申请表所要求的所有文件。委员会可酌情要求对申请表中列出的任何信息请求作出更详细或完整的回应，作为考虑申请的条件。

E. 向委员会提交的每份申请均应附有本规则第 1 章规定的适当费用。

第三节 执业针灸师和针灸戒毒专家认证；提名和督导人员的任职条件

2111 本节的适用范围

本节规定了获得针灸执照、针灸戒毒专家认证，以及路易斯安那州督导医师和督导执业针灸师执照所需的资格和程序。

2113 获得针灸执照的资格

A. 为获得针灸执照，申请人应当具备以下条件：

1. 应年满二十一岁。

2. 应具有第 2103.A 条所定义的良好品德。

3. 应在高中或同等学力中顺利完成四年制教学课程。

4. 应为美国公民或拥有由美国公民及移民服务局（USCIS）国土安全部根据《移民和国籍法》(66 Stat. 163)及其下的专员条例(8 CFR)正式颁发的在美国居住和工作的有效和现行法律授权。

5. 应当满足以下两项要求：

a. 在国家针灸与东方医学认证委员会维持执业状态。

b. 已顺利通过国家针灸与东方医学认证委员会（NCCAOM）或其继受机构给予的认证考试，包括生物医学部分的考试。

6. 应确认他或她在从事针灸实践时始终与本规则第 5106.A 条所定义的医生建立并保持关系。

B. 申请人应承担向委员会证明其任职条件和资格的责任，按照委员会规定的方式提供证据证明该资格，并获得委员会认可。

2114 针灸戒毒专家资格认证；督导医师或督导执业针灸师的注册条件

A. 要获得针灸戒毒专家认证资格，申请人：

1. 应年满二十一岁。

2. 应具有本章第 2103.A 条所定义的良好品德。

3. 应在高中或同等学力中顺利完成四年制教学课程。

4. 应为美国公民或拥有由美国公民及移民服务局（USCIS）国土安全部根据《移民和国

籍法》(66 Stat. 163)及其下的专员条例(8 CFR)正式颁发的在美国居住和工作的有效和现行法律授权。

5. 应已:

a. 顺利完成 NADA 注册培训师的 NADA 培训。

b. 持有 NADA 颁发的现行针灸戒毒执照。

6. 应确认他或她只能在本规定 5106.B 所定义医生或执业针灸师的一般监督下提供针灸戒毒治疗。

B. 在接受针灸戒毒专家的监督之前,执业针灸师应在委员会注册。为获得资格注册以监督 ADS,拟任督导医师应在申请之日:

1. 持有在路易斯安那州行医不受限制的现行执照。

2. 目前未参加任何研究生住院医师培训。

C. 在接受针灸戒毒专家的监督之前,执业针灸师应在委员会注册。为获得资格注册以监督针灸戒毒专家,提名的督导执业针灸师应在申请之日:

1. 持有不受限制的 LAc 现行执照。

2. 在申请日期之前,已获得委员会颁发的 LAc 认证或执照,且已在本州执业至少两年。

D. 耳穴戒毒专家、拟任督导医师或拟任督导执业针灸师的申请人应当以委员会规定和认可的方式提供证据,证明其自身具备规定的任职条件和资格。

2115　执业针灸师的申请程序

A. 执业针灸师的认证申请应以委员会批准的格式提出。

B. 根据本节提出的申请应包括:

1. 以委员会认可的形式证明申请人具备本章规定的资格。

2. 申请人出具的证明文件,证实完整申请中包含或随同该申请提交的所有信息、陈述和文件的真实性及可靠性。

3. 委员会可能要求的其他信息和文件。

C. 采用英语以外语言提交的文件,应附有由申请人以外的翻译人员核证的英文译本。翻译人员应证明该译本的准确性,并遵循伪证相关的法律条款。

D. 委员会可以拒绝或拒绝考虑任何细节不完整的申请,包括提交申请表要求的所有文件。委员会可酌情要求对申请表中列出的任何信息请求作出更详细或完整的回应,以此作为考虑申请的条件。

E. 向委员会提交的每份申请均应附有本规则第 1 章规定的适当费用。

F. 在申请人提交完整申请,随附申请所需文件,并支付申请费后,若委员会对申请人的资格有疑问,则申请人应按照要求出现在委员会或其指定人员面前。

2116　针灸戒毒专家申请程序

A. 针灸戒毒专家的认证申请应当以委员会规定的格式提出,包括以委员会规定的格式提出的执业意向告知书,并由已注册或已向委员会申请注册的拟任督导医师或督导拟任执业针灸师签署。

B. 根据本节申请认证和批准,应包括:

1. 以委员会认可的形式证明申请人具备本章规定资格的证明。

2. 申请人出具的证明文件,证实在行使本部分执照赋予的特权时,应遵守本规定第5106B 条的要求。

3. 申请人出具的证明文件,证实完整申请中包含或随同该申请提交的所有信息、陈述和文件的真实性及可靠性。

4. 委员会可能要求的其他信息和文件。

C. 采用英语以外语言提交的文件,应附有由申请人以外的翻译人员核证的英文译本。翻译人员应证明该译本的准确性,并遵循伪证相关的法律条款。

D. 委员会可以拒绝或拒绝考虑任何细节不完整的申请,包括提交申请所需的所有文件。委员会可酌情要求对申请表中列出的任何信息请求作出更详细或完整的回应,以此作为考虑申请的条件。

E. 向委员会提交的每份申请均应附有本规则第 1 章规定的适用费用。

2117 督导医师或督导执业针灸师的注册申请程序

A. 督导医师或督导执业针灸师的注册申请,应当以委员会规定的格式提出,包括令委员会认可的证明,证实申请人具备本章规定的资格,并包含委员会可能要求的其他信息和文件。

B. 委员会可以拒绝或拒绝考虑任何细节不完整的申请,包括提交申请所需的所有文件。委员会可酌情要求对申请表中列出的任何信息请求作出更详细或完整的回应,以此作为考虑申请的条件。

C. 注册或批准督导 LAc 或督导 ADS 时,不得另行收费。

第四节 委员会批准成立针灸院校

2118 适用范围

A. 本节规定了委员会批准成立针灸院校的方法和程序。

2119 批准的适用性

A. 如本章所述,顺利完成经委员会批准的学校或学院的针灸正规培训,是获得针灸医师或执业针灸师资格所必需的限定条件之一。若申请人完成针灸院校的培训之日起,该院校获得委员会批准,则视为申请人满足此项条件。

2121 批准成立针灸院校

A. 目前获得针灸及东方医学教育审核委员会(ACAOM)或其前身国家针灸和东方医学院校认证委员会(NACSCAOM)认证的针灸培训学校或学院,应同时视为获委员会批准。

B. 若 ACAOM 或其前身 NACSCAOM 授予提供针灸培训的学校或学院候选资格,则应同时视其为获得委员会的附条件批准,但若在授予其候选资格之日起三年内,ACAOM 未授予认证,则委员会的批准将自动撤销。

C. 委员会在应申请人要求或任何此类学校或计划的申请,并在此类学校或计划向委员会提交文件,说明其提供的针灸培训标准与 ACAOM 规定的认证标准基本同等后,可另外批准提供针灸培训的学校或计划。

第五节　证书和执照的颁发；批准注册为督导医师或督导执业针灸师；终止；续期和恢复

2125　颁发证书和执照，批准注册

A. 若申请人符合本章规定的针灸医师的资格、要求和程序及委员会要求，委员会应当认证其为针灸医师。

B. 若申请人符合本章规定的执业针灸师资格、要求和程序及委员会的要求，委员会应当认证其为执业针灸师。

C. 若申请人符合本章规定的针灸戒毒专家的资格、要求和程序及委员会的要求，委员会应认定其为针灸戒毒专家。根据本章向申请人颁发证书，即构成对拟任督导医师或拟任督导执业针灸师的注册批准。

D. 虽然医师或执业针灸师每次对针灸戒毒专家进行一般监督时，都必须通知委员会，但只需在委员会注册一次。若针灸戒毒专家根据本章第2127.F条向委员会提交执业意向告知书，则视注册督导医师或督导执业针灸师对新任针灸戒毒专家发出的监督通知已提交。

E. 若医师或执业针灸师已完成注册，以监督一名针灸戒毒专家，则一旦所需的任何信息发生变化，每位注册医师、执业针灸师和针灸戒毒专家都有责任在十五日内向委员会更新信息。

2127　认证和执照的到期和终止；修改

A. 委员会根据本章颁发的每份证书和执照，均应在颁发年份的最后一日到期、失效或者归于无效。

B. 根据本章第2129条的规定，按时提交认证或执照续期申请，将在续期或拒绝续期认证或执照之前，使即将到期的认证或执照保持完全效力。

C. 无论执业针灸师的执照是初始执照还是续期执照，均将在到期后而未能及时续期的任何一日终止、失效或者归于无效。

D. 除本节F小节规定的情况外，无论针灸戒毒专家的执照是首次颁发的执照还是续期执照，均将在到期后而未能及时续期的任何一日终止、失效或者归于无效：

1. 督导医师或督导执业针灸师不再具有不受限制的现行医师执照，即不能在路易斯安那州作为医师或执业针灸师执业。

2. 督导医师或督导执业针灸师自愿或非自愿地停止从事医疗活动或作为执业针灸师执业。

3. 针灸戒毒专家与督导医师或督导执业针灸师的关系终止。

4. 针灸戒毒专家执照因未能及时续期而失效。

E. 如满足以下条件，督导执业针灸师或督导医师与针灸戒毒专家的关系终止时，执照并不终止：

1. 针灸戒毒专家目前与另一名督导医师或督导执业针灸师之间存在监督关系；或者，针灸戒毒专家将停止执业，直到以委员会规定格式向委员会提交通知，告知其已与符合任职条件、要求和程序的新任督导医师或督导执业针灸师建立监督关系。该通知自委员会收到之

日起生效,以下次委员会会议最终批准为准。

2. 若针灸戒毒专家的督导医师或督导执业针灸师有任何变化或补充,则针灸戒毒专家应在十五日之内,将变动情况通知委员会。

2129 证书和执照的续展;注册验证

A. 委员会根据本章颁发的每份证书或执照,应于颁发证书或执照当年的最后一日或之前续期,续期的具体方式是按照委员会规定的格式向委员会提交正确填写的续期申请,附带提交第 1 章规定的十五学时专业继续教育和续期费用的证明。

B. 续期申请和说明可以通过委员会的网页、当面要求或书面请求委员会获得。

C. 每位注册督导医师和督导执业针灸师应当每年以委员会规定的格式向委员会确认注册信息的准确性。

2130 到期执照的恢复

A. 自届满之日起两年内因未续期而到期的执照,可以由委员会根据如下规定的条件和程序恢复。

B. 恢复申请应以委员会规定的格式提交,并附有:

1. 委员会提供的统计宣誓书。

2. 申请人近照一张。

3. 本章提及或规定的或委员会可能要求的证明执照资格的其他信息和文件。

4. 第一章规定的执照到期后每一年的续期费和逾期费。

a. 若申请自到期之日起不足一年,则罚款相当于执照的续期费。

b. 逾期一年但不足两年提出申请的,罚款为执照续期费的两倍。

C. 执照已失效并逾期超过两年的个人不具备考虑恢复执照的资格,但可以根据本章的适用规则向委员会申请初始执照。

D. 可以根据法案或本规则规定的任何拒绝执照的理由拒绝恢复请求。

E. 申请人有责任向委员会证明其资格,以申请恢复针灸执照。除非申请人按照委员会规定的方式提供证据证明该资格,并获得委员认可,否则不得视申请人为符合此类任职条件。

第六节 受限执照,许可

2131 紧急临时许可

A. 针灸戒毒专家。委员会可以向一名针灸戒毒专家颁发紧急临时许可,有效期不超过六十日,以便在该州公共卫生紧急情况期间,以及路易斯安那州卫生部(LDH)认为有必要在其指定或经委员会批准的地点继续提供紧急服务的期间内,提供自愿、无偿的针灸戒毒服务。此种许可的申请应根据本编 412 条提出,并囊括在督导医师或督导执业针灸师监督下执业的执业意向告知书,该告知书应以委员会批准的方式提交。

B. 前述针灸戒毒专家的服务仅限于针灸戒毒,由督导医师或督导执业针灸师批准并在其一般监督下进行。所有服务均应由针灸戒毒专家存档,并由其督导医师或督导执业针灸师进行审核。

C. 执业针灸师。委员会可以根据本编第 412 条向执业针灸师颁发紧急临时许可,以便在公共卫生紧急情况期间，以及路易斯安那州卫生部认为需要继续提供紧急服务的期间内，在本州提供自愿、无偿的针灸服务。

第七节　针灸咨询委员会

2139　本节适用范围

为协助医学委员会处理与针灸有关的事务，特设立针灸咨询委员会，承担如下职责。

2141　咨询委员会的构成、职能和职责

A. 州医学委员会应当按照本节的规定，组建和任命一个针灸咨询委员会。

B. 组成。该委员会应由委员会选出的五名成员组成，其中四名应为执业针灸师，其中一名应为针灸医师。咨询委员会的所有成员都将获得委员会的许可，并在本州执业和居住。

C. 在可能或切实可行的范围内，委员会在任命咨询委员会成员时应保持地域多样性，以便为居住在本州各个地区的居民选拔出具有代表性的咨询委员会成员。

D. 服务期限。委员会每位成员的任期为四年，或直到继任者被任命并合格。委员会成员为委员会服务。委员会成员可连任两届，任期四年。

E. 委员会的职能。该委员会将向州医学委员会提供有关以下方面的建议：

1. 执照申请。

2. 与获取执照有关的教育要求。

3. 有关法规、规章的变化。

4. 履行州医学委员会可能要求的其他职能并提供相应的意见和建议。

F. 委员会会议。委员会应当在每个日历年至少开会一次，或在委员会或委员会的法定人数认为必要时更频繁地开会。三名委员会成员构成法定人数。委员会应从其成员中选举一名主席。主席应召集会议、指定日期、时间和地点，并主持委员会的所有会议。主席应当记录或促使记录咨询委员会所有会议的准确和完整的书面会议记录，并将其副本提供给州医学委员会。

G. 保密。在履行本节授权的职能时，咨询委员会及其成员在该权力范围内行事时，应当被视为委员会的代理人。未经州医学委员会的书面授权，咨询委员会成员不得向州医学委员会以外的任何人传达、披露或以任何方式向任何人披露在担任委员会代理人时获得的任何机密信息或文件。

第八节　继　续　教　育

2149　本节适用范围

本节规定每年续期针灸执照所需的继续专业教育标准，以及适用的程序和文件。

2151　继续教育的要求

为符合年度执照续期资格，执业针灸师应当以州医学委员会规定的格式证明自己顺利完成规定的十五学时继续专业教育。

2153　合格的计划和活动

一项活动或计划若要根据此类规定确定为合格的继续专业教育，则必须具有重要的知

识或实践内容,并主要解决与针灸有关的问题,其主要目标必须是保持或提高参与者作为针灸师的能力。

2155 计划发起人的批准

任何获得国家针灸与东方医学认证委员会或其继任者认可或美国教育部认可的教育计划、课程、培训会或活动,均应被视为州医学委员会认可其作为专业继续教育的计划。

2157 文件编制程序

A. 州医学委员会规定的用于记录和证明完成继续专业教育的格式或方法应由持证人填写,并与年度续期申请一起或作为年度续期申请的一部分交回。

B. 任何未经州医学委员会根据本规则批准的继续专业教育活动,应当提交咨询委员会进行评估和建议。若委员会裁定某项继续教育活动不符合其规定的标准,或不符合申请人要求的继续教育单位的数量,应当将此类情形通知申请人,以便其续期执照。委员会关于批准和认可任何此类活动的决定应为最终决定。

2159 未能满足继续教育要求

A. 州医学委员会应当书面通知未能证明符合继续专业教育要求的执照续期申请人。申请人的执照在六十日内保持完全效力。州医学委员会在此六十日内的通知载明:本执照将被视为到期、未续期,并可被撤销,恕不另行通知。除非申请人在六十日内书面声明提供符合委员会要求的证据,即:

1. 申请人已满足继续专业教育要求;或者

2. 申请人未能满足继续专业教育要求的原因是残疾、疾病或委员会可确定的其他正当理由。

B. 针灸执照因不再续期或因不符合本规则继续教育要求而被吊销的,可以由州医学委员会在规定的时间内按照本规则规定程序予以恢复。

2161 豁免要求

A. 如果有执业针灸师提出书面申请并提供符合委员会要求的证据,证明其存在永久性身体残疾、疾病、经济困难或其他类似减责情形,以致不能满足继续专业教育的要求,州医学委员会可酌情放弃本规则要求的全部或部分继续专业教育。

密西西比州

密西西比州针灸法①

第 73-71-1 条　简称

本章应称为《针灸服务法案》。制定法中任何条款凡提及《针灸服务法案》,均应按照本章规定解释。

第 73-71-3 条　立法目的和意图

(1)考虑到根治疾病以及对患者采取整体治疗的必要性,立法机构制定本条例,旨在通过针灸构建医学艺术和科学实践的框架。

(2)本章的目的是鼓励希望获得针灸服务的公民有效利用针灸从业者相关技能;消除不必要的阻碍有效提供医疗服务的现有法律限制;并将针灸作为一种基本的、独立的卫生保健职业,对其进行管理和控制。

第 73-71-5 条　定义

用于本章时,除文意另有所指外,下列术语应具有以下含义:

(a)"经认证的针灸学院"系指提供东方医学理学硕士学位(Master of Science in Oriental Medicine, MSOM)或同等学位并经针灸及东方医学教育审核委员会(Accreditation Commission of Acupuncture and Oriental Medicine, ACAOM)认证的任何学院、学校或分部。

(b)"针灸师"系指获得针灸和东方医学学院专业学位的人。

(c)"针灸医患关系"系指针灸师承担对患者的健康状况和医疗需要作出临床判断的责任,患者已同意遵循针灸师的指示。

(d)"针灸医师"系指根据本章获得执照,可在本州从事针灸实践的医师,并包括"针灸师"一词。

(e)"咨询委员会"系指本章设立的密西西比州针灸咨询委员会。

(f)"委员会"系指第 73-43-1 条及其后各条中设立的州医疗许可委员会。

(g)"补充和综合疗法"系指一组不同的预防、诊断、治疗理念和实践,在实施时可能与

---

① 根据《密西西比州法典》注释版第 73 卷第 71 章"针灸服务法案"译出。

当前的科学知识不同,或者其理论基础和技术可能与在认证医学院常规教授的西医不同,或者两者兼而有之。这些疗法包括但不限于针灸、穴位疗法和穴位按压。

(h)"残障针灸师"系指由于身体或精神上的残疾而无法在保证患者安全的情况下采用适当方法从事针灸实践的针灸师,其残疾情况由主管部门的书面决定或基于临床证据的书面同意书证明,包括脑力功能退化、丧失运动能力或滥用药物或酒精,其程度足以削弱为患者提供有效医疗的能力。

(i)"知情同意"系指针灸医生以正常人能够理解的方式将诊断和治疗方案、风险评估和预后告知患者,并告知患者应给予的治疗费用估计数,并且患者已同意建议的治疗。

(j)"NCCAOM"系指国家针灸与东方医学认证委员会。

(k)"医师"系指在密西西比州获得法律授权从事医学工作的内科医生或骨病医生。

(l)"针灸实践"系指:

(i)通过针灸技术治疗、纠正、改变、减轻或预防疾病、疾病、疼痛、畸形、缺陷、损伤或其他身体或精神病症,包括:

1. 本章所定义的设备或其他治疗技术的管理或应用;或

2. 使用本章所定义的补充和综合疗法;或

3. 通过包括电话和其他电子通信在内的任何方式就任何上述事项提供意见或建议。

(ii)直接或间接、公开或非公开地声明其有能力和意愿从事本段所述行为。

(iii)使用任何头衔、单词、缩写或字母,其方式或情形应使人相信使用这些头衔、单词、缩写或字母的人有资格从事本款所述的任何行为。

(m)"针灸技术"包括针灸、艾灸或加热方式、拔罐、磁铁、离子泵送线,包括皮肤电活动评估在内的电针、冷敷、饮食、营养和生活方式咨询、手法疗法(推拿)、按摩、呼吸和功法技术、使用任何草药及营养补充剂和经络疗法。本款所用术语定义如下:

(i)"针灸"系指在身体的特定位置插入并操作针头,并在身体的特定位置应用东方药物及其他方式和程序,以预防或纠正任何疾病、病症、损伤、疼痛或其他情况。

(ii)"拔火罐"系指加热杯中的空气或通过机械方式产生吸力,将其施加到身体的特定位置以引起局部血管舒张和皮下组织的机械膨胀。

(iii)"离子泵线"系指将包含二极管的导线放置在应用于人体的针灸针上。

(iv)"磁疗"系指将磁铁应用于人体的特定位置。

(v)"电针,包括皮肤电活动评估"系指使用电子生物反馈和电刺激仪器。

(vi)"冷敷袋"系指将冷敷袋和冰敷在人体的特定位置,以减少身体表皮组织的发热或炎症。

(vii)"饮食,营养和生活方式咨询"系指对患者进行深入的访谈和咨询,以确定不良的饮食,生活方式或营养习惯是否是导致患者疾病的因素,并进行健康的生活方式教育。

(viii)"手法疗法(推拿)和按摩"系指松动骨骼和软组织。

(ix)"呼吸和功法技术"系指使用气功和其他治疗性呼吸和功法。

(x)"使用草药和植物源物质"系指使用动物、植物或矿物质来源的草药,以维持健康和治疗疾病。

(xi)"维生素,矿物质或营养补充剂"系指营养物质,包括此类物质的浓缩物或提取物。

(xii)"经络治疗器械"系指用于针灸经络的所有评估和/或治疗器械。

第 73‑71‑7 条　实践要求;医师评估;免责条款;知情同意;从业者信息;不做诊断

以下所有规定均适用于在密西西比州取得针灸执照的针灸从业者:

(a)除(c)款另有规定外,只有在针灸治疗前六个月内对患者进行适当评估时,针灸从业者才能对患者进行针灸治疗。州医疗许可委员会在密西西比州针灸咨询委员会的建议下,可以根据规则修改本款规定的评估范围或必须根据本款规定开始治疗的时间。

(b)针灸从业者必须按照州医疗许可委员会规定的表格获得患者签署的书面陈述,表明该患者已在规定的时间内由医师进行了评估。该表格必须包含明确声明,即患者应由医师对针灸从业者正在治疗的疾病进行评估。

(c)尽管(a)款另有规定,针灸从业者可在未经医师评估的情况下,针对以下情况对患者进行针灸疗法:

(i)烟瘾。

(ii)减肥。

(iii)滥用药物,须在州医疗许可委员会通过的法规允许的范围内,并听取密西西比针灸咨询委员会的建议。

(d)在治疗患者之前,针灸从业者应告知患者针灸不能替代常规医学诊断和治疗,并应征得患者的知情同意。

(e)在最初与患者亲自会面时,医师应以书面形式提供其姓名,营业地址和营业电话号码,以及有关针灸的信息,包括所使用的技术。

(f)在治疗患者时,针灸从业者不得做出诊断。如患者的病情没有改善或需要紧急医疗,针灸从业者应立即咨询医师。

第 73‑71‑9 条　被 2017 年法典第 391 章废止,2017 年 7 月 1 日失效

第 73‑71‑11 条　密西西比州针灸咨询委员会;创建;会员资格法定人数;赔偿;报告

(1)特此设立密西西比州针灸咨询委员会,以协助州医疗许可委员会管理本章的规定。

(2)委员会应由州医疗许可委员会行政主管任命的三人组成,并应从密西西比东方医学协会的六名候选人中选出。委员会的成员应为非内科医生,整骨或整脊医生或外科医生的针灸从业者,或经注册从事针灸实践或有资格作为针灸从业者的医生。

(3)委员会的初始成员应由州长按以下交错任期任命:任命一名成员,任期至 2011 年 7 月 1 日,任命两名成员,任期至 2012 年 7 月 1 日。初始任期届满后,每位继任者的任期为三年。未届满任期的空缺应当由州长委任填补。委员会成员在继任者上任并胜任工作之前,不得结束任期。

(4)任何委员会成员的任期均不得连任超过两届,并且在委员会给予适当通知后连续三次未参加会议的任何成员,应自动解除其委员会成员职务。但因委员会条例所述原因予以免责者除外。

(5)在下列情况下,州长可罢免任何委员会成员的职务:对法律规定的任何职责失职、存在不称职行为、做出委员会条例规定的不当或违反职业道德的行为、有利益冲突,或任何可以吊销或撤销针灸执照的理由。

（6）委员会成员的多数构成处理事务的法定人数。应要求出席会议的多数成员投赞成票，以采取任何行动或通过任何动议。委员会应不迟于 2009 年 9 月 1 日及其后每年 7 月举行会议，并从其成员中选出主席和副主席。委员会应在主席，多数成员或州长认为必要或适当的其他时间召开会议。所有会议的合理通知均应按照《公开会议法》（第 25－3－41 条及其后各条）规定的方式进行。委员会成员对其在履行职责期间善意执行的任何行为不承担民事诉讼责任。

（7）委员会成员应按照第 25－3－41 条的规定报销费用和里程，但不得在委员会上获得其他报酬、补贴或服务津贴。

（8）委员会应每年向立法机关报告有关上一年度持证人的数量，许可检查的结果以及所调查的违规情况的统计数据。

第 73－71－13 条　州医疗许可委员会；监管权和责任

（1）特此授权，授权和指示州医疗许可委员会通过，修改，颁布和执行规范针灸实践的规则，法规和标准，以进一步实现本章的目的，并在此基础上以咨询委员会的相应建议为基础。

（2）委员会的权限和职责包括：

（a）根据本章或其他适用的州法律授予、拒绝颁发、续期、限制、吊销或撤销针灸执照。

（b）按照既定协议审查本州针灸执照申请人的资格和适当性。

（c）对涉嫌违反本章规定的行为进行调查，以确定是否有充分的理由开启纪律处分程序。

（d）每三年检查一次场地舍和设备，每次检查收取一百美元的检查费，为受检查机构雇用的每位执业针灸师额外收取五十美元的费用。

（e）就适当向委员会提交的所有事项举行听证会，以宣誓、接受证据、作出必要的决定并根据调查结果作出命令。委员会可以传票要求证人出席并作证，并出示文件，记录或其他文件证据和委托书。委员会可以指定一名或多名成员担任听证官。委员会应通过在委员会面前进行听证的规则和条例，并且该规则应为出席委员会的任何人提供程序上正当程序的保障。正式的证据规则不适用于此。

（f）根据本章规定，与独立顾问或其他适当机构签订合同，安排执照考试，并确定该等考试费用不超过五百美元。

（g）制定并公布一份年度执照、认证和续期的费用表，每年不超过四百美元。

（h）根据州法律保存并维护所有委员会事务的准确记录。

授予本节中所列权力旨在使委员会能够有效地监督针灸实践，并为实现这一目标对该等权力进行宽松解释。

第 73－71－15 条　禁止无执照从事针灸实践

除非根据本章获得针灸执照，或根据本章的规定免予豁免执照要求，否则任何人不得以有偿或无偿方式从事针灸实践。

第 73－71－17 条　执照的效力；本章的构成

（1）针灸执照授权持证人从事针灸实践。

（2）本章不应解释为限制、干扰或阻止任何其他类型的持证卫生保健专业人员在各执业的州执照法规所定义的执业范围内从事相关实践。

（3）本章不得解释为将由联邦或州监管的研究机构主持下的从事研究的人员的活动定为非法。

（4）针灸的实践和技巧不应包括《1972 年密西西比州法典》第 73 编第 23 章所定义的物理疗法。

第 73－71－19 条　执照要求；教育；考试

（1）任何人除非通过考试和/或被证明具备委员会通过的条例中规定的必要资格，否则没有资格获得针灸执照。

（2）在任何申请人有资格参加考试或取得资格之前，他或她应提供充分证据，证明他或她：

（a）是美国公民或永久居民。

（b）熟练掌握英语。

（c）年满二十一岁。

（d）具有良好品德。

（e）已按照本章规定完成针灸课程，并获得委员会批准的机构的证书或文凭。

（f）完成了委员会批准的临床实习培训。

（g）接受了心肺复苏术（CPR）的培训。

（3）委员会可每年至少举行一次考试，并应以书面形式将所有考试的日期和时间通知所有申请人。如果委员会认为全国统一考试足以使从业者有资格在本州获得执照，则可以使用 NCCAOM 考试。在任何情况下，州考试都不得低于国家认可的考试。

（4）除笔试外，如果国家认可的考试没有提供与委员会标准相当的实践考试，则委员会应对申请人的东方医学诊断和治疗技术的实际应用进行考核，考核的方式和方法应能够体现申请人的技能和知识。

（5）委员会须要求所有符合资格的申请人接受下列学科的考核：

（a）解剖学和生理学。

（b）病理学。

（c）诊断。

（d）卫生，卫生设备和灭菌技术。

（e）所有主要的针灸原则，实践和技术。

（f）洁针技术考试。

（6）为协助委员会进行执照调查，所有申请人应接受密西西比州中央犯罪数据库和联邦调查局犯罪史数据库的指纹犯罪记录检查。每位申请人应以委员会规定的表格和方式提交申请人指纹，该指纹应提交给密西西比州公共安全部（部门）和联邦调查局身份识别司。委员会获得的任何及所有州或国家犯罪历史记录，如尚未公开记录事项，应视为非公开和机密信息，仅限于在评估申请人资格或取消执照资格时，由委员会、委员会成员、官员、调查员、代理人和律师使用，该信息不受 1983 年《密西西比州公共记录法》的限制。除在委员会的听证会上为确定执照资格提出证据外，除非事先征得申请人的书面同意或有管辖权的法院的命令,否则委员会不得向任何其他人或机构披露或以其他方式披露此类信息或记录。委员会应向部门提供申请人的指纹、该部门可能需要的任何补充信息,以及申请人签署的同意检查犯罪记录和使用州或国家存储库所需的指纹和其他识别信息的表格。委员会除收取所有其他适用费用外,还应向申请人收取委员会在请求获取关于申请人的州和国家犯罪历史记录时可能产生的金额。

(7)若申请人已向委员会提出申请并获批,且已缴付规定费用,并符合下列条件之一,委员会须向其颁发执照:

(a)通过委员会的笔试和实践考试,每次考试成绩均不低于百分之七十;或

(b)在委员会承认的国家认可的考试中达到及格分数,该考试包括委员会确定的笔试和实践部分;或

(c)已从委员会承认的国家认证程序中获得认证;或

(d)在委员会承认的国家认可的笔试中取得及格分数,并且通过了委员会的实践考试,分数不低于百分之七十。

(8)委员会应记录举行的所有考试,参加考试的所有人员的姓名、地址及考试结果。考试后四十五日内,委员会应将考试结果书面通知每位申请人。

第 73‐71‐21 条　互惠许可

如果符合以下三项条件,委员会可酌情向在任何州或准州获得执照、认证或其他形式的法律认可的针灸师或针灸从业者免试颁发执照:

(a)申请人符合其获得针灸师或针灸从业者执照、认证或注册所在州或准州的执业要求。

(b)申请人获得针灸师或针灸从业者执照、认证或注册所在州或准州的执业要求至少与本州一样严格。

(c)申请人获得针灸师或针灸从业者执照、认证或注册所在州或准州,允许获得本州执照的针灸师通过资格考试在其管辖区从事针灸实践。

通过互惠原则向接受军事训练申请人、军人配偶或在本州居住的人员颁发执照,应遵守第 73‐50‐1 条或第 73‐50‐2 条的规定。

第 73‐71‐23 条　继续教育要求

(1)委员会应通过条例为在该州获得执照的针灸从业者制定强制性继续教育要求,包括以下内容:

(a)每个根据本章获得执照的人员,无论是否居住在州内,都应在每个两年期的续期内完成三十学时的继续教育,但最初的两年期续期除外。

(b)每个未达到继续教育所需学时数的人员,经委员会决定,有正当理由的,可以对其执照续期,条件是委员会要求,在下一续期内,除满足当前续期的继续教育要求外,还应补足缺乏的继续教育学时数和所有未缴纳的费用。如果任何针灸从业者未能补足缺乏的学时数,并完成随后续期内的继续教育要求,或未能补足任何未缴纳的费用,则不得续期执照,直至支付所有费用,且完成所有所需学时,并向委员会提供记录。

(2)委员会须按照条例制定继续教育提供者的教育标准和记录保存要求。继续教育课程的提供者应向委员会提出申请,在委员会制定的表格上列明满足上述要求的继续教育课

程,并支付一笔费用,用于委员会对提供者的批准及监督。提供继续教育的机构,协会和个人应保存出勤记录,包括签到表,保存期为三年。

第73－71－25条　针灸机构;委员会批准标准

(1)委员会须制定标准,批准提供针灸实践教育和培训的学校和学院。

(2)委员会在批准针灸学院之前,应确定该机构符合职业教育标准。这些标准应规定针灸机构:

(a)作为毕业的前提条件,要求学员参加至少两千五百学时的学习计划。

(b)符合委员会承认的国家认证机构的最低要求。

(c)要求学员参加严格监督的临床或实习计划。

(d)只有在本人出勤课堂和临床教学后,方可颁发针灸证书、文凭或学位。

第73－71－27条　不受规定限制条款;禁止无资格执业;责任保险要求

(1)任何根据本州先前法律获得执照、认证或注册的针灸师,均应视为根据本章规定获得的执照。

(2)所有根据本条获得执照的针灸师,在知悉或应当知悉的情况下,不得履行其培训、经验或认证资格以外的专业职责。如违反本条规定,持证人的执照应被撤销或吊销。委员会应就这些要求制定条例,并应根据具体情况为先前获得执照、认证或注册的针灸师授予执业资格。

(3)委员会应要求每位持证人获取并保有足够数量的职业责任保险,并向委员会提供该保险的证明。

第73－71－29条　报告和记录保存要求

(1)根据本章获得执照的人员应遵守以下报告要求:

(a)本州的所有发病率、死亡率、传染病、滥用药物和忽视报告要求。

(b)向委员会报告其已完成所需的继续教育学习并续期其执照。

(c)在地址变更后三十日内,以书面形式通知委员会。

(d)如预计停业时间超过九十日,或以其他方式限制查阅病历,则以书面形式通知委员会终止或暂停持证人的执业资格。持证人应在恢复执业时通知委员会。

(e)始终将其执照张贴在其执业地点的醒目位置。

(2)根据本章获得执照的人应遵守以下记录保存要求:

(a)保存他或她治疗的每位患者的准确记录。记录应包括患者姓名、病史、主观症状、客观诊断结果和治疗情况。

(b)将病历保存七年。

(c)保存已完成所需继续教育学习的证明文件,保存期为三年。

第73－71－31条　健康与卫生要求

(1)针灸从业者应遵守本州所有适用的公共卫生法律。

(2)卫生措施应包括:

(a)治疗不同患者之间,应使用肥皂和水或其他消毒剂洗手。

(b)在插入针头之前,应先用酒精或其他杀菌溶液擦拭施针区域的皮肤。

(c) 应对针灸实践中所用的针头和其他设备进行消毒。

(d) 针头和其他危险废物应按照法律规定的方式处理。

(e) 应遵守委员会规定的其他卫生措施，以确保患者的健康和安全。

第 73 - 71 - 33 条　纪律处分的依据

以下行为构成委员会可采取纪律处分的依据：

(a) 试图通过贿赂或曲解的方式获得或续期针灸执照。

(b) 持有被撤销、吊销或以其他方式受到处分的针灸执照，包括被另一州或准州的发证机构以妨碍本州执照颁发的原因拒绝颁发执照。

(c) 无论判决如何，在任何司法管辖区内被判犯有重罪、道德败坏罪或与针灸直接有关的罪行。为本款之目的，法院接受的有罪答辩或不抗辩答辩都将视为有罪。

(d) 以他人名义进行广告宣传、执业或者企图执业。

(e) 进行虚假或误导性的广告宣传或患者招揽。

(f) 帮助、协助、促成、雇用或宣传无执照的人违反本章或委员会规则从事针灸实践。

(g) 没有履行针灸从业者的法定或法律义务。

(h) 制作或提交持证人已知虚假的报告，故意或过失地未能提交州或联邦法律要求的报告，故意妨碍或阻碍提交报告或诱使他人这么做。这些报告应仅包括以针灸从业者身份签署的报告。

(i) 通过胁迫、恐吓或施加不当影响的方式与患者发生性关系，或与存在性关系的患者继续保持患者-医师关系（如此类性关系导致持证人无法称职地提供服务）。本款不适用于针灸从业者与其配偶之间的性关系。

(j) 在针灸实践中作出欺骗性、不真实或欺诈性的陈述。

(k) 通过使用欺诈、恐吓或不当影响或以某种过分的行为亲自或通过代理人招揽患者。

(l) 未能保留书面医疗记录，证明患者的治疗过程是正当的。

(m) 对患者施加不当影响以剥削患者，从而获取持证人或第三方的经济利益。

(n) 由于生病或过度使用酒精、药物、麻醉剂、化学药品或任何其他类型的物质，或由于任何精神和身体病症而无法在保证患者安全的情况下采取合理手段为患者提供针灸服务。

(o) 渎职，或未能达到合理谨慎的针灸从业者认为在类似条件和情况下可接受的治疗水平。

(p) 在知悉或应当知悉其培训、经验或认证不符合执业资格的情况下，在法律许可的范围之外从事针灸实践或提出从事针灸实践，或接受或履行专业职责。

(q) 持证人在知悉或应当知悉某人的培训、实践或认证不符合执业资格的情况下，将专业职责委托给该人。

(r) 违反本章的任何规定、委员会的规定或委员会先前在纪律听证会中发布的合法命令，或不遵守委员会依法向其发出的传票。

(s) 串谋实施、胁迫、恐吓或阻止另一持证人合法地宣传或提供其服务。

(t) 在学习过程中的欺诈或欺骗、重大过失、不称职或违反职业道德的行为。

(u) 未遵守州、县、市有关公共卫生和传染病控制的法规或报告要求。

（v）未遵守委员会制定的健康和安全的任何规则,包括但不限于设备消毒和潜在感染性材料的处置。

（w）针灸实践中不称职、重大过失或其他渎职行为。

（x）协助非法从事针灸实践。

（y）申请或报告任何疾病检测时存在欺诈或不诚实行为。

（z）未能依法报告或对任何传染性疾病作出虚假或误导性报告。

（aa）未能保存准确的病历;或

（bb）未能允许委员会或其代理人进入并检查委员会颁布的规则中规定的针灸场所和设备。

第 73-71-35 条　纪律处分程序;处罚;精神或体格检查;恢复执照

（1）根据本章进行的纪律处分程序,应与州医疗许可委员会进行的其他纪律程序相同。

（2）当委员会裁定任何人犯有第 73-71-33 条中规定的任何行为时,可以发布命令给予以下一项或多项处罚:

（a）拒绝向委员会证明其执照申请。

（b）撤销或吊销执照。

（c）限制执业。

（d）对每项罪名或单独违法行为处以不超过一千美元的行政罚款。

（e）发出谴责。

（f）根据委员会规定的条件,将针灸从业者列入一段时间的察看期。

（3）在执行本章规定时,如委员会发现存在合理根据,认为持证人由于实施第 73-71-33 条所述的任何行为或第 73-71-37 条所述的任何罪行,不能担任针灸从业者,则委员会必须发布命令,迫使持证人接受委员会指定医生的精神或体格检查。如持证人拒绝遵守该命令,则委员会指导检查的命令可向任何有管辖权的法院申请强制执行。在任何公开法庭记录或文件中,不得提及被申诉的持证人的姓名或首字母,除非持证人另有规定,否则诉讼应不向公众开放。委员会应有权采用所适用的州法律规定的简易程序。应在合理的时间间隔内,向受到本款影响的针灸从业者提供机会,以证明其能够以合理的技能水平恢复针灸实践,并确保患者的安全。在根据本款进行的任何诉讼程序中,无论是诉讼记录还是委员会的命令,均不得在任何其他诉讼程序中用于反对针灸从业者。

（4）委员会不得恢复针灸从业者的执照,或向其认为不合格的人颁发执照,直至委员会确信其遵守了最终命令中规定的所有条款和条件,且能够安全地从事针灸实践。

第 73-71-37 条　非法行为;罚款

（1）任何人进行以下行为均属违法:

（a）声称自己为针灸从业者,除非根据本章规定获得执照。

（b）未获有效执照或根据本章授权设立的委员会规则允许,从事针灸实践或试图从事针灸实践。

（c）通过欺诈或谎报获得或试图获得针灸执照;或

（d）除本章另有规定外,允许受雇人员从事针灸实践,除非该人员持有有效的针灸执照。

（2）违反本条任何规定的，即属轻罪，一经定罪，可处一千美元以下罚款，或处县监狱六个月以下监禁，或两罪并罚。

第73－71－39条　残障针灸师计划；诚信报告要求

（1）委员会应为残障针灸师制定护理、咨询或治疗计划。

（2）护理、咨询或治疗计划应包括一份符合委员会要求的有组织的治疗、护理、咨询、活动或教育的书面时间表，旨在使残障针灸师可以在保证患者安全的情况下采用适当方法从事针灸实践，以提供合格的医疗服务。

（3）所有被委员会授权执业的人，如合理认为任何针灸师为第73－71－5条定义的残障针灸师，应诚信报告。

第73－71－41条　披露特权信息；条件；免责；豁免

（1）任何执业针灸师不得披露任何关于其患者的医疗信息，除非获得其患者的书面授权或弃权，或法院命令、传票或本节另有规定。

（2）任何执业针灸师根据患者的书面授权和弃权，或法院命令、传票或本节规定的其他方式发布信息，不对患者或任何其他人承担责任。

（3）如果执业针灸师的患者在任何民事刑事诉讼中，对执业针灸师的护理和治疗或对患者造成的伤害的性质和程度存在争议，则应放弃本节规定的特权。

第73－71－43条　支付执照续期费和继续教育费用

每位持证人都必须支付两年一次的执照续期费并满足本章规定的继续教育要求。

第73－71－45条　执照续期；时限；新执照的要求

（1）已到期执照可在执照到期后九十日的任何时间通过委员会提供的表格提交续期申请，并在最后一个常规续期日支付有效的续期费。如果执照在到期后九十日内未续期，作为续期条件，针灸从业者应支付续期费以及委员会规定的滞纳金。

（2）未在到期后四年内续期执照的，不得续期，并且在此期限后不得补发或恢复执照；但符合下列条件的，可以申请领取新的执照：

（a）参加并通过适当的考试，或证明参加了委员会认可的持续针灸实践和继续教育。

（b）支付首次申请执照时所需的所有费用。

第73－71－47条　非执业执照状态；恢复要求

在执照有效或到期但未失效的任何时候，持证人可以要求将其执照列为非执业状态。在非执业状态下，持证人无须缴纳费用或满足继续教育要求。作为恢复执照的条件，持证人必须满足以下要求：

（a）证明他或她未实施任何本章规定中可导致不予颁发执照的行为或犯罪。

（b）支付委员会指定的恢复状态所需费用。

（c）满足与前两年相同的继续教育要求。

（d）在充分考虑公众利益的前提下，以符合委员会要求的方式，确定其有资格作为针灸从业者从事针灸实践。

第73－71－49条　吊销和撤销执照

（1）吊销的执照到期后，应按照本章规定进行续期，但续期后执照仍处于吊销状态。在执照恢复前,针灸师不得违反吊销命令从事针灸实践及其他活动或行为。

(2)据本条规定,撤销的执照到期后不得续期。如原持证人在执照到期后恢复使用,则持证人应支付续期费,以此作为恢复使用的条件,该续期费的金额相当于执照恢复日期前最后一个正常续期日应付的续期费,加上到期时累计的逾期费(如有)。

第 73－71－51 条　费用

(1)委员会可就以下各项收取合理的费用:

(a)执照的初始申请费。

(b)笔试和实践考试,不包括国家认可的考试的费用。

(c)为针灸从业者每两年续期一次执照。

(d)执照到期后,逾期超过三十日,但不超过一年,除其他费用外还需缴纳滞纳金。

(e)互惠许可费。

(f)继续教育提供者年度注册费。

(g)任何及所有费用,针灸咨询委员会确定的合理且必要的行政费用。

(2)所有费用须在委员会正式通过的条例中列明。

(3)根据本章收取的所有费用和其他资金,应存入州医疗许可委员会的专项资金。

第 73－71－53 条被 2017 年法典 391 章废止,2017 年 7 月 1 日失效

密西西比州针灸行政法①

第一节　范　　围

以下规则适用于实施针灸技术的针灸从业者。除下文另有规定外,只有在针灸从业者对患者进行针灸之日前六个月内对患者的病情进行了适当的评估后,针灸从业者才能对患者实施针灸。根据密西西比州针灸咨询委员会的建议,委员会可以根据规则修改本段规定的评估范围或本段规定的必须开始治疗的期限。

针灸从业者必须取得由患者在委员会规定的表格上签名的书面陈述,说明患者已由医师在规定的时间内进行评估。该表格必须包含明确声明,即患者应由医师对其所治疗的疾病进行评估。

针灸从业者可以不由医师评估,对患者进行针灸治疗:

A. 吸烟成瘾。

B. 减肥;或

C. 药物滥用,在委员会允许的范围内,由密西西比州针灸咨询委员会提供建议。

在治疗患者时,针灸医师不得进行医学诊断,但可根据中医理论提供辨证。若患者的病情没有改善或需要紧急医疗,针灸从业者应立即咨询医师。

---

① 根据《密西西比州行政法典》第 30 卷第 17 编第 2625 篇第 1 章"针灸服务"译出。

针灸可以在密西西比州由持执业医师证且接受过针灸技术和科学培训的医师进行。接受过充分培训的人员定义为在针灸领域接受过至少二百学时的 AMA 或 AOA 批准的 I 类 CME。希望在临床实践中使用针灸的此类持证人可以这么做,前提是针灸治疗的任何及所有部分均由具备相应资质的医师执行,并且在此情形下不得指定他人代替其提供服务。医师从事针灸实践应遵循该医师或其社区中的任何其他医生在提供任何其他医疗服务时相同的标准。适用的医疗标准应包括医患关系的所有要素。此有效关系的要素包括:

A. 核实要求治疗的人确实是他们声称的那个人。

B. 对患者进行适当检查,以使其符合适用的医疗标准,并足以证明鉴别诊断和建议的治疗方法是正确的。

C. 通过使用公认的医学惯例,即患者病史,精神状态检查,身体检查以及适当的诊断和实验室检查,来建立鉴别诊断。

D. 与患者讨论各种治疗方案的诊断、风险和益处,并获得知情同意。

E. 确保提供适当的随访护理,包括使用传统药物。

F. 保持完整的病历。

在任何密西西比州获得许可的医生被批准提供针灸治疗之前,州医疗许可委员会必须拥有所需 CME 的文件副本。经密西西比州医疗许可委员会规定在 2011 年 1 月之前进行针灸的持证人无须满足上述 CME 的要求。

第二节　定　义

为第 2625 卷第一章之目的,下列术语含义如下:

A. "委员会"系指密西西比州医疗许可委员会。

B. "咨询理事会"系指密西西比州针灸咨询委员会。

C. "NCCAOM"系指国家针灸与东方医学认证委员会。

D. "ACAOM"系指针灸及东方医学教育审核委员会。

E. "CCAOM"系指针灸与东方医学行业协会。

第三节　获得执照的资格条件

在 2009 年 7 月 1 日当日或之后,针灸执照申请人必须满足以下要求:

A. 符合委员会标准,他或她须年满二十一岁,并且品德良好。

B. 符合委员会标准,他或她是美利坚合众国的公民或永久居民。

C. 递交执照申请,使用委员会提供的表格,详细填写,并附近照一张(钱包大小/护照类型)。不得提交拍立得或非正式快照。

D. 支付委员会确定的适当费用。

E. 出示出生证明或有效的当前护照的核证副本。

F. 若适用,请提交合法的姓名变更证明(婚姻或其他法律程序的公证或认证副本)。

G. 如申请人目前或曾经作为针灸师获得注册或执照,提供该申请人在所有其他州的注册或执照信息。

H. 提供申请人曾经与其一起工作或接受培训的两名在美执业针灸师出具的有利介绍信。

I. 直接从机构提供证明,证明其顺利完成了具有候选资格或得到 ACAOM、NCCAOM 或其前身或继受机构认可的针灸师教育课程,该课程为期至少三年,并包括受监督的临床实习,以确保在美国以外接受教育的申请人通过 NCCAOM 对外国申请人的审查程序取得认可。

J. 通过 NCCAOM 管理的认证考试,并且在针灸或东方医学领域中拥有 NCCAOM 的当前文凭身份,并符合以下条件之一:

1. 若在 2004 年 6 月 1 日之前参加考试,则应通过综合笔试(CWE)、洁针技术部分(CNTP)和点位技能实践考试(PEPLS)。

2. 若在 2004 年 6 月 1 日或之后,且在 2007 年 1 月 1 日之前,则应通过 NCCAOM 中医基础课程、针灸模块、穴位模块和生物医学模块。

3. 若在 2007 年 1 月 1 日或之后,则应通过 NCCAOM 东方医学基础课程、包含穴位定位模块的针灸模块和生物医学模块。

K. 若申请人是国际教育课程的毕业生,请提供以下证明之一,证明申请人能够用英语交流:

1. 通过英语版的 NCCAOM 考试。

2. 通过 TOEFL(托福考试),笔考成绩应达到 560 分或以上,机考成绩应达到 220 分或以上。

3. TSE(英语口语考试)成绩应达到 50 分或以上。

4. TOEIC(托业考试)分数应达到 500 分或以上。

L. 提供顺利完成 NCCAOM 规定的洁针技术课程的证明,该课程直接由课程提供者发送给委员会。

M. 提供美国心脏协会或美国红十字会的现行心肺复苏(CPR)认证证明。

N. 提供至少一百万美元保额的医疗事故保险证明。

O. 提交指纹以供州和国家犯罪历史背景检查。

第四节　针灸执业标准

在治疗患者之前,针灸师(若不是密西西比州执业医师)应确保执业医师在过去六个月内对患者的病情进行了评估。在征求密西西比州针灸咨询委员会建议的情况下,委员会可以按规定修改本段所述的评估范围或根据本段规定必须开始治疗的时间,并应审核患者当前治疗的疾病诊断。

针灸师在告知患者针灸治疗计划的潜在风险和益处后,应征得患者的知情同意。

针灸师应获取一份由患者在委员会规定的表格上签署的书面声明,表明该患者在规定的时间内接受了医师的评估。

针灸师应详细询问患者的病史,以确定是否有针灸禁忌证,如出血性疾病。

针灸从业者应使用已按照美国疾病预防控制中心(CDC)标准进行消毒的消毒设备。

针灸师应遵守州和市政府关于公共卫生的所有适用要求。

第五节　病　　历

执业针灸师应保存每位患者完整及准确的病历。该病历应足以证明有效的针灸师-患者关系：

A. 证实要求治疗的人确实是他们声称的那个人。

B. 获取一份由患者在委员会规定的表格上签署的书面声明,表明该患者在规定的时间内接受了医师的评估。

C. 对患者进行适当的检查,以达到适用的医疗标准,并足以证明鉴别诊断和建议疗法合理。

D. 通过使用公认的医疗实践来建立鉴别诊断,即患者病史,精神状态检查,体格检查以及适当的诊断和实验室检查。

E. 与患者讨论各种治疗方案的诊断、风险和益处,并获得知情同意。

F. 确保提供适当的随访护理,包括使用传统药物。

G. 保存完整的病历。

从最后一次治疗之日起,病历必须保存七年,若将来的法规有要求,则必须保存更长时间。

应患者的要求,针灸师应向患者或其他授权人员提供针灸记录的副本。请参阅《行政法规》第 2635 卷第十章,病历的发布。

针灸师必须接受咨询委员会进行的同行评审程序。

第六节　监　　督

针灸师在治疗患者前,应告知患者针灸不能替代常规医疗的诊断和治疗,并须取得患者的知情同意。

针灸师在初次与患者见面时,应以书面形式提供针灸师的姓名、营业地址和业务电话号码,以及针灸从业信息,包括所用技术。

在治疗患者时,针灸师不得作出诊断。若患者的病情没有好转或患者需要紧急治疗,针灸师应及时咨询医师。

第七节　通知委员会地址变更的责任

任何在该州获得执照的针灸师并更改其执业地点或邮寄地址的,应立即以书面形式将更改信息通知委员会。在三十日内未通知可能会受到纪律处分。

委员会定期向执业针灸师发送信息。无论是通过 U.S.Mail 还是通过电子方式,持证人都必须接收此信息。持证人的执照记录应包括实际执业地点,邮寄地址,电子邮件地址和电话号码,委员会可以直接与持证人联系。委员会不鼓励使用办公室人员的邮件和电子邮件地址以及电话号码。未向委员会提供直接联系方式可能会受到纪律处分。

第八节　继　续　教　育

A. 每位针灸师必须接受超过三十个学时与针灸有关的继续教育课程,作为在下一个财政年度续期执照的前提条件。这三十个学时是每两年一个周期。超出的学时不可延续到另一个两年周期。为本法规之目的,两年周期自 2010 年 7 月 1 日开始,此后每两年一个周期。继续教育课程必须由以下组织之一赞助或批准:

1. 密西西比州针灸咨询理事会

2. 密西西比东方医学协会

3. 美国针灸师协会

4. 国家针灸与东方医学认证委员会

5. 美国针灸理事会

6. 美国东方生殖医学委员会

B. 所有获得针灸师执照的人必须遵守以下继续教育规则,作为执照续期的前提条件。

1. 6 月 30 日之后,在密西西比州获得初始针灸执照的针灸师在获得执照后两年可豁免最低继续教育要求。三十学时的继续教育认证将在下一个两年周期内到期。

2. 无论个人参加或完成课程或活动的次数如何,每两年内,任何单个课程或活动的批准学时数计入所需总学时,均不得计算超过一次。

3. 如持证人因病、兵役、伤残或其他过度困境而未能取得所需的继续教育学时,委员会可对其豁免或以其他方式修改本条规定。豁免或修改申请必须在继续教育续期到期前以书面形式发送给行政主管。

第九节 违 规 行 为

任何针灸师未如实证明其完成所需继续教育的,可根据《密西西比州法典》第 73 - 71 - 33 条和第 73 - 71 - 35 条的规定给予纪律处分。

任何未能完成所需继续教育的针灸师可根据《密西西比州法典》第 73 - 71 - 33 条和第 73 - 71 - 35 条的规定受到纪律处分,并且可能不被允许续期执照。若对持证人进行审核时,发现继续教育方面存在问题,应吊销其执照,吊销时间为(i)三个月或(ii)直至问题得到纠正(以两者中时间较长者为准)。由于继续教育审核而被吊销执照的任何持证人,可以请求听证会,对吊销提出申诉。若因伪造继续教育认证而吊销执照,则吊销时间应在确认其伪造认证后开始,不再按下列规定进行通知或听证。

因在任何纪律处分中遵守委员会命令的条款而获得的继续教育,不得计入在任何两年期间必须获得的继续教育中。

第十节 执照续期日程安排

获得密西西比州针灸执照的人员,应每年续期执照。

每年的 5 月 1 日或之前,州医疗许可委员会应通知在当前执照期限内获得或续期执照的每位针灸即将进行的年度执照续期。该通知应提供获取和提交续期申请的说明。申请人应在 6 月 30 日之前,以委员会在通知中规定的方式获取并填写申请,并将其提交委员会,随附委员会规定的续期费。所有七十岁以上的针灸师都可以选择支付年度执照续期费。收到申请和费用后,委员会应核实申请的准确性,并在接下来的一年期间(自下一个执照周期的

7月1日起至6月30日）向申请人颁发续期执照。

在密西西比州执业的针灸师如未按照前款规定续期执照而导致执照失效，经向委员会作出未能续期执照的满意解释，在填写恢复执照的表格并支付当年的续期费用后恢复执照。若执照在到期后的九十日内未续期，则应收取二百美元的滞纳金。

任何致使执照失效的针灸师，应在执照失效后的三十日内通知委员会。

针灸师在执照到期后四年内未续期的，不得续期该执照。该执照将失效，针灸师必须申请并获得新的执照。

在执照失效期间从事针灸实践的任何人应视为非法从业者，并应遵守《密西西比州法典》第73-71-33条和第73-71-35条的规定。

第十一节　职业道德

所有持证人均应遵守NCCAOM通过的道德规范，但与密西西比州法律或委员会规则相冲突的除外。若NCCAOM道德规范与州法律或规则相冲突，则以州法律或规则为准违反道德规范、州法律或规则的，可能会使持证人根据2625卷第一章10节规则受到纪律处分。

第十二节　纪律处分程序

A. 听证程序和申诉

不得拒绝颁发、吊销、撤销或限制任何个人的执照，除非该执业针灸师已得到通知并有机会进行听证。为通知、纪律听证和申诉之目的，委员会特此通过并援引纳入委员会目前对持有密西西比州医师执照的个人使用的"程序规则"的全部规定。

B. 恢复执照

1. 针灸执照被撤销、吊销或以其他方式限制执业的人员，可以在撤销或吊销之日起一年后，向密西西比州医疗许可委员会呈请恢复其执照。因不遵守第93-11-153条所定义的支持令而被吊销执照的恢复程序，应遵从第93-11-157或93-11-163条的规定。

2. 该呈请须附有至少两份来自执业医师或针灸师的经核实的推荐信，其执照由听取呈请的医疗许可委员会颁发，以及至少两份公民的推荐信，每个公民都应了解呈请人自纪律处分以来的活动以及医疗许可委员会可能需要的事实。

可以在医疗许可委员会的下一次定期会议中听取呈请，但不得早于呈请书提出后的三十日。在呈请人因任何刑事犯罪而被判刑时，包括在其缓刑或假释期间，均不得考虑呈请。医疗许可委员会认为有必要时，听证会可继续进行。

3. 在确定是否应废除纪律处分以及是否应废除纪律处分施加的条款和条件时，医疗许可委员会可以调查并考虑呈请人自纪律处分以来的所有活动、对其处以纪律处分的事由、在其执照信誉良好期间的活动，在诚实、职业能力和品德上的普遍声誉；并可能要求呈请人通过口头讯问。

第十三节　残障针灸师

因以下一种或多种原因而致残的执业针灸师，应被限制、吊销或撤销执照：

A. 精神疾病，或

B. 身体疾病，包括但不限于老化导致的身体退化或运动技能丧失。

C. 过度使用或滥用毒品，包括酒精。

若委员会有合理的理由认为，由于上述一种或多种情况，针灸师无法在保证患者安全的情况下采取合理手段为患者提供针灸服务，则应转送该针灸师，并按照 73－25－55 条至第 73－25－65 条规定的方式采取相关行动（如有），包括转送至由密西西比州医学协会发起的密西西比专业人员健康计划。

第十四节　使用专业头衔

持证人应使用"针灸师""执业针灸师""Lic.Ac.""L.Ac."的头衔，在与持证人的针灸实践有关的任何广告或其他对公众可见的材料上都紧随其名。只有获得针灸师资格的人才能使用这些头衔。在密西西比州还获得医师、牙医、整脊疗法医师、验光师、足科医生和/或兽医执照的持证人可免除持证人的针灸头衔紧随其名的要求。

第十五节　针灸广告，误导或欺骗性广告

针灸师不得授权或使用虚假、误导或欺骗性广告，且不得从事下列任何活动：

A. 自称为内科医生或外科医生，或使用这些术语的任何组合或派生词，除非获得州医疗许可委员会颁发的《密西西比州医学实践法》所定义的执照。

B. 使用"委员会认证"一词。针灸师可使用"认证"一词，但必须在广告中注明授予上述认证的委员会的完整名称。

C. 若宣传的认证已到期，且在有关广告发布、传播或以其他方式宣传时未续期，仍使用"认证"或任何类似词语或短语来传达相同含义。

第十六节　在执业场所销售商品

由于在销售商品时可能会侵害患者权利，因此针灸师应注意与患者的适当界限，应避免在其诊所出售商品时施加胁迫，且不应从事独家经销和/或个人品牌化。

针灸师应披露与任何商品销售相关的信息，以告知患者其经济利益。

针灸师可以免费或以成本价分发商品，以便患者随时获得这些商品。

针灸师可以在办公室出售对患者治疗必不可少的耐用医疗用品，以及与慈善组织有关的非健康用品。

第十七节　规则生效日期

上述有关针灸师执业的规则将于 2009 年 10 月 17 日生效。

第十八节　废　　止

南卡罗来纳州

南卡罗来纳州针灸法[①]

第 40‑47‑700 条　条款引用

本节可被引用为"南卡罗来纳州针灸法案"。

第 40‑47‑705 条　定义

为本条之目的:

(1)"针灸"系指一种从东方传统和现代保健观念发展而来,采用东方医学技术、治疗和辅助疗法,旨在促进、维持和恢复健康并预防疾病的医疗保健形式。针灸实践不包括:

(a)整骨医学和整骨疗法。

(b)第 40‑9‑10 条中定义的"整脊疗法"。

(c)第 40‑45‑20 条中定义的"物理疗法"或为物理疗法实践所允许的治疗方式。

(2)"耳穴戒毒疗法"系指将一次性无菌针灸针插入由国家针灸戒毒协会(NADA)规定的五个耳穴中的疗法,其目的是治疗化学依赖、戒毒和药物滥用。

(3)"委员会"系指州医学考试委员会。

(4)"咨询委员会"系指本节设立的针灸咨询委员会,指对委员会负责的咨询委员会。

(5)"NADA"系指国家针灸戒毒协会。

(6)"NCAAOM"系指国家针灸与东方医学认证委员会。

(7)"ACAOM"系指针灸及东方医学教育审核委员会。

(8)"耳穴疗法"系指将一次性针头插入耳朵,并仅限于耳朵,以治疗有限的病症的疗法。

第 40‑47‑710 条　针灸咨询委员会;成员资格;术语;填补职位空缺;开除成员;会议安排;理事

(A)针灸咨询委员会由五名成员组成,成员由州医学考试委员会任命,任期四年,直至其继任者获得任命并合格。根据本节规定,必须有三名成员获针灸执照,其中一人从事针灸

---

① 　根据《南卡罗来纳州法典》第 40 卷第 47 章第 6 节"针灸法案"译出。

实践至少三年,一人必须根据本章获得针灸执照,一人必须来自本州。咨询委员会成员享有的旅费、每日津贴和生活津贴应与法律规定的州委员会、委员会、政府机关成员一致,并承担本节规定的委员会可能承担的职责。

(B)必须按照原始任命方式填补任期内未届满的职位空缺。委员会在通知并给予听证机会后,可因任何委员会成员的失职、玩忽职守、不称职、撤销或吊销执照,或因其他不光彩的行为将其开除。任何成员不得连任超过两届四年任期,但可在上一个四年任期届满之日起四年内重获委任。

(C)咨询委员会每年应至少召开两次会议,并在必要时召开其他会议。四名委员会成员构成法定人数。咨询委员会应在其首次会议以及此后的每年年初,从其成员中选出一名主席、副主席和秘书,任期一年。

(D)咨询委员会应根据本节的规定收取和结算所有款项,并应将收集到的所有款项按法律规定支付给委员会,以便存入州财政部。

第40-47-715条 权力与责任

(A)咨询委员会可以:

(1)向委员会提出有关职业行为的法规,以执行本节规定,包括但不限于职业认证以及建立本州针灸师、耳穴治疗师及耳穴戒毒专家的执业道德标准。

(2)向委员会提出对针灸师、耳穴治疗师及耳穴戒毒专家继续教育的要求。

(3)请求并接受州教育机构或其他州机构的协助,并向委员会推荐与消费者利益相关的信息,此类信息应说明咨询委员会的监管职能,以及委员会接收及处理消费者投诉的程序。委员会应向公众和有关的州机构提供这些信息。

(B)咨询委员会应:

(1)举行听证会并保留履行其职能所需的记录和会议记录。

(2)根据《行政程序法》,提供根据本节授权的所有听证会的通知。

(3)确定合格针灸师、耳穴治疗师和耳穴戒毒专家获发执照的资格,并就颁发执照提出建议。

(4)根据本节规定的条件,向委员会建议是否颁发或续期执照。

(5)保存其程序记录和所有持证人的注册记录,包括姓名及最新的就业和居住地点。委员会应每年编制并提供一份经授权在本州执业的针灸师、耳穴治疗师和耳穴戒毒专家的名单。有兴趣的人士可向委员会申请并缴付足以支付印刷及邮寄费用的款项,以取得该名单的副本。

(6)每年向委员会报告所履行的职责、采取的行动和提出的建议。

(7)听取纪律案件,并向委员会说明事实调查结果、法律结论和制裁。委员会应举行最终听证会,并作出最终决定。

(8)执行委员会可能委派给咨询委员会的职责和任务。

第40-47-720条 针灸执照;要求和资格;临时执照

(A)每个针灸执照申请人应:

(1)按照委员会的规定提交一份完整的申请。

（2）按照第 40－47－800 条的规定缴纳费用。

（3）持有 NCCAOM 的现行针灸认证。

（4）具有良好品德。

（5）没有认罪、不抗辩、被判重罪或道德败坏罪。

（B）申请必须详细填写后才能获得批准。若委员会行政工作人员已审查全部申请的完整性、正确性，认为申请人符合条件并已向咨询委员会或者指定的委员会成员提出申请，则可以向其颁发临时执照。在下次咨询委员会会议上必须审查该申请，若符合条件，咨询委员会可向委员会建议颁发永久执照。若咨询委员会拒绝建议颁发永久执照，咨询委员会可以延长或撤回临时执照。

第 40－47－725 条　现行针灸从业者的执照

（A）（1）若针灸师已获委员会批准在本州从事针灸实践，且拥有良好信誉，并顺利完成经委员会批准且全国认可的洁针技术课程，则必须在提交下列材料后按照本节规定取得初始执照：

（a）按照委员会的规定提交一份完整的申请。

（b）按照第 40－47－800 条的规定缴纳费用。

（2）但根据第（A）（1）项颁发的执照有效期仅为两年。有效期后，个人若欲续期执照，则必须持有 NCCAOM 的现行证书，并符合本节规定的执照和续期要求。

（B）自 1980 年以来一直在本州持续从事针灸实践，并一直保持良好信誉的个人，提交下列材料后不需符合本章的要求即可获发和续期执照：

（1）按照委员会的规定提交一份完整的申请。

（2）按照第 40－47－800 条的规定缴纳费用。

第 40－47－730 条　耳穴治疗执照；资格；临时执照

（A）耳穴疗法执照的申请人：

（1）必须年满二十一岁。

（2）按照医疗委员会的规定提交一份完整的申请。

（3）按照第 40－47－800 条的规定缴纳费用。

（4）应提供证明文件，证实除戒毒专家所使用的耳穴外，还接受过使用耳穴的培训。

（5）顺利完成针灸咨询委员会和医疗考试委员会批准的国家认证项目。

（6）顺利完成委员会批准的洁针技术课程。

（B）申请必须详细填写后才能获得批准。若委员会行政工作人员已审查全部申请的完整性、正确性，认为申请人符合条件并已向咨询委员会或者指定的委员会成员提出申请，则可以向其颁发临时执照。在下次咨询委员会会议上必须审查该申请，若符合条件，咨询委员会可向委员会建议颁发永久执照。若咨询委员会拒绝建议颁发永久执照，咨询委员会可以延长或撤回临时执照。

第 40－47－735 条　耳穴戒毒疗法执照；资格；临时执照

（A）耳穴戒毒治疗执照的申请人：

（1）须年满二十一岁。

（2）应按照委员会的规定提交一份完整的申请。

（3）应按照第 40－47－800 条的规定缴纳费用。

（4）应顺利完成经委员会批准且国家认可的耳穴戒毒培训计划，内容为治疗化学依赖、戒毒和药物滥用。

（5）顺利完成委员会批准且国家认可的洁针技术课程。

（B）申请必须详细填写后才能获得批准。若委员会行政工作人员已审查全部申请的完整性、正确性，认为申请人符合条件并已向咨询委员会或者指定的委员会成员提出申请，则可以向其颁发临时执照。在下次咨询委员会会议上必须审查该申请，若符合条件，咨询委员会可向委员会建议颁发永久执照。若咨询委员会拒绝建议颁发永久执照，咨询委员会可以延长或撤回临时执照。

第 40－47－740 条　现行耳穴治疗师或耳穴戒毒专家的执照

（A）若耳穴治疗师或耳穴戒毒专家已获委员会批准在本州从事针灸实践，且拥有良好信誉，并顺利完成经委员会批准且全国认可的洁针技术课程，则必须在提交下列材料后按照本节规定取得初始执照：

（1）按照委员会的规定提交一份完整的申请。

（2）按照第 40－47－800 条的规定缴纳费用。

（B）但根据第（A）项颁发的执照有效期仅为两年。有效期后，若个人续期执照，则必须顺利通过委员会批准且全国认证的耳穴疗法或耳穴戒毒培训计划，并符合本节规定的执照要求。

第 40－47－745 条　未经授权的服务；处罚；停止令和禁令；特权通信

（A）未根据本节获得执照而自称为针灸师、耳穴治疗师和耳穴戒毒专家为非法行为。"执业针灸师"和"针灸师"的头衔仅限于根据本节取得针灸执照的人使用。此外，持有耳穴疗法或耳穴戒毒执照的人不得从事针灸实践或自称针灸师。"耳穴戒毒专家"的头衔仅限于根据本节取得耳穴戒毒执照的人使用。持有耳穴治疗师或耳穴戒毒专家的执照本身并不赋予个人针灸师的身份。在执照吊销或撤销期间，若未根据本节获得执照而自称为针灸师、耳穴治疗师和耳穴戒毒专家的，即属轻罪，一经定罪，可处三百美元以下罚款或九十日以内监禁，或二罪并罚。

（B）为根据本节进行的任何调查或诉讼之目的，委员会或由其指定人员可以主持宣誓和申明、传唤证人、收集证言，并要求出示委员会认为与调查有关的任何文件或记录。

（C）若委员会有充分证据证明某人违反本节的规定，除采取所有其他补救办法外，委员会可命令该人立即停止并结束这种行为。委员会可以依照第 1 卷第 23 章第 5 节的规定，向行政法官申请禁令，禁止该人从事此种行为。行政法官可以单方面发布临时禁令，经通知和充分听证后，可酌情发布其他命令。行政法官不得要求委员会提供任何承诺，作为发布本节规定所述禁令或命令的条件。

（D）由个人或公司或代表个人或公司的人对委员会或委员会指定人员进行的每次口头或书面沟通，以调查或听取有关撤销、吊销执照的其他限制或持证人其他的纪律处分，无论是以投诉还是证词的方式，均有权在任何理由下免于披露，在委员会审议的程序中披露除外。除非有证据证明提交投诉或证词是出于恶意,否则不得对提交的个人或公司采取民事或刑事诉讼或程序。

(E)本节的任何规定均不得解释为禁止被告人或其法律顾问根据正当的法律程序行使被告人的宪法权利,或禁止被告人根据正当的法律程序获得对他的指控和证据。

第 40-47-750 条　耳穴疗法;监督

耳穴疗法可以在执业针灸师或根据本章获得医师执照的人的监督下进行。耳穴治疗师的治疗严格限于将针头插入耳朵。将针头插在身体的任何其他位置都被认为是在没有执照的情况下从事针灸实践。

第 40-47-755 条　耳穴戒毒疗法;监督

耳穴戒毒疗法可以在执业针灸师或根据本章获得医师执照的人的直接监督下进行。耳穴戒毒专家的治疗严格限于 NADA 规定的五点耳穴疗法方案,以治疗药物滥用、化学依赖或戒毒。

第 40-47-760 条　豁免活动

本节不适用于:

(1)作为参与针灸教学计划的学生的学习计划中不可或缺的一部分开展的针灸实践,该教学计划在具有至少五年临床经验的执业针灸师的监督下开展,并且是 ACAOM 已认证、待认证或积极寻求认证的教学计划。

(2)美国政府聘用的针灸师或戒毒专家(若此类服务仅在美国政府的指导或控制下提供)

第 40-47-765 条　撤销、吊销或拒绝颁发执照的理由

针灸师、耳穴治疗师和耳穴戒毒专家具有以下不当行为时,可以吊销、撤销、惩戒、限制、拒绝颁发执照或将执照列入察看状态:

(1)故意使人误认其为医师。

(2)已经或曾经向委员会提交任何虚假、欺诈或伪造的声明或文件。

(3)执行任何超出执照执业范围的工作、任务或其他活动。

(4)滥用酒精或药物,以致不适合执业。

(5)被判犯有重罪或涉及道德败坏或毒品的罪行。

(6)有任何身体或精神上的残疾,令其继续执业会对公众构成危险。

(7)从事任何可能欺骗或伤害患者的不光彩或不道德的行为。

(8)在与执业或执照相关的任何文件中使用或作出任何具有虚假性或欺诈性的陈述。

(9)在不光彩、虚假或欺诈手段获取或协助他人获取费用。

(10)违反或串谋他人违反本节的任何规定。

(11)缺乏执业所需的道德或专业能力。

(12)如患者的医疗状况已被确定为超出执业范围,而并未向执业医师或牙医进行转介。

(13)持证人每月一次、连续三个月为患者提供针灸、耳穴戒毒治疗或耳穴疗法服务,并未出现临床改善,除非持证人在第三个月到期时或到期前向患者提供书面通知,告知其可能需要继续接受针灸、耳穴戒毒治疗或耳穴疗法服务。在此之前应寻求执业医师或牙医的医

疗诊断,除非患者由执照医师或牙医转介至持证人处。

委员会在发现不当行为后,有权根据本章实施制裁。

第 40‐47‐770 条　视察

委员会或委员会指定的人员可不定期视察任何雇用针灸师或耳穴戒毒专家的诊所或执业场所。

第 40‐47‐775 条　执照的展示

持有根据本节颁发的执照并且积极从事针灸、耳穴疗法或耳穴戒毒治疗实践的人,应在其执业地点适当且显眼的位置展示该执照。

第 40‐47‐780 条　执照续期

（A）根据本节颁发的执照,持证人必须每两年续期一次:

（1）按照委员会规定提交一份完整的续期申请。

（2）提交第 40‐47‐800 条规定的适用费用。

（3）在提交续期申请时并不处于违反本节规定的状态。

（4）符合委员会条例所规定的继续教育及专业发展的要求。

（5）处于 NCCAOM 的有效认证状态。

（B）持证人必须每两年续期一次根据本节颁发的耳穴疗法或耳穴戒毒专家执照:

（1）按照委员会规定提交一份完整的续期申请。

（2）提交第 40‐47‐800 条规定的适用费用。

（3）在提交续期申请时不处于违反本节或根据本节颁布的任何条例的状态。

（4）符合委员会规章所规定的继续教育及专业发展的要求。

（5）积极从事耳穴治疗或耳穴戒毒治疗实践。

第 40‐47‐785 条　申请非执业状态

根据委员会制定的程序和条件,持证人可以申请将其执照列为非执业状态。持证人可随时申请将执照列为执业状态,并在符合委员会在规章中订立的条件后,恢复为执业状态。

第 40‐47‐790 条　持证人不得声称自己获授权行医

任何根据本节获发执照的人,均不得宣传或向公众声称自己获授权行医。

第 40‐47‐800 条　执照费用

必须根据 40‐1‐50（D）每两年重新制定并调整针灸师、耳穴治疗师和耳穴戒毒专家的执照费用,确保金额足够且不过量,并能涵盖南卡罗来纳州为委员会的事务所承担的直接和间接费用总额:

（1）初始执照费。

（2）执照续期费。

（3）超期续期费。

（4）重新激活申请费。

第 40‐47‐810 条　第三方补偿

本节中的任何内容均不得被解释为要求第三方直接向针灸师、耳穴治疗师或耳穴戒毒专家支付服务费用。

田 纳 西 州

田纳西州针灸法[①]

第 63－6－1001 条　定义

除文意另有所指外,下列定义适用于本节:

(1)"ACAOM"系指针灸及东方医学教育审核委员会。

(2)"针灸"系指由传统和现代东方医学概念发展而来的一种保健形式,采用东方医学诊断、治疗及辅助疗法和诊断技术,旨在促进、维持和恢复健康并预防疾病。

(3)"ADS"系指接受过五点耳穴戒毒治疗训练,并且只开展五点耳穴戒毒疗法的针灸戒毒专家。

(4)"医学委员会"系指田纳西州医学委员会。

(5)"NADA"系指国家针灸戒毒协会。

(6)"NCCAOM"系指国家针灸与东方医学认证委员会。

(7)"针灸实践"系指在东方医学诊断基础上,在人体特定部位实施针刺或灸法为主的治疗方法。针灸范围内的辅助疗法可包括穴位按压、拔火罐、热疗和电疗法,以及基于东方传统医学理念的膳食指南、补充剂以及治疗性运动建议。

第 63－6－1002 条　法律适用

(a)本节不适用于以下情形:

(1)据本章或本编第 9 章获得执照的医生,也不得解释为禁止此类医生从事针灸实践或禁止此类医生使用"针灸师"的头衔。

(2)经国家认证为全科护士并顺利完成针灸认证教育课程的注册护士;或

(3)根据本编第 4 章获得许可的整脊医师。本编各节也不得解释为禁止完成二百五十小时认证针灸课程并通过国家整脊检查师委员会针灸考试的整脊医师从事针灸实践。

(b)除非获得本节认证,有偿或无偿从事针灸实践都是非法的。此限制不适用于以下情形:

---

① 　根据《田纳西州法典》注释版第 63 卷第 6 编第 10 章"针灸"译出。

（1）学生在认证针灸师的监督下从事针灸实践,该针灸实践作为委员会批准的学习课程的一部分。

（2）对于不具备本节或委员会据此颁布的条例所要求的证书的个人,如果符合下列条件,可作为 ADS 获授有限认证,将针灸用于治疗酗酒、药物滥用或化学依赖:

（A）提供文件证明其顺利完成了获得委员会批准的耳穴戒毒针灸培训计划,该计划达到或高于国家针灸戒毒协会设定的培训标准。

（B）在认证针灸师或医务主任的监督下,在提供全面酒精和药物滥用或化学依赖性服务(包括咨询)的医院、诊所或治疗机构开展耳穴戒毒疗法。

（C）满足第 63－6－1007 条中规定的所有适当道德标准。

（D）将执业范围限制在五点耳穴戒毒治疗。

（c）违反本条规定的,构成 C 类轻罪。违反本条规定的应同时受第 63－6－1007 条规定的制裁。

第 63－6－1003 条　田纳西州针灸咨询委员会、组成、职责和会议

（a）为协助委员会履行其职责,现成立田纳西针灸咨询委员会。

（b）委员会由州长任命的五名成员组成。三名成员应为执业针灸师,一名成员应为在田纳西州执业的针灸戒毒专家,一名成员应为既不受雇于卫生保健专业或行业,也未与卫生保健专业或行业有任何其他直接或间接关系的消费者。最初任命的三名针灸师在任命时无须获得认证,但必须符合所有认证的资格条件。

（c）（1）尽管第 3－6－304 条或其他法律有相反的规定,除了委员会对于成员资格的补充要求之外:

（A）根据第 3 编第 6 章的登记要求登记为说客的任何人,如随后被任命或提名为委员会成员,在担任委员会成员之前,应当与任何商业活动和专业活动受委员会监管的主体终止一切雇佣关系以及作为说客的商业往来。本条(c)(1)(A)目适用于 2010 年 7 月 1 日之后任命或以其他方式提名到委员会的所有人员。

（B）任何委员会成员在其任职期间,不得根据第 3 编第 6 章,为从事商业活动或专业活动受委员会监管的任何主体进行注册或担任说客。本条第(c)(1)(B)目适用于 2010 年 7 月 1 日之后任命或以其他方式提名为到委员会的所有人员,以及在该日期未登记为说客的所有委员会成员。

（C）担任委员会成员的任何人在其于委员会的服务期结束后一年内,不得在商业活动或专业活动受委员会监管的主体中担任说客。本条第(c)(1)(C)目适用于截至 2010 年 7 月 1 日在委员会任职的人员,以及该日期之后被委任为委员会成员的人员。

（2）违反本(c)款的应根据第 3 编第 6 章的规定受到处罚。

（3）为本(c)款之目的,伦理和竞选资金管理局有权颁布规章制度。所有此类规章制度,均应依据《统一行政程序法》第 4 编第 5 章以及第 4－55－103 条中规定的伦理委员会向伦理和竞选资金管理局发起和提出规章制度的程序予以颁布。

（d）除了对委员会成员资格的其他要求外,2010 年 7 月 1 日后任命或以其他方式提名为委员会成员的所有人应为本州居民。

（e）在委员会的首届任命中,两名成员任期三年,两名成员任期两年,一名成员任期一年。此后每届定期任命的任期为四年。任何人不得连续担任委员会委员两届以上。每名成员应在委员会任职,直至任命继任者为止。未届满任期的空缺应当由州长委任填补。

（f）在委员会每年任命新成员后的第一次会议上,新成员中应选择一名成员担任委员会当年主席,另一名成员担任联席主席。任何人不得连续担任委员会主席五年以上。

（g）（1）委员会应在新成员任命的四十五日后,每年至少召开一次会议。委员会应根据需要在其他时间开会以履行其职责。

（2）（A）任何成员在一个日历年内缺席预定会议超过百分之五十的,应免去其委员会成员的职务。

（B）委员会主席应及时通知或安排通知未达到第（g）（2）（A）目规定的出席要求的成员。

（h）每名成员应领取处理委员会事务所需的一切必要费用,此外,在处理委员会事务期间,每日有权领取五十美元的日津贴。所有差旅费的报销应按照由财政部和行政部颁布并经总检察长和报告人批准的综合差旅条例执行。

（i）委员会应根据第 63－1－101 条的规定,从卫生部卫生相关委员会处获取所有行政、调查和文书服务。委员会的经费从针灸师和针灸戒毒专家的认证费中支出。

第 63－6－1004 条　医学委员会的职责

（a）咨询委员会应当与州医学委员会商讨确定如下事项:

（1）确立申请人认证的资格和适当性、认证续期和相互认证的条例。

（2）确立撤销、暂停或拒绝认证的条件。

（3）确立将证书持有人列入察看期的情形。

（4）确定与认证有关的费用类别和可能征收的费用数额。

（5）根据《统一行政程序法》第 4 编第 5 章发布宣告令。

（6）如果咨询委员会认为确有必要,制定继续教育标准。

（7）采用印章对咨询委员会的正式文件进行验证。

（b）根据本节采取的任何行动只有在咨询委员会成员以多数票通过后才有效。医学委员会可在下次审议行政事项的医学委员会会议上,以其成员的多数票,撤销咨询委员会采取的任何行为。

第 63－6－1005 条　认证要求

（a）任何人要获得委员会的针灸执业认证,须证明:

（1）以下两项其中之一:

（A）当前处于执业状态的 NCCAOM 针灸专家;或

（B）当前具有其他州颁发的基本同等或更高标准的执照,且信誉良好。

（2）顺利完成获得 ACAOM 认证、处于候选状态或符合 ACAOM 标准的继续高等教育三年培训课程或针灸学院课程;且

（3）顺利完成 NCCAOM 批准的洁针技术课程。

（b）对于 2001 年 7 月 1 日前居住在田纳西州的申请人,委员会应免除第（a）款的要求,

如果该申请人向委员会提供充分的证据,证明其顺利完成了符合 NCCAOM 标准的获批学徒或辅导计划,则委员会应予以认证。

(c)对于向委员会提供充分的证据,证明其在田纳西州执业前持有另一州的信誉良好的执照,且此后一直在田纳西州执业的申请人,委员会应免除第(a)款的要求,并予以认证。

(d)符合第 63-6-1002 条要求的 ADS 应予以受限的针灸认证。

第 63-6-1006 条　执照的续期

针灸执照每两年续期一次。续期执照时,须提交现行有效的 NCCAOM 针灸认证或符合第 63-6-1005 条的文件。续期 ADS 执照时,须提交经咨询委员会确认的现行有效的耳穴戒毒疗法执业证明。

第 63-6-1007 条　纪律处分

申请人或认证针灸师存在下列情形的,咨询委员会经与医学委员会协商后,可以拒绝、吊销或撤销认证,要求其接受补救教育或向其发出谴责信:

(1)从事违背针灸执业规范的虚假或欺诈行为,包括:

(A)在申请认证或委员会调查相关事项中存在谎报行为。

(B)试图提前收费。

(C)虚假广告,包括承诺针灸疗法可以治愈疾病。

(D)分割或同意分割费用,目的是将患者转诊至针灸治疗。

(2)未能适当控制自己的执业行为:

(A)在针灸师知情或应当知情的情况下,将专业职责委托给不具备资格的人员;或

(B)对于未经认证参与本机构工作的人员,未能进行适当的管理。

(3)未能以适当的方式保存记录:

(A)未对每一个患者的治疗过程进行书面记录。

(B)在患者提出要求的情况下,拒绝向其提供为患者准备的记录或患者付费记录。

(C)未经同意泄露患者的个人身份信息,但法律另有授权的除外。

(4)未能对患者实施适当的医疗行为,包括发生性行为、提出性行为请求或将服从此类行为作为治疗条件,从而对针灸师-患者关系施加不当影响。

(5)表现出药物滥用或精神障碍,且足以影响其提供安全有效治疗的能力。

(6)被判有罪或认罪,或对任何证明其不适合从事针灸实践的罪行不予抗辩。

(7)由于疏忽而在执业过程中未能以专业认可的技术水平从事针灸实践。

(8)故意违反本节或委员会的任何规定。

(9)其执照或证书在另一个司法管辖区内被拒绝、吊销或撤销,且相关行为在田纳西州也应受到同样处理。

第 63-6-1008 条　卫生要求

(a)所有根据本节获得认证的个人在进行针灸治疗时,只能使用预消毒的一次性针头。禁止使用其他任何针头。

(b)卫生要求应包括:

（1）在处理针头之前以及治疗不同患者之间,应使用肥皂和水或其他消毒剂洗手。

（2）在插入针头之前,应使用酒精或其他杀菌溶液彻底擦拭施针区域的皮肤。

（3）个人获准从事针灸实践和相关技术之前,应通过国家认可的洁针技术课程。

第 63－6－1009 条　费用

（a）医学委员会应与咨询委员协商,确定与申请、认证和续期有关的费用,该费用应足以支付认证费和咨询委员会履行本节职责直接导致的所有费用。

（b）所有存款和支出应按照第 63－1－137 条处理。

第 63－6－1010 条　头衔

（a）根据本条获得认证的人可使用"执业针灸师"或"针灸戒毒专家"的头衔。任何人未经适当许可从事医学或整骨疗法的,均不得使用本节规定的证明以自称为医生或医师。

（b）每名获准执业的针灸师,应将该执照展示在其执业地点的显著位置。

田纳西州针灸行政法[①]

第 0880－12－01 条　定义

本章条例中,下列术语和缩写词的含义如下:

（1）ACAOM：针灸及东方医学教育审核委员会。

（2）行政办公室：田纳西州医学委员会和针灸咨询委员会的行政办公室位于田纳西州纳什维尔市,主流大道 665 号,37247。

（3）ADS：接受过五点耳穴戒毒治疗训练,并且只开展五点耳穴戒毒疗法的针灸戒毒专家。

（4）委员会：田纳西州医学委员会。

（5）咨询委员会：针灸咨询委员会。

（6）资格证书：准许执业的文件。该术语在本章出现,同时适用于受限和正式的证书持有人。除非本章条例明确指明该术语仅适用于受限证书。

（7）管理处：田纳西州卫生部的卫生相关委员会管理处,咨询委员会从该处获得行政支持。

（8）NADA：国家针灸戒毒协会。

（9）NCCAOM：国家针灸与东方医学认证委员会。

第 0880－12－02 条　执业范围

（1）针灸师执业范围由《田纳西州行政程序法》（T.C.A.）第 63－6－1001 条第（7）款管理。

（2）所有针灸戒毒专家的执业范围均由《田纳西州行政程序法》（T.C.A.）第 63－6－1001 条第（3）款和第 63－6－1002 条（b）款（2）（B）和（D）项管理。

---

① 根据《田纳西州行政法》第 0880 卷第 12 章"针灸服务总则"译出。

第0880-12-03条　保留

第0880-12-04条　针灸认证程序

在田纳西州获得针灸执业资格证书,必须遵守以下程序和要求:

(1)祖父条款。任何人如符合第(2)款所载除(e)(i)及(j)项外的所有款项,并进一步提供充分证据,证明符合下列其中一项,均可获发证书:

(a)2001年1月1日在田纳西州居住,并顺利完成符合NCCAOM标准的学徒或辅导计划。

1.田纳西州的居民身份可以通过提交选民登记卡复印件来证明,该登记卡应表明其在2001年1月1日或之前居住在田纳西州,或通过提交2001年1月1日或之前签发的田纳西州驾照复印件来证明。

2.所有支持学徒或辅导计划的文件,以及它如何符合NCCAOM标准,都必须直接由该计划或NCCAOM发送到行政办公室。

(b)自2001年1月1日起,在田纳西州持续从事针灸实践,并在该州进行实践之前持有在他州信誉良好的执照/证书。

1.自2001年1月1日起在田纳西州持续从事针灸实践,可通过提交下列任何一项来证明:

(i)工资单、工资单存根或美国国税局(IRS)表格W-2、1099-Misc或IRS表格1040的附表C或C-EZ的复印件,以核实针灸实践的收入证明。

(ii)由家庭成员以外的两人出具的证明申请人持续执业的公证书。

2.在其他州信誉良好的执照/证书必须直接从该州的执照/证书机构提交给行政办公室,颁发日期须先于申请人在田纳西州开始从事针灸实践的日期。

(2)学历证明。申请人应执行以下操作进行学历证明:

(a)向行政办公室索取一份申请书。

(b)对申请表中提出的每一个问题和要求应如实、完整地作出答复,并将其连同申请表和规则要求的所有文件、费用一并提交行政办公室。本规则的目的为,完成所需文件归档的必要活动应在提交申请之前完成,并同时提交所有文件。

(c)提交一张清晰、可识别、近期拍摄的半身照片,显示肩部以上正脸及完整头部。

(d)提交具有良好道德品质的证明。该证明应为两份最近(在过去12个月内)由医学专业人员出具的原件,在签署的信笺上证明申请人的个人品质和职业道德。

(e)已直接从NCCAOM向行政办公室提交当前针灸学历证明。

(f)披露与下列任何一项有关的情况:

1.对违反任何国家,州或市的任何刑法行为的定罪,情节轻微的交通违法行为除外。

2.其他州拒绝其专业执照/证书申请或在任何州受到执照/证书的处分。

3.执照/证书的丢失或限制。

4.申请人作为被告方的任何民事诉讼判决或民事诉讼和解,包括但不限于涉及医疗事故、违约、反垄断活动或根据国家或州的成文法、普通法或判例法认可的任何其他民事诉讼补救措施。

5. 未通过任何专业执照或证书考试。

（g）申请人应直接向委员会行政办公室提交来自委员会认证申请材料中确定的提供方提供的犯罪背景调查结果。

（h）提交与田纳西州背书证明（执照/证书的验证）同等的各州或各国执照/证书委员会的证明，在该州或该国申请人持有或曾经持有任何职业的执业执照/证书，证明其持有或曾经持有现行的执照/证书且证明其现在或在其进入非执业状态前是否信誉良好。申请人有责任要求各执照/证书委员会将此材料直接送至行政办公室。

（i）完成由培训计划或学院直接送至行政办公室的三年高等专科针灸培训计划或大学针灸项目的证明。此证明还必须包括以下内容：

1. 高校学习或培训计划证明：

（i）持有 ACAOM 证书；或

（ii）处于 ACAOM 候选状态；或

（iii）符合 ACAOM 标准。

2. 顺利完成或毕业于针灸培训计划或大学针灸项目并加盖单位公章的证明。

（j）顺利完成 NCCAOM 批准的洁针技术课程的证明，该证明直接从课程提供者发送至行政办公室。

（k）提交第 0880－12－06 条规定的费用。

（3）互惠认证。如果要基于其他州的执照或认证来获得田纳西州的证书，申请人必须：

（a）除（e）项外，遵守本条第（2）款的所有规定。

（b）持有一州执照或证书的证明，根据委员会确定，该执照或证书与《田纳西州行政程序法》（T.C.A.）第 63－6－1001 条及其后的要求基本同等，该州执照/证书机构须将该证明与本章规则直接送至行政办公室。

（4）申请评审和认证决定应遵从第 0880－12－07 条规则。

第 0880－12－05 条 针灸戒毒专家（ADS）认证程序

（1）要在田纳西州作为针灸戒毒专家（ADS）获得受限的针灸证书，必须遵守以下程序和要求：

（a）向行政办公室索取一份申请书。

（b）对申请表中提出的每一个问题和要求应如实、完整地作出答复，并将其连同申请表和规则要求的所有文件、费用一并提交行政办公室。本规则的目的为，完成所需文件归档的必要活动应在提交申请之前完成，并同时提交所有文件。

（c）提交一张清晰、可识别、近期拍摄的半身照片，显示肩部以上正脸及完整头部。

（d）提交具有良好道德品质的证明。该证明应为两份最近（在过去 12 个月内）由医学专业人员出具的原件，在签署的信笺上证明申请人的个人品质和职业道德。

（e）提交由培训计划或学院直接送至行政办公室的顺利完成委员会认可的耳穴戒毒培训计划文件。要获得委员会批准，培训计划必须达到或超过 NADA 设定的培训标准。

（f）披露与下列任何一项有关的情况：

1. 对违反任何国家，州或市的任何刑法行为的定罪，情节轻微的交通违法行为除外。

2. 其他州拒绝其专业执照/证书申请或在任何州受到执照/证书的处分。

3. 执照/证书的丢失或限制。

4. 申请人作为被告方的任何民事诉讼判决或民事诉讼和解，包括但不限于涉及医疗事故、违约、反垄断活动或根据国家或州的成文法、普通法或判例法认可的任何其他民事诉讼补救措施。

5. 未通过任何专业执照或证书考试。

（g）申请人应直接向委员会行政办公室提交来自委员会认证申请材料中确定的提供方提供的犯罪背景调查结果。

（h）提交与田纳西州背书证明（执照/证书的验证）同等的各州或各国执照/证书委员会的证明，在该州或该国申请人持有或曾经持有任何职业的执业执照/证书，证明其持有或曾经持有现行的执照/证书且证明其现在或在其进入非执业状态前是否信誉良好。申请人有责任要求各执照/证书委员会将此材料直接送至行政办公室。

（i）提交第 0880–12–06 条规则要求的费用。

（2）申请评审和认证决定应遵从第 0880–12–07 条规则。

（3）开始执业之前，针灸戒毒专家证书的持有人应当向委员会行政办公室提供以下文件：

（a）合格的书面确认，以证明耳穴戒毒疗法将在可提供综合性酒精和药物滥用或化学依赖性服务（包括咨询）的医院、诊所或治疗机构进行。

（b）其所在的机构、设施或主体的督导执业针灸师或医学主任（即根据《田纳西州法典注释版》第 63 编第 6 章或第 9 章获得许可的医生）出具的证明，以证明受其雇佣并同意承担监管责任。

第 0880–12–06 条　费用

本规则规定的所有费用概不退还。

项　　目	针 灸 师	针灸戒毒专家
（1）申请时须缴纳申请费	五百美元	七十五美元
（2）首次认证费用须于申请时缴纳	二百五十美元	二十五美元
（3）两年一次的续期费，每两年在证书续期到期时缴纳一次	三百美元	五十美元
（4）逾期续期费	一百美元	五十美元
（5）证书激活和/或恢复费	一百美元	五十美元
（6）证书复印费	二十五美元	十美元
（7）申请时须提交两年一次的国家监管费	十美元	十美元
（8）所有费用均可通过亲自提交、邮寄或电子方式支付，支付方式为现金、支票、汇款单或卫生相关委员会管理处接受的信用卡和/或借记卡。若费用是通过认证支票、个人支票或公司支票支付的，则必须从美国银行的账户中支取，并支付给针灸咨询委员会	—	—

第 0880 - 12 - 07 条　申请审查、批准和拒绝

（1）审查所有申请以确定申请文件是否完整,可委托委员会行政主任处理。

（2）《田纳西州行政程序法》(T.C.A.)第 63 - 1 - 142 条中描述的临时执业授权书可根据医学委员会和针灸咨询委员会指定人员的初步决定授予申请人,指定人员已对申请人完整的申请进行审查并确定申请人满足认证、续期或恢复的所有要求。临时执业授权书有效期为自临时执业授权书颁发之日起六个月,不得延期或续期。若随后医学委员会和针灸咨询委员会确定申请人未满足认证、续期或恢复的要求,因而拒绝、制约或限制其认证、续期或恢复,或对其附加条件,那么因颁发临时执业授权书后对认证的拒绝、制约、附加条件或限制,而对本州提起的法律诉讼中,申请人不得援引禁止反言原则。

（3）若行政办公室收到的申请不完整,或审查委员会和/或委员会成员或医学委员会和针灸咨询委员会指定人员认为在作出初步决定之前需要申请人提供更多的信息,则委员会（第0880 - 12 - 07 条规则,续）管理员应将所需信息通知申请人。申请人应于通知所需资料的函件发出后九十日内,将所要求的资料送交行政办公室。

（4）若未及时收到所需信息,该申请文件可以被视作放弃,并可能被管理者关闭。若发生这种情况,应通知申请人,根据该程序的规则,在未收到新的申请之前,医学委员会和针灸咨询委员会将不会考虑发放证书,新的申请应包括需另外支付适用于申请人情况的所有费用并提交医学委员会和针灸咨询委员会要求的新的证明文件。

（5）如果医学委员会和/或咨询委员会的成员,或其指定人员初步决定,一项申请应被拒绝、制约、附加条件或限制,则不得颁发临时授权书。应告知申请人初步决定,医学委员会和针灸咨询委员会将在后续适当的会议上对申请作出最终裁定。若医学委员会和针灸咨询委员会对初步决定的拒绝、制约、附加条件或限制予以批准,则该决定应为最终决定,并应采取以下行动:

（a）行政办公室应通过挂号邮件发送拒绝、制约、附加条件或限制的通知,其中应包含拒绝、制约、附加条件或限制的具体原因,例如信息不完整、非官方认证、考试失败或认证不足,且应包括所有有关拒绝、制约、附加条件或限制的法令或规则,要求回执。

（b）在适当情况下,通知还应包含根据《田纳西州行政程序法》(T.C.A.)第 4 - 5 - 301 条及其后申请人具有对有争议案件进行听证的权利的声明,以对拒绝、制约、附加条件或限制以及完成该行动所需的程序提出抗辩。

1. 申请人只有在证书被拒绝、制约、附加条件或限制是基于主观或酌定标准的情况下,才有权就有争议的案件进行听证。

2. 若证书被拒绝、制约、附加条件或限制是基于客观、明确定义的标准,只有在委员会行政人员经过审查并试图解决后,申请不能获得批准,且继续被拒绝、制约、附加条件或限制的理由为适合上诉的事实和/或法律问题,申请人才能获准进行有争议案件的听讯。听证请求必须在收到医学委员会和针灸咨询委员会的拒绝、制约、附加条件或限制通知后三十日内以书面形式向行政办公室提出。

（6）若医学委员会和针灸咨询委员会发现其证书发放有错误,将通过挂号邮件发出书面通知,说明撤销或取消证书的意图。该通知将允许申请人有机会在收到通知之日起三十

日内满足证书要求。若申请人不同意所述理由以及撤销或取消认证的意图，有权依照本条第（5）款的规定起诉。

第 0880 - 12 - 08 条　保留

第 0880 - 12 - 09 条　证书续期

须续期证书方可继续执业。续期证书须遵从以下规定：

（1）根据卫生相关委员会管理处按照第 1200 - 10 - 1 - 10 条规则的"每两年续期一次的制度"，证书续期的截止日期为证书持有人生日所在月份的最后一日。

（2）续期方法。证书持有人可采用以下任意一种方法完成续期：

（a）网上续期。个人可在网上进行续期。申请人可访问以下网站进行续期：www.tennesseeanytime.org。

（b）纸质材料续期。证书持有人如未能通过互联网在网上续期证书，会收到一份续期申请表格，该表格将邮寄至其向委员会提供的最新地址。如未能收到该通知，并不免除个人应及时满足所有续期要求的责任。

（3）要获得续期资格，个人必须在截止日期或之前向卫生相关委员会管理处提交以下内容：

（a）一份填妥并签署的续期申请表格。

（b）第 0880 - 12 - 06 条规定的续期费和州监管费用。

（c）根据《田纳西州行政程序法》（T.C.A.）第 63 - 6 - 1005 条的祖父条款颁发证书的除外。

1. 对于认证针灸师，需提供现行有效的 NCCAOM 认证。

2. 对于针灸戒毒专家（ADS）证书持有人，需证明其当前积极从事耳穴戒毒疗法。

（4）任何在证书到期日之后、且在证书到期日后一个月的最后一日之前收到的续期申请，必须附带第 0880 - 12 - 06 条规定的超期续期费用。

（5）未遵守续期规定和/或未及时续期通知的个人，应根据第 1200 - 10 - 1 - 10 条规定办理证书。

（6）到期证书续期。因未能根据第 1200 - 10 - 1 - 10 条规定及时续期而到期的证书，可在符合下列条件后完成：

（a）对于证书到期未满两年的人：

1. 提交一份完整的恢复申请。

2. 按照第 0880 - 12 - 06 条规定提交续期费和超期续期费。

3. 对于证书已到期的针灸师，应在要求恢复证书的日历年之前的两个日历年（1 月 1 日至 12 月 31 日）期间，顺利完成第 0880 - 12 - 12 条规定的继续教育要求，并提交证明文件，该文件连同申请表一并提交。

（b）对于证书已到期两年及以上的人：

1. 根据第 0880 - 12 - 04 或第 0880 - 12 - 05 条提交一份新的证书申请。

2. 根据第 0880 - 12 - 06 条规定提交申请、初始证书和证书恢复费用。

3. 对于证书已到期的针灸师，应在要求恢复证书的日历年之前的两个日历年（1 月 1

至 12 月 31 日)期间,顺利完成第 0880－12－12 条规定的继续教育要求,并提交证明文件,该文件连同申请表一并提交。

(7)如在续期过程中收到贬低性的资料或讯息,若医学委员会和/或针灸咨询委员会或其正式授权代表提出要求,续期申请人必须出席医学委员会和/或针灸咨询委员会的面试,主要包括委员会正式小组、一名医学委员会和/或针灸咨询委员会成员、委员会筛选小组。面试须先于申请人接受调查或准备接受委员会认为保护公众必要之条件或限制。

(8)可由行政机关根据本规定作出续期证书的决定,也可由医学委员会和针灸咨询委员会或其指定人员审议。

第 0880－12－10 条　监督

所有持受限证书、作为针灸戒毒专家(ADS)从事针灸实践的人,均应在认证针灸师或来自医院、诊所或医疗机构的临床主管的监督下提供全面的酒精和药物滥用或药物依赖服务,包括咨询。

第 0880－12－11 条　证书失效和重新激活

(1)希望保留证书但无法积极执业的证书持有人为避免遵守续期程序,可获取一份闲置宣誓书、填妥后提交至行政办公室,同时提交表格所要求的任何文件。

(2)医学委员会和针灸咨询委员会收到所有填妥且符合要求的适当文件,并批准证书失效申请后,证书注册为失效状态。任何失效证书持有人均不得在田纳西州执业。

(3)重新激活－任何失效证书可以通过以下方式进行重新激活:

(a)向行政办公室提交重新激活申请的书面请求。

(b)将重新激活申请填妥后提交至行政办公室,随附第 0880－12－06 条规定的续期费。若在失效之日起的一年内要求重新激活证书,则委员会可要求支付第 0880－12－06 条规定的证书恢复费和逾期续期费。

(c)对于针灸师,提交顺利完成第 0880－12－12 条规定的十五学分继续教育的证明文件,该文件连同申请表一并提交。

(d)向行政办公室提交表格可能要求的任何文件。

(e)如有要求,在医学委员会和针灸咨询委员会或其指定人员进行审查后,应出席医学委员会和/或针灸咨询委员会,或由委员会正式组成的小组,或另一名医学委员会和针灸咨询委员会成员或其指定人员就继续执业问题组织的面谈。

(f)若失效时长超过两年或在激活过程中收到负面信息,申请人应准备面临或接受医学委员会和针灸咨询委员会为了保护公众而施加的限制。

(g)若失效超过五年,申请人可能需要顺利完成医学委员会和针灸咨询委员会认为必要的教育和/或测试要求,以确定目前的能力水平。

(4)证书重新激活的申请、评审和决定应遵从第 0880－12－07 条的规定。

第 0880－12－12 条　继续教育

所有经认证为针灸师的人员须遵从以下继续教育规则,作为证书续期的先决条件。

(1)所有认证针灸师必须在证书续期前的两个日历年(1 月 1 日至 12 月 31 日)内获得 NCCAOM 规定的三十个职业发展活动(PDA)学分。

（2）新证书持有人的继续教育。根据第 0880 - 12 - 04 条规则，提交顺利完成田纳西州证书要求的所有教育和培训要求的证明，应视为已完成充分的预科教育的证明，以满足在完成该教育和培训要求的两个日历年(1月1日至12月31日)内顺利完成继续教育要求。

（3）无论个人参加或完成课程或活动的次数如何，每两个日历年(1月1日至12月31日)内，任何单个课程或活动的批准学时数在计入所需总学分时，均不得计算超过一次。

（4）如证书持有人因病、伤残或其他过度困境而未能取得所需的继续教育学分，医学委员会和针灸咨询委员会可对其豁免或以其他方式修改本条规定。豁免或修改申请必须在继续教育续期到期前以书面形式送至行政办公室。

（5）可接受的继续教育课程和活动。以下专业课程和活动符合继续教育职业发展活动（PDA）学分：

（a）课程。每一学时课程为一学分，直接提高针灸师知识和/或针灸实践能力。东方医学理论和技术课程，如人体工学、营养学和草药学，以及与针灸实践相关的西方科学课程，均可加分。学习太极和气功也可加分。

（b）研究。每两学时的书面研究为一学分。可接受的研究项目包括与针灸相关的知识和实践。

（c）写作出版。每篇文章为十学分；一本著作或主要作品为三十学分。出版物包括与针灸知识和实践有关的文章、研究、报告、书籍等。

（d）教学/诊所监督。每一学时的针灸指导或监督为一学分。教学或监督指持续进行理论和/或实践教育的责任。若有适当的文件证明，学分可以通过各种教学职务获得，包括正规学校或师承制的教学或临床监督。

（e）监督下的临床经验。在一名高级针灸师的监督下每积累一学时经验可获 1.5 学分，该针灸师至少有五年经验且持有 NCCAOM 针灸文凭。临床经验可包括观察、病例讨论和/或在监督下开展的服务。

（6）合规证明

（a）完成所需继续教育的截止日期为证书续期前的两个日历年的 12 月 31 日。

（b）所有针灸师必须在证书续期表上输入电子或其他方式的签名，表明在证书续期前的两个日历年(1月1日至12月31日)期间已完成所需的继续教育。

（c）所有针灸师必须保留完成所有继续教育课程和活动的独立文件。文件必须在接受继续教育的两个日历年(1月1日至12月31日)结束后保留四年。若部门在核查过程中提出书面要求，则必须编制本文件以供核查。证明针灸师完成继续教育的文件可以包括以下任意一项或更多：

1. 课程。继续教育课程的日期、地点、学时、课程名称/内容及导师姓名，须载于经公证的结业证书原件影印本或由课程提供者出具的官方原件信笺。

2. 研究。研究的日期、地点和主题/标题，由学校、医院或其他官方机构出具的经公证的宣誓书影印本。

3. 写作出版。出版日期、书名和出版商名称，须载于书名页的影印本。

4. 针灸相关课程教学。课程的日期和地点、教学大纲、课程名称和学时，须载于目录、计算机记录或证明活动和学时的公证证书复印件和其他官方声明。

5. 师承制。临床或学徒活动的日期、时间和地点,须载于指导医师出具的经公证的宣誓书影印本。

(d) 若针灸师提交的继续教育文件不能明确认定为符合要求的继续教育,医学委员会和/或针灸咨询委员会将要求提供关于继续教育内容的以及它如何运用于针灸师执业的书面描述。

(7) 违规行为

(a) 任何针灸师未如实证明其完成所需继续教育的,可根据第 0880 - 12 - 15 条的规定给予纪律处分。

(b) 任何未能完成所需继续教育的针灸师可根据第 0880 - 12 - 15 条的规定受到纪律处分,并且可能不被允许续期证书。

(c) 在任何纪律处分中,因服从医学委员会和/或针灸咨询委员会处分命令中的相关条款而参加的继续教育,不得计入任何两个日历年(1 月 1 日至 12 月 31 日)期间应完成的继续教育。

第 0880 - 12 - 13 条　职业道德

(1) 所有证书持有人应遵守 NCCAOM 通过的道德规范,但与田纳西州法律或医学委员会和/或针灸咨询委员会规则相冲突的除外。若 NCCAOM 道德规范与州法律或规则相冲突,则以州法律或规则为准。违反道德规范、州法律或规则的,可能会使证书持有人根据第 0880 - 12 - 15 条规则受到纪律处分。

(2) NCCAOM 道德规范的副本可以从美国弗吉尼亚 22314,亚历山德里亚,运河中心广场 11 号 300 号房或致电(703)548 - 9004 或从 http://www.nccaom.org 网站上获得。

第 0880 - 12 - 14 条　保留

第 0880 - 12 - 15 条　纪律处分及民事处罚

(1) 医学委员会和针灸咨询委员会在发现证书持有人违反任何《田纳西州行政程序法》(T.C.A.)第 63 - 6 - 1001 条及其后的规定,或根据其颁布的任何规定,可采取以下任何一项或多项与证书持有人罪行相适用的行动:

(a) 警告信。针对轻微或近乎违规行为作出的书面行动。其为非正式和建议性质,不构成正式的纪律处分。

(b) 警告处分。针对一次性和不太严重的违规行为作出的书面行动,是一项正式的纪律处分。

(c) 察看处分。是一项正式的纪律处分,证书持有人将在一段固定时期内处于严格审查之下。该处分可能伴有取消察看处分前必须满足的条件和/或在察看期间限制个人活动的条件。

(d) 证书吊销。是一项正式的纪律处分,暂停在一定时期内的执业权利。根据先前颁发的证书考虑是否允许重新执业。

(e) 因故被撤销。是一项最严厉的纪律处分,将把个人从专业实践中移除,并终止先前颁发的证书。医学委员会和/或针灸咨询委员会可酌情决定在其认为适当的条件下及时间后恢复撤销的证书。证书因故被撤销的人员,自撤销令生效之日起至少六个月期满前,不得受理其恢复证书的申请和新的证书的申请。

(f) 限制。医学委员会和/或针灸咨询委员会认为适当的,在察看或吊销期间对受纪律处分的证书持有人采取的任何行动,或作为解除察看或吊销或恢复撤销证书的先决条件的任何行动。

(g) 民事处罚。医学委员会和针灸咨询会根据本条第(5)款采取的罚款纪律处分。

(2) 一旦下令,除非证书持有人根据本条第(3)款提交申请书且向委员会证明,其在经过最初的察看、吊销、撤销或其他限制条件之后,满足解除关于察看、吊销、撤销处分的所有条件,并且已支付任何经评估的民事罚款,否则不得解除察看、吊销、撤销、民事处罚评估或任何其他形式的纪律处分。

(3) 遵守令。这一程序是对先前发出纪律处分命令的必要补充,只有当申请人完全遵守先前纪律处分命令的规定,包括未经认证的民事处罚命令,并希望或需要获得反映其遵守规定的命令时,才可使用这一程序。

(a) 医学委员会和针灸咨询委员会将仅在以下三种情况下,严格遵守(b)项规定的程序,受理对遵守令的申请,作为先前发布的命令的补充:

1. 申请人能够证明已遵守先前发出的命令的所有条款,并请求寻求发布一项命令,反映其遵守先前的规定;或

2. 申请人能够证明已遵守先前发出的命令的所有条款,并请求发布一项命令,解除先前发出的吊销或察看处分;或

3. 申请人能够证明已遵守先前发出的命令的所有条款,并请求发布一项命令,恢复先前撤销的证书。

(b) 程序

1. 申请人应向委员会行政办公室提交(c)项所载的遵守令申请书,其中应载有以下所有内容:

(i) 先前发出的命令的副本。

(ii) 一份声明,说明申请人依据第(a)项中的哪条规定要求遵守令。

(iii) 所有证明其遵守先前发出的命令的所有条款或条件的副本。如证明需要个人证词,包括申请人证词,则申请人须提交其所要依据的全部人员的签署声明,以宣誓证明其遵守规定。委员会的顾问和行政工作人员可酌情要求对签署的声明进行公证。除提交的文件或证词外,在对申请书作出初步决定或最后的答复命令前,将无须采纳其他任何文件或证词。

2. 委员会授权其顾问和行政工作人员对申请书作出初步决定,并采取下列行动之一:

(i) 证明其遵守规定,并安排将该事项作为无争议事项提交医学委员会和针灸咨询委员会。

(ii) 在与法律工作人员协商后,若无法证明申请人已遵守先前命令的所有规定,则拒绝该申请,并通知申请人仍有哪些条款需要履行和/或哪些相关证据不充分或未提交。

3. 若提交申请书至医学委员会和针灸咨询委员会,申请书所载文件和证词应与最初提交时相同,不得提交任何额外文件或证词。

4. 若医学委员会和针灸咨询委员会认为申请人已遵守先前命令的所有条款,则应签发

遵守令。

5. 若申请书最初是由行政人员拒绝或在向医学委员会和针灸咨询委员会提交后被拒绝,并且申请人认为其遵守该命令已得到充分证明,申请人可以根据法律授权,按照《田纳西州行政程序法》(T.C.A.)第 4-5-223 条和第 1200-10-1-11 条规则提交申请,要求作出宣告性命令。

(c)申请格式

医学考试委员会和针灸咨询委员会遵守令申请书

申请人姓名:_____

申请人邮寄地址:_____

申请人电子邮箱地址:_____

电话号码:_____

申请人律师:_____

律师邮寄地址:_____

律师电子邮箱地址:_____

电话号码:_____

如所附文件证实,本人谨声明已遵守所附纪律处分命令的所有规定,本人谨此请求:

1. 一份反映本人遵守规定的命令。

2. 一份反映本人遵守规定,并解除先前发出的吊销或察看处分的命令。

3. 一份反映本人遵守规定,并恢复先前撤销证书的命令。

注:您必须附上证明您的请求所需的所有文件,包括原始命令的副本。若您证明遵守规定所依据的证明为个人(包括您自己在内)证词,必须附上所要依据的全部人员的签署声明,并宣誓证明遵守规定。委员会的顾问和行政工作人员可酌情要求对签署的声明进行公证。除提交的文件或证词外,在对申请书作出初步决定或最后的答复命令前,将不采纳其他任何文件或证词。

谨于____日提交_____,20

_____申请人签名

(4)修改命令。本程序不允许任何人根据先前发布的纪律处分命令,包括未经认证的民事处罚命令,修改命令中包含的任何事实调查结果、法律结论或作出决定的理由。医学委员会和针灸咨询委员会所作所有此类规定均需根据《统一行政程序法案》(《田纳西州行政程序法》第 4-5-301 条及其后)进行重新审议和上诉。此程序不能代替复议和/或上诉,只能在所有复议和上诉权利用尽或没有及时行使之后才适用。同时其不适用于已判警告处分的个人。

（a）医学委员会和针灸咨询委员会将严格遵守（b）项规定的程序，只有在申请人能够证明先前发出的命令中有一项或多项规定无法遵守的情况下，才受理关于修改先前发出的纪律处分命令的申请。为本条之目的，术语"无法"并不表示由于个人、财务、日程安排或其他原因，不便遵守或不切实际。

（b）程序

1. 申请人应就（c）项所载表格，向委员会行政办公室提交关于一份经签署的修改命令的申请书，其中应载有以下所有内容：

（i）先前发出命令的副本。

（ii）申请人认为无法遵守已发布的命令的说明。

（iii）所有证明无法遵守规定的文件副本。若无法遵守规定的依据需要个人证词，包括申请人证词，则申请人须提交其所要依据的全部人员的签署声明，以宣誓解释无法遵守规定的理由。除提交的文件或证词外，在对申请书作出初步决定或最后的答复命令前，将无须采纳其他任何文件或证词。

2. 委员会授权其顾问和行政工作人员对申请书作出初步决定，并采取下列行动之一：

（i）证明其无法遵守规定，并将申请书转交总法律顾问办公室，作为无争议事项提交医学委员会和针灸咨询委员会。

（ii）在与法律工作人员协商后，若不能证明其无法遵守先前命令的规定，则应拒绝申请书，并通知申请人，证明无法遵守规定的证据不充分或未提交。

3. 若提交申请书至医学委员会和针灸咨询委员会，申请书所载文件和证词应与最初提交时相同，不得提交任何额外文件或证词。

4. 若申请书获得批准，应发布一项新命令，反映医学委员会和针灸咨询委员会授权对先前命令中发现的违规行为所作的适当和必要的修改。

5. 若申请书最初是由行政人员拒绝或在向医学委员会和针灸咨询委员会提交后被拒绝，并且申请人认为无法遵守该命令已得到充分证明，申请人可以根据法律授权，按照《田纳西州行政程序法》（T.C.A.）第4-5-223条和第1200-10-1-11条规则提交申请，要求作出宣告性命令。

（c）申请格式

医学考试委员会和针灸咨询委员会修改命令申请书

申请人姓名：_____

申请人邮寄地址：_____

申请人电子邮箱地址：_____

电话号码：_____

申请人律师：_____

律师邮寄地址：_____

律师电子邮箱地址：_____
电话号码：_____

如所附文件所证实，本人谨声明，由于下列理由，无法遵守所附纪律处分命令中已明确的规定：_____

注：您必须附上证明您的请求所需的所有文件，包括原始命令的副本。若您证明无法遵守规定所依据的证明为个人（包括您自己在内）证词，必须附上所要依据的全部人员的签署声明，并宣誓无法遵守。委员会的顾问和行政工作人员可酌情要求对签署的声明进行公证。除提交的文件或证词外，在对申请书作出初步决定或最后的答复命令前，将不采纳其他任何文件或证词。

谨于____日提交_____，20
_____申请人签名

（5）民事处罚

（a）目的。本规则的目的为制定一个附表，规定根据《田纳西州行政程序法》（T.C.A.）第 63－1－134 条可评定的最低和最高民事处罚。

（b）民事处罚表

1. 医学委员会和针灸咨询委员会发现需要其颁发执照、认证、许可或授权的人故意违反《田纳西州行政程序法》（T.C.A.）第 63－6－1001 条及其后的部分或据其颁布的条例，对患者或公众的健康、安全和福利造成或可能造成即时、重大的威胁，可以对其处以"A 类"民事处罚。为本条之目的，未经医学委员会和针灸咨询委员会颁发执照、认证、许可或授权，故意地作为针灸师或针灸戒毒专家（ADS）执业，属于"A 类"民事处罚。

2. 当医学委员会和针灸咨询委员会发现需要其颁发执照、认证、许可或授权的人违反《田纳西州行政程序法》（T.C.A.）第 63－6－1001 条及其后的部分或据其颁布的条例，对患者的护理或公众造成直接影响，可对其处以"B 类"民事处罚。

3. 当医学委员会和针灸咨询委员会发现需要其颁发执照、认证、许可或授权的人违反《田纳西州行政程序法》（T.C.A.）第 63－6－1001 条及其后的部分或据其颁布的条例，虽未对患者或公众有直接的伤害或影响他们的护理，但对患者的护理或公众造成间接影响，可对其处以"C 类"民事处罚。

（c）民事处罚金额

1. "A 类"民事处罚的数额应不少于五百美元且不高于一千美元。

2. "B 类"民事处罚的数额应不少于一百美元且不高于五千美元。

3. "C 类"民事处罚的数额应不少于五十美元且不高于一百美元。

（d）民事处罚评定程序

1. 卫生相关委员会部门可提交民事处罚评定备忘录，以启动民事处罚评定。部门应在备忘录中说明其指控一项违法行为所依据的事实和法律、拟议的民事处罚数额以及该等处罚的依据。部门可将民事处罚评定备忘录与指控通知书一并发出。

2. 民事处罚也可由医学委员会和针灸咨询委员会在审议任何指控通知时启动和评定。此外,如有充分理由,医学委员会和针灸咨询委员会可评定部门未建议的民事处罚的种类和数额。

3. 在根据本规则评定民事处罚时,医学委员会和针灸咨询委员会可考虑下列因素:

(ⅰ)所征收金额是否会对违法者产生实质性的经济威慑。

(ⅱ)导致违法的情形。

(ⅲ)违法行为的严重程度和危害公众的风险。

(ⅳ)违法者因违规行为而获得的经济利益。

(ⅴ)公众的利益。

4. 所有民事处罚评定程序均应遵从《田纳西州行政程序法》(T.C.A.)第4编第5章有争议案件的条款。

第0880-12-16条　证书补发

具有艺术设计的证书遗失或者毁坏的,证书持有人经向行政机关书面申请,可以补发证书。该要求应随附一份宣誓书(经签署和公证),说明有关原始文件遗失或毁坏的事实,以及根据第0880-12-06条规则要求支付的费用。

第0880-12-17条　姓名和/或地址变更

(1)姓名变更。证书持有人变更姓名应当在三十日内以书面形式通知行政机关,并提供新旧姓名。姓名变更通知还必须包括所涉及的官方文件的副本,并提及个人的职业、医学委员会或针灸咨询委员会、社会保障和证书号码。

(2)地址变更。证书持有人变更地址应以书面形式向行政机关提交新旧住址。此类申请必须在变更生效后三十日内送达行政办公室,并注明个人姓名、职业、社会保障号码、证书号码。

第0880-12-18条　保留

第0880-12-19条　委员会官员、顾问、记录、宣告令和筛查小组

(1)委员会应每年从其成员中选出下列官员:

(a)主席。主持委员会所有会议。

(b)联席主席。主席缺席时主持会议,和委员会署长共同负责委员会的信件。

(2)委员会有权挑选一名委员会顾问担任部门顾问,并有权采取下列行动:

(a)审查投诉,并就部门收到投诉或进行调查后,是否采取纪律处分,以及采取何种纪律处分提出建议。

(b)就投诉、案例或纪律处分是否可获解决以及根据什么条款解决提出建议。任何提议解决的事项随后都必须由医学委员会和针灸咨询委员会审查、评估和批准,才能生效。

(c)处理经医学委员会和针灸咨询委员会多数表决通过的任何其他事项。

(3)记录和投诉

(a)委员会会议记录和所有记录、文件、申请书和信件将保存在行政办公室。

（b）所有请求、申请、通知、其他通信和信件均应直接送交行政办公室。任何要求委员会作出决定或采取正式处分的请求或询问，除与纪律处分或听证要求有关的文件外，必须在预定会议前十四日收到，并将保留在行政办公室，在委员会会议上提交委员会。此类文件未及时收到的，应提交下届委员会会议进行审议。

（c）除依法要求保密的记录外，正常办公时间内，委员会所有记录在行政办公室的一名工作人员的监督下可供查阅。

（d）公共记录的副本经付费后可提供给任何人。

（e）所有投诉应直接送至部门的调查科。

（4）委员会成员或顾问有权采取以下行为：

（a）审查并确定申请证书、续期和重新激活，但须遵守管理这些申请的规则，并须经医学委员会和针灸咨询委员会随后批准。

（b）担任部门顾问，并决定以下事项：

1. 在部门收到投诉或进行调查后，是否采取纪律处分，以及采取何种纪律处分。

2. 投诉、案件或纪律处分是否可获解决以及根据什么条款解决。任何提议解决的事项随后都必须由医学委员会和针灸咨询委员会审查、评估和批准，才能生效。

（5）委员会授权主持委员会有争议案件的成员作为机构成员，根据第 1360‐4‐1‐18 条规则作出关于复议请求和搁置该案件的决定。

（6）要求在其他州执业的针灸师或针灸戒毒专家（ADS）的执照验证请求必须以书面形式向行政办公室提出。

（7）宣告令。委员会已通过卫生相关委员会部门第 1200‐10‐1‐11 条规则，已在此悉数列出，并可能不时予以修改，作为其对宣告令程序的管理规则。凡涉及委员会管辖范围内的法例、规则或命令的宣告性命令申请，均须由委员会根据该规则处理，而非由部门处理。宣告令申请表可以从行政办公室获得。

（8）筛查小组。委员会已通过卫生相关委员会部门第 1200‐10‐1‐13 条规则，已在此悉数列出，并可能不时予以修改，作为其对筛查小组程序的管理规则。

第 0880‐12‐20 条　广告

（1）政策声明。许多公众对针灸缺乏了解，而针灸师的选择会影响重要的公众利益，且针灸师无限制的宣传会造成可预见的后果，并被认为特别有可能构成欺骗，这些问题要求针灸师特别小心，避免误导公众。针灸师须注意，广告的效益取决于其可靠性和准确性。由于针灸师投放广告需经过仔细考虑，不可随意发布，因此，为促使针灸师遵守适当标准，而不阻碍有用、有意义和相关的信息流向公众，制定合理的规章制度符合公众利益。

（2）定义

（a）广告。以任何方式向公众传达信息，旨在引起公众对田纳西州执业针灸师的关注。

（b）证书持有人。任何持有田纳西州针灸执业证书的人。如适用，应包括合伙企业和/或公司。

（c）重要事实。理性谨慎的普通人士需要了解或依赖的任何事实，以便作出关于选择医师以服务其特定需要的知情决定。

（d）诱导转向广告。一种诱人但不真实产品或服务推销，而推广人实际上并不打算或想要出售该产品或服务。它的目的是使消费者从购买广告宣传的服务或商品转向购买其他商品，通常价格更高或对推广人更有利。

（e）折扣费用。指个人或产品或服务提供或收取的费用，低于该个人或组织通常为该产品或服务收取的费用。明确免费提供的产品或服务不应视为以折扣费用提供。

（3）广告费用和服务

（a）固定费用。可在广告中提及任何服务的固定费用。除非在广告中另有说明，否则假定一项服务的固定费用应包括所有专业人员的在普遍接受的标准下完成服务公认所需的费用。

（b）其他费用。可在广告中提及服务的其他费用，广告必须披露决定实际收费的因素，以防止欺骗公众。

（c）折扣费用。在以下情形中，可在广告中提及折扣费用：

1. 折扣费用实际上低于证书持有人通常收取的服务费用。

2. 证书持有人以折扣费用提供的服务和材料的质量和内容与该服务通常以正常、非折扣费用提供的相同。

（d）相关服务及附加费用。与广告中所提服务可能需要一起提供的、需额外收费的服务应在广告中提及指明。

（e）广告费的时间段。

1. 凡寻求广告服务的，均应在广告所述时间段支付广告费，无论广告服务是否在该时间内实际提供或完成。

2. 若广告费没有固定时间段，则广告费应在发布之日起三十日内或下一次预定发布时间之前支付，以较晚者为准，不论服务是否在该时间内实际提供或完成。

（4）广告内容。任何证书持有人在广告中所作的下列行为或不作为，均构成虚假或欺诈行为，并根据《田纳西州行政程序法》（T.C.A.）第 63－6－1007 条第（1）款给予证书持有人纪律处分：

（a）在无法证明的情况下，声称其提供的服务、所雇用的人员、所使用的材料或办公设备在专业上优于通常的服务、人员、材料或设备，或表明该证书持有人优于其他证书持有人。

（b）在广告中误导性地使用未获得的或非医疗卫生学位。

（c）在证书持有人知悉或应当知悉的情况下，推广其能力范围以外的专业服务。

（d）使用沟通技巧对潜在客户造成恐吓、施加过度压力或不当影响。

（e）任何过度或不合理地引起个人焦虑的行为。

（f）使用任何无法合理验证的个人证明，证明证书持有人所提供的服务或治疗质量合格。

（g）利用基于过去表现的任何统计数据或其他信息来预测未来的服务，从而对证书持有人能够实现的结果产生不合理的预期。

（h）未经患者同意而传播有关患者可识别的个人事实、数据或信息。

（i）重大事实的谎报。

（j）故意淡化、遗漏或隐瞒重要事实或者法律，导致广告具有欺骗性或误导性。

（k）有关涉及重大风险的针灸流程或产品的好处或其他属性的陈述，但不包括：

1. 对这些流程或产品的安全性和效率的现实评估。

2. 可选择的替代方案。

3. 必要时为避免欺骗，对这些替代方案的好处或其他属性进行描述或评估。

（l）对任何治疗的潜在结果产生不合理预期的任何沟通。

（m）未遵守关于广告费用、服务或记录的规定。

（n）使用"诱导转向"广告。如相关情况表明存在"诱导转向"的广告宣传，委员会可以要求证书持有人提供与广告宣传产品和其他销售产品有关的数据或其他证据。

（o）谎报证书持有人的证书、培训、经验或能力。

（p）未在任何广告中包含公司、合伙企业或个人证书持有人的姓名、地址和电话号码。任何通过使用商标名称做广告或未能列出在特定地点执业的所有证书持有人的公司、合伙企业或协会应：

1. 根据要求提供在该地点执业的所有证书持有人的名单。

2. 在证书持有人的办公室内保留并醒目地展示含在该地点执业的所有证书持有人的名录。

（q）为刊登广告（如报纸文章）而给报刊、广播、电视或其他通信媒体的代表提供报酬或馈赠，但未披露该事实。除非此类广告的性质、格式或媒介足以说明已给予报酬的事实。

（r）在证书持有人离开后三十日，在证书持有人先前执业或合伙执业的广告地点、办公室标牌或建筑使用其姓名。本条不适用于已退休或已亡故的，且曾与一名或多名在任人员共同执业的前合伙人（第0880－12－20条，续），其身份应在任何广告或标志中披露。

（s）声明或暗示某证书持有人可提供所有服务，实际上其中有些服务由其他证书持有人提供。

（t）向第三方直接或间接提供、给予、收取或同意收取费用或其他报酬，以转诊其专业服务相关患者。

（5）广告记录和责任

（a）任何证书持有人如担任广告中指明的公司或实体的主要合伙人或高级人员，均须对任何广告的形式及内容负连带责任。本规定还应包括作为该公司或实体代理人的任何持有执照或经认证的专业雇员。

（b）所有广告均假定为经过广告中出现的证书持有人批准。

（c）电子媒体传播的每个广告的记录，印刷媒体传播的每个广告的副本，以及任何其他形式的广告的副本，均应由证书持有人自最后的广播或出版之日起保留两年，并按照委员会或其指定人员的要求提供审查。

（d）在投放任何类型的广告时，证书持有人必须拥有并依赖于所提供的资料，这些资料在公布时可证实广告或公众资料所载的任何断言、遗漏或陈述的重要事实的真实性。

（6）可分割性。特此声明，本规则的条、款、句和部分均可分割，不是相互具有实质因果关系的事项,若本规则违反宪法或变得无效,则任何一项均应予以撤销。若任一或多个条、款、句或部分出于任何原因在法庭上受到质疑,并且被判定为违宪或无效,则该判决不得影响、损害余下条款或使得余下条款无效,而应限于违宪或无效的具体条款,任何一个或多个情况下,任何条、款、句或部分的不适用或无效不得以任何方式影响或损害它在任何其他情况下的适用性或有效性。

西弗吉尼亚州

西弗吉尼亚州针灸法[①]

第 30 - 36 - 1 条　从事针灸实践所需执照

为了保护公众的生命、健康和安全,任何人以针灸师身份从事或提供针灸实践,都需要提交他或她具备资格的证据,并按照本条的规定获得执照。1997 年 6 月 30 日之后,任何未根据本条规定获得许可的人在本州从事针灸实践,或使用任何头衔、标志、卡片或装置来表明他或她是针灸师,都属违法行为。本条款的规定并非旨在限制、排除或以其他方式干扰在任何场所工作并由西弗吉尼亚州的适当机构或委员会许可的其他卫生保健提供者的实践行为,该等卫生保健提供者的实践行为和培训可能包含与执业针灸师的实践行为性质相同的要素。

第 30 - 36 - 2 条　定义

(a) 除非上下文明确规定不同含义,下列定义适用于本节:

(1)"针灸"系指一种基于能量生理学理论的卫生保健形式,该理论描述身体器官或功能与相关穴位或穴位组合的相互关系。

(2)"耳穴戒毒"系指经委员会批准或由国家针灸戒毒协会(NADA)规定的耳穴戒毒疗法,用于治疗药物滥用、酒精中毒、化学依赖、戒毒、行为疗法或创伤恢复。

(3)"委员会"系指西弗吉尼亚州针灸委员会。

(4)"证书持有人"系指由委员会向接受耳穴戒毒训练的人员颁发的授权,这些人员符合根据本条和委员会规则所确定的资格,可认证为耳穴戒毒专家(ADS)。

(5)"执照"系指由委员会颁发的从事针灸实践的执照。

(6)"艾灸"系指艾蒿在皮肤上或皮肤附近燃烧,刺激穴位。

(7)"NADA"系指国家针灸戒毒协会。

(8)"NADA 方案"系指国家针灸戒毒协会耳穴戒毒疗法方案。

(9)"从事针灸实践"系指采用东方医学疗法,使包括疼痛控制在内的精神生理功能正常化,旨在促进、维持和恢复健康。

[①]　根据《西弗吉尼亚州注释版法典》第 30 章第 36 节"针灸师"译出。

（b）（1）"针灸实践"包括：

（A）通过插入针灸针来刺激身体的穴位。

（B）艾灸的应用。

（C）手动、机械、热或电疗法只有在符合东方针灸医学理论的原则下才能进行。

第30－36－3条　委员会成立

特此设立一个名为"西弗吉尼亚州针灸委员会"的州委员会。

第30－36－4条　委员会成员

（a）委员会由五名成员组成，由州长任命，并得到参议院的建议和同意。

（1）根据本条（c）款的规定，从提交的名单中指定三名执业针灸师。

（2）一人应为公众人士。

（3）一人应为在西弗吉尼亚州执业的医生。

（b）每名执业针灸师应：

（1）为本州居民。

（2）在任命前至少三年在本州从事针灸实践。

（c）委员会应编制一份针灸师成员的空缺名单，以下列方式提交给州长：

（1）委员会应将空缺情况通知该州所有执业针灸师，以征求填补空缺的提名。

（2）本州的每个针灸师专业协会应为每个空缺至少提名两人。

（3）在本州提供针灸培训的每个教育机构应为每个空缺至少提名两人。

（d）公众成员：

（1）不得为针灸师，不得曾经是针灸师，不得正在接受培训成为针灸师。

（2）不得有针灸师或者正在接受针灸师培训的家庭成员。

（3）不得参与或曾经参与过与针灸相关的商业或专业领域。

（4）不得有参与针灸相关商业或专业领域的家庭成员。

（5）在任职之前的两年内，不得与受委员会监管的人员存在重大经济利益关系。

（e）担任委员会成员期间，公众成员不得与受委员会监管的人员存在重大经济利益关系。

（f）在就职之前，委员会的每一位被委任人应宣誓并签署本州宪法第四节第5条规定的誓言。

（g）任职；空缺。

（1）成员任期为三年。

（2）成员的任期从1996年7月1日开始错开。首次任命的成员的任期届满日期应在提名时由州长指定，第一年年底有一名成员任期届满，第二年年底两名，第三年年底两名。在原任期届满后，以后的每一任任期应为三年。

（3）在任期结束时，该成员继续任职，直到继任者被任命并合格。

（4）一名成员不得连任两届以上。

（5）在任期开始后被任命的成员只在任期的剩余时间内任职，直到继任者被任命并合格为止。

(h)州长可因任何成员玩忽职守或不称职或不道德或不光彩的行为而将其从委员会中开除。

第30－36－5条 管理人员

委员会应从其成员中选举管理人员,选举方式和任期由委员会决定。

第30－36－6条 法定人数;会议;报销;工作人员

(a)委员会正式授权成员的多数构成法定人数。

(b)委员会每年至少召开两次会议,时间和地点由委员会决定。

(c)委员会的每一名成员都有权报销参加委员会活动时实际发生的旅费和其他必要费用。所有费用的报销应由本条规定设立的针灸委员会基金支付。

(d)委员会可雇用履行委员会职能所需的人员,包括一名行政秘书,并根据国家预算从针灸委员会基金中支付所有人员的工资。

(e)委员会可与其他州委员会或州机构签订合同,根据本条的授权共享办公室、人员和其他行政职能。

第30－36－7条 制定规则的权力;其他权力和职责

(a)委员会可根据第29A－3－1条及其后各条的规定,提议颁布实施本条规定的法规。

(b)委员会可采纳执业道德守则。

(c)除本节其他条款中列明的权力外,委员会还应保存:

(1)有序开展事务所必需的记录和会议纪要。

(2)每个当前的执业针灸师名单。

(d)委员会可在2019年立法会常会期间,在本节重新生效之日提出紧急立法性规章,以实施必要的规定,向接受耳穴戒毒培训的人员颁发证书,并根据本条规定为持证人确定费用。

第30－36－8条 针灸委员会基金;费用;开支;资金处置

(a)特此在州财务办公室设立针灸委员会基金。

(b)委员会可为执照的发放和续期及其其他服务设定合理的费用。支付委员会成员或员工薪酬和支出的所有资金应由本款规定的费用产生。

(c)委员会应将根据本条规定收取的所有费用支付给州财政部。

(d)该基金应专门用于支付在履行本条规定的委员会法定和监管职责过程中,实际记录的直接和间接成本。该基金是一个持续的、非失效的基金。基金的任何未用部分不得转移或归还给国家一般收入基金,而应留在基金中用于本条规定的目的。

(e)立法审计员应审计基金的账目和交易。

第30－36－9条 需要执照或证书;豁免

(a)除本节另有规定外,个人在本州从事针灸或耳穴疗法之前,应获得委员会颁发的执照或证书。

(b)本条不适用于:

(1)受雇于联邦政府担任针灸师,并在该职业范围内执业的个人;或

(2)被指定在经委员会或州教育委员会批准的项目中,同时在执业针灸师的监督下参

加学习或培训课程的学生、学员或客座教师。

第 30 - 36 - 10 条　执照申请人的资格；和证书持有人的资格

（a）要取得执照，申请人应：

（1）品德良好。

（2）年满十八岁。

（3）通过或满足下列教育、培训或经验证明标准之一，证明自己有能力从事针灸实践：

（A）从至少一千八百学时（包括三百个临床学时）的培训课程毕业，即：

（i）经国家针灸和东方医学院校认证委员会批准；或

（ii）经委员会认定相当于国家针灸和东方医学院校认证委员会批准的课程。

（B）考试成绩合格，即：

（i）由国家针灸师认证委员会颁发；或

（ii）由委员会确定等同于国家针灸师认证委员会进行的考试。

（C）在该司法管辖区已正式批准针灸执业的个人指导下，在五年内顺利完成至少二千七百学时的学徒期；或

（D）在申请之前的五年内，根据另一个或多个司法管辖区的法律从事至少三年的针灸实践，包括每年至少五百次患者就诊。

（4）达到委员会在条例中规定的任何其他资格。

（b）尽管本法典中有任何其他相反的规定，为获得耳穴戒毒专家证书，申请人应：

（1）年满十八岁。

（2）在本州获授权从事以下任何一项活动：

（A）医师助理，根据本法规第 30 - 3E - 1 条及其后各条。

（B）牙医，根据本法规第 30 - 4 - 1 条及其后各条。

（C）注册专业护士，根据本法规第 30 - 7 - 1 条及其后各条。

（D）实习护士，根据本法规第 30 - 7A - 1 条及其后各条。

（E）心理学家，根据本法规第 30 - 21 - 1 条及其后各条。

（F）职业治疗师，根据本法规第 30 - 28 - 1 条及其后各条。

（G）社会工作者，根据本法规第 30 - 30 - 1 条及其后各条。

（H）专业顾问，根据本法规第 30 - 31 - 1 条及其后各条。

（I）紧急医疗服务提供者，根据本法规第 16 - 4C - 1 条及其后各条；或

（J）矫正医疗服务提供者，根据本法规第 15A - 1 - 1 条及其后各条。

（3）提供顺利完成委员会批准的耳穴戒毒计划的证据。

（4）提交委员会规定的完整申请。

（5）按照法律规定交纳适当的费用。

（c）按照本法典第 30 - 36 - 10（b）款的规定，满足以下要求，可向退休或非现役专业人员颁发证书：满足该专业人员符合证书持有人的资格要求，并且在过去三年的专业活动中信誉良好。但是，在公共卫生紧急情况或紧急状态期间，持有其他司法管辖区的耳穴戒毒专家证书或同等证书的人员经委员会批准可以从事耳穴戒毒疗法，具体期限将由委员会的立

法性规章规定。

第 30‑36‑11 条　申请执照

申请执照时,申请人应当:

(a) 按委员会提供的格式向委员会提交申请。

(b) 向委员会支付委员会规定的申请费。

第 30‑36‑12 条　执照的发放

委员会应向符合本节要求,以及符合委员会根据本节通过的规定的任何申请人发放执照。

第 30‑36‑13 条　执照的范围

除本节另有规定外,持证人须在执照有效期内从事针灸实践。

第 30‑36‑14 条　执照和证书的期限和续期;限制;广告

(a) 执照和证书的条款:

(1) 委员会应根据本条对执照和证书的期限和续期进行规定。

(2) 执照或者证书的期限不得超过三年。

(3) 执照或证书在其期限结束时到期,除非按委员会规定续期执照或证书。

(b) 续期通知。在执照或证书到期前至少一个月,委员会应通过一级邮件向执照或证书持有人发送一份续期通知,邮件地址为持证人的最后一个已知地址,通知内容为:

(1) 当前执照或证书到期的日期。

(2) 在执照或证书到期之前,委员会必须收到续期申请的日期,以便发出并邮寄该续期申请。

(3) 续期费金额。

(c) 续期申请。在执照或证书到期之前,执照或证书持有人可定期将其续期一段时间,如果该执照或证书持有人:

(1) 有资格取得执照或证书。

(2) 向委员会支付由委员会设定的续期费用。

(3) 向委员会提交:

(A) 符合委员会格式要求的续期申请。

(B) 充分的证据,证明其符合本条规定的针对执照或证书续期的任何继续教育要求。

(d) 除了委员会规定的任何其他资格和要求外,委员会还可以规定继续教育要求,作为本条中续期执照和证书的一项条件。

(e) 委员会应当为符合本条要求的每个执照和证书持有人续期执照,并颁发续期证书。

(f) 持证人只可在委员会通过的规则所准许的情况下刊登广告。

(g) 被认定为耳穴戒毒专家的持证人不得在耳穴戒毒范围之外针刺任何身体穴位,也不得宣传自己是针灸师:但本条中的任何内容不得禁止个人在法律授权的范围内执业。

第 30‑36‑15 条　来自其他州或国家的针灸师的互惠许可

(a) 如满足下列条件,针灸委员会可通过互惠原则,为本州合法注册或另一州的执业针灸师颁发执照:此类执照的申请人应符合委员会根据本法典第 29 章 a 节的规定颁布的互惠条例的要求：但是，当其他州不允许西弗吉尼亚州的持证针灸师享有互惠待遇时，则互惠原则不适用。

（b）除非申请人符合委员会颁布的外国申请人执照条例，否则委员会可拒绝对来自其他国家的针灸师实行互惠待遇。

（c）本条规定的执照申请人应在提出申请时向委员会交纳规定的费用。

第30－36－16条　非执业状态；恢复到期执照

（a）如果持证人向委员会提交以下文件，委员会应将持证人列入非执业状态：

（1）以委员会要求的格式提交非执业状态申请书。

（2）委员会规定的非执业状态费用。

（b）如果处于非执业状态的个人符合从非执业状态变为执业状态时存在的续期要求，委员会应向该个人颁发执照。

（c）如果原持证人符合以下条件，委员会应恢复因任何原因未能续期执照的原持证人的执照：

（1）符合本节第14条的续期要求。

（2）向委员会支付由委员会规定的恢复费。

第30－36－17条　执照或证书持有人放弃执照或证书

（a）除非委员会同意注销执照或证书，否则执照或证书持有人不得注销执照或证书，在执照或证书持有人正在接受调查期间，或对执照或证书持有人提出指控期间，执照或证书也不得因法律的实施而失效。

（b）委员会可设定条件，与受调查或受指控的执照或证书持有人达成一致，同意其注销执照或证书。

第30－36－18条　谴责、察看、吊销和撤销；理由

执照或证书持有人存在下列情形的，委员会经其全体授权成员的多数赞成票，可对任何执照或证书持有人进行申诉，将任何执照或证书持有人列入察看期，或吊销或撤销其执照或证书：

（1）申请人、执照持有人、证书持有人或其他人通过欺诈或欺骗手段获得或试图获得执照或证书。

（2）通过欺诈或欺骗手段：

（A）使用执照或证书；或

（B）招标或宣传。

（3）在针灸或耳针实践中存在不道德或违反职业道德的行为。

（4）由于专业、身体或精神原因不具备执业能力。

（5）提供专业服务过程中：

（A）受酒精影响；或

（B）使用本法规第60A－1－101条中定义的任何麻醉剂或管制药品，或超过治疗量或无有效医学指征的其他药品。

（6）故意违反本节的任何规定或委员会根据本节通过的任何规定。

（7）被判犯有重罪或涉及道德败坏的罪行，或承认有罪，或对重罪或涉及道德败坏的罪行不抗辩，无论是否有任何上诉或其他诉讼有待撤销定罪或抗辩。

（8）与未经许可的人员共同从事针灸或者耳穴戒毒疗法，或者协助未经许可的人员从事针灸或者耳穴戒毒疗法。

（9）受到本州或任何其他州或国家的许可或纪律部门的纪律处分，或被任何州或国家的法院判定有罪或采取纪律处分，根据本条规定，其行为构成采取纪律处分的行为。

（10）在针灸、耳穴戒毒疗法实践中，故意作出虚假报告或者记录的。

（11）故意不按照法律规定归档或者记录报告，故意妨碍或者阻挠报告归档或者记录，或者诱导他人不进行报告归档或者记录的。

（12）交纳虚假陈述从而收取费用；或

（13）根据医生、牙医和其他执业卫生保健专业人员在该类型情况下所制定的治疗标准，持有执照且符合资格的人员在提供专业服务方面抵制、拒绝、否认或歧视艾滋病毒阳性者。

第30-36-19条　正当程序

（a）委员会收到书面申诉书，指控某人犯有本节第16条所述的任何行为时，委员会的行政秘书或其他授权雇员应向被申诉人提供一份申诉书副本或指控清单。此人将有二十日时间对申诉书作出书面答复。如果指控成立，委员会应展开调查。如果委员会认为申诉有合理的理由，应确定听证的时间和地点，并应在听证日期前至少十五个日历日将通知送达持证人或申请人。通知应直接送达或通过挂号邮件发送至该人的最后已知地址。

（b）委员会可向举行听证所在县的巡回法院提出呈请，要求其发出传票，让证人出庭，并在任何听证中出示必要的证据。应答辩人或其律师的请求，委员会应呈请法院代表答辩人发出传票。巡回法院可根据呈请发出其认为必要的传票。

（c）除本条另有规定外，听证程序应根据本法典第29-a章规定的本州行政程序颁布，对委员会的裁定不满的，可根据该行政程序提起上诉。

第30-36-20条被2010年法典第32章废止，2010年6月11日失效

西弗吉尼亚州针灸行政法[①]

第一节　针灸委员会会议

第32-1-1条　总则

1.1　范围：本规则规定了所有定期会议的时间和地点以及委员会所有特别会议的时间、地点和目的。

1.2　权限：《西弗吉尼亚州法典》第30-36-7条。

1.3　提交日期：1998年8月3日。

---

① 根据《西弗吉尼亚州行政法典》第32章"针灸委员会"译出。

1.4　生效日期：1998 年 9 月 2 日。

第 32 - 1 - 2 条　申请和执行

本程序规则适用于西弗吉尼亚州针灸委员会。规则的执行权属于委员会主席。

第 32 - 1 - 3 条　定义

3.1　委员会：西弗吉尼亚州针灸委员会。

3.2　主席：由委员会成员选举其中一人担任委员会主席。

3.3　委员会副主席兼财务主管：由委员会成员选举其中一人担任委员会副主席。

3.4　秘书：由委员会成员选举其中一人担任委员会秘书。

3.5　决定：在法定人数出席的任何会议上，需要委员会表决的议案、提案、决议、命令或措施的任何决定、行动、表决或最终处置。

3.6　会议：召开委员会会议，需要到法定人数才能就任何事项做出一项决定或商议一项决定，但该术语不包括：

　　a. 在任何准司法行政程序中为做出裁决性决定而召开的任何会议；或

　　b. 对任何针灸或东方医学医师、诊所或教育计划的任何现场检查。

3.7　法定人数：委员会成员的多数。

第 32 - 1 - 4 条　会议

4.1　主席可召开委员会会议，且主席应在两名委员会成员的书面请求下召开会议。

4.2　主席应在会议召开前至少七日以书面形式通知委员会成员，说明会议的时间和地点以及拟考虑的事项，但如果时间、地点和拟考虑的事项是在所有成员都出席的会议上确定的，则不需要再发出通知。

4.3　主席应至少提前七日向州务卿办公室提交会议公告，通知公众和新闻媒体。公告应载明时间、地点和拟考虑的事项。

4.4　本条规定不适用于需要委员会立即正式批准的紧急情况。

4.5　经与会表决的委员会成员多数票通过，特别会议可在下一个工作日的规定时间和地点继续举行。

4.6　如无委员会成员反对，主席可取消特别会议。

第 32 - 1 - 5 条　公开程序；例外情形；允许召开执行会议

5.1　委员会的所有会议均应向公众开放，但委员会可在审裁官根据《西弗吉尼亚州法典》第 6 - 9A - 4 条的规定授权，并提交委员会和公众后，在定期会议、特别会议或紧急会议期间举行不对公众开放的执行会议。委员会不得在执行会议上作出决定。

5.2　委员会只有在出席会议的成员根据《西弗吉尼亚州法典》第 6 - 9A - 4 条及其后各条提出的理由以多数赞成票的情况下，才能召开执行会议。

第 32 - 1 - 6 条　会议记录

6.1　委员会应准备其所有会议的书面记录。所有会议记录应在会议后的合理时间内向公众开放，并应包括以下信息：

　　a. 会议的日期、时间和地点。

　　b. 出席或缺席的每位委员会成员的姓名。

c. 提议的所有动议、建议、决议、命令、法令和措施,提议人的姓名及其处理方式。

d. 所有投票结果以及每位成员的投票结果(应成员要求按姓名列出)。

6.2 执行会议的会议记录仅限于披露不违反《西弗吉尼亚州法典》第6-9A-4条中规定的材料。

第32-1-7条 要求多数票;禁止代理投票

采取任何行动都必须获得出席委员会任何会议的所有成员的多数票通过。禁止代理投票。

第32-1-8条 委员会记录公开

委员会的记录是可根据《法典》第29B-1-3条进行检查的公开记录,并且复印一页收费25美分(0.25美元)。《法典》第29B-1-3条规定的情况例外。

第三节 针灸执照申请表

第32-3-1条 总则

1.1 范围:本规则适用于针灸执照的申请。

1.2 权限:《西弗吉尼亚州法典》第30-36-7条。

1.3 提交日期:1999年5月21日。

1.4 生效日期:1999年5月21日。

第32-3-2条 申请

本立法规则适用于向委员会申请执照的人。

第32-3-3条 定义

3.1 学徒制:由委员会批准的一名讲师指导一名学生的学习课程或辅导计划,以使申请人在顺利完成该课程或计划后满足《法典》第30-36-10条规定的针灸执照要求。

3.2 CCAOM:针灸和东方医学学院委员会。

3.3 培训课程:在针灸或东方医学学校或学院学习针灸的系统课程,可获得针灸或东方医学学位或文凭。

3.4 NACSCAOM:国家针灸与东方医学学院认证委员会。

3.5 NCCA:国家针灸认证委员会或其继受机构国家针灸与东方医学认证委员会。

第32-3-4条 委员会准许颁发执照

4.1 如果申请人已经提交了委员会资格审查所要求的申请表和证明文件,且申请人符合《法典》第30-36-1条及其后各条规定的要求和委员会颁布的规则,则委员会应向申请人颁发针灸执业执照。

4.2 如果委员会确定申请人符合取得针灸执照的要求,则应向申请人颁发有效期为两年的执照。委员会可自行决定是否颁发执照,并可规定额外的培训、临床经验或国家针灸与东方医学认证委员会(NCCAOM)考试作为执照要求。

第32-3-5条 颁发执照的条件

5.1 执照申请人应:

5.1.1 具备良好品德。

5.1.2　年满十八岁。

5.1.3　证明具备针灸执业能力。

5.2　申请人应向委员会提交三个人对其的品德证明，以证明其具备良好品德，这三个人应均可证明申请人诚实可信的声誉。品德证明应包括以下内容：

5.2.1　两人与申请人无亲属关系，且在申请人提交申请前五年内认识该申请人。

5.2.2　一人为执业针灸师或东方医学医生，与申请人无亲属关系，并在申请人提交申请前三年内认识该申请人。

5.3　执照申请人应向委员会提供一份政府正式文件、护照或显示出生日期的出生证明的核证副本，以证明其年龄。

5.4　执照申请人应在提交申请时提供培训、学徒制、考试成绩合格的文件，或在另一个司法管辖区的执照，从而向委员会证明他或她有能力实施针灸疗法。

5.4.1　他或她的针灸或东方医学学校或学院的正式成绩单。

5.4.2　针灸或东方医学导师出具的正式成绩单。

5.4.3　NCCAOM 对其资格考试成绩的正式记录；或

5.4.4　另一个司法管辖区的许可委员会颁发的执照的正式副本，证明申请人先前获得的执照。

5.5　申请人应在申请上贴一张本人近期签名的护照规格的照片。

第 32－3－6 条　证明文件的认证

由申请人或代表申请人提交的证明文件应由适当的官员或政府机关盖章证明，如果是外国培训的申请人，当确定无法通过尽职调查实现该要求时，委员会可自行决定免去该要求。

第 32－3－7 条　查证

所有由申请人或代表申请人提交的声明须遵循虚假宣誓的相关的法律条款。申请人或持证人作出虚假陈述将受到纪律处分，包括但不限于立即撤销或吊销执照。

第 32－3－8 条　翻译要求

采用英语以外语言提交的申请文件，应附有由申请人以外的翻译人员核证的英文译本。翻译人员应证明该译本的准确性，并遵循虚假宣誓相关的法律条款。

第 32－3－9 条　申请截止日期

9.1　新申请人应使用委员会提供的表格提交执照考试申请，并应附上所有要求的声明和文件。所有申请必须在委员会对其申请进行资格审查之日前至少三十日送达委员会办公室。委员会应每年举行两次资格审查。

9.2　续期执照申请人须以委员会提供的表格提交续期执照申请，并须附上所有要求的声明及文件。所有申请必须在委员会对其续期申请进行资格审查之日前至少三十日送达委员会办公室。

9.3　由具有相关资质的教育机构或辅导教师出具的所有成绩单和证明文件必须在委员会资格审查之日前至少三十日内送达委员会办公室。

9.4　如在资格审查或其他方面的管理上存在困难，委员会可自行决定宽限上述提交日期。

第 32 - 3 - 10 条　申请的审查和处理

10.1　在收到申请后的合理时间内,委员会应通知申请人该申请是否填妥并通过委员会的资格审查,以及完成该申请需要哪些具体信息或文件。

10.2　在收到完整申请后的合理时间内,委员会应通知申请人其口试的日期、时间和地点。

10.3　在完成委员会资格审查和口试后的合理时间内,委员会应通知所有申请人其获得执照资格,并在支付本章第四节《针灸委员会费用》中规定的费用后通知申请人。

第 32 - 3 - 11 条　委员会审查资格证书和能力证明

11.1　委员会资格审查。在根据法典第 30 - 36 - 12 条颁发执照之前,委员会应审查每个申请人的资格证明文件和申请表。

11.2　地点。委员会应公布举行资格审查的时间和地点。

11.3　语言。委员会应管理英文资格审查。

11.4　内容。资格审查应包括资格文件审查和口试。口试应测试和审查申请人通过针灸从事东方医学实践的知识和能力。

11.5　额外培训。如果委员会确定申请人符合针灸执照的要求,则应颁发为期两年的执照。委员会有权自行决定是否颁发临时执照,并规定额外的培训、临床经验或 NCCAOM 考试作为执照要求。

第 32 - 3 - 12 条　培训证明文件

12.1　每个参加辅导或学徒计划的申请人应已完成法典第 30 - 36 - 10 条中规定的最低教育或辅导要求,由申请人就读的各所学校的教务主任或申请人的导师出具证明文件。

12.2　所有从已批准的教育计划毕业,并参加 NCCA 或 NCCAOM 的考试作为其执照要求一部分的申请人,应已完成了法典第 30 - 36 - 10 条中规定的课程学习和培训。

12.3　所有执照申请人都应在委员会对其申请进行资格审查之日前满足《法典》第 30 - 36 - 1 条及其后各条规定的最低教育或辅导要求。

第 32 - 3 - 13 条　放弃申请

如果申请人在完成其申请、提供所需的补充信息或文件或支付任何所需费用时没有尽职尽责,委员会可以在不损害申请人利益的情况下拒绝其申请。

第 32 - 3 - 14 条　未能参加口试-撤回申请

委员会口试申请人如未能参加两次口试,且未提交符合委员会要求的书面解释,委员会将撤回其申请。如果申请人后来决定重新申请执照,他或她应提出新的申请,并支付全额申请费。

第 32 - 3 - 15 条　拒绝申请

15.1　任何申请被拒绝的申请人可在收到回复之日起三十个日历日内提交书面请求,要求将其申请提交给委员会,以便在委员会下一次例会上进行进一步评估。

15.2　作为评估程序的一部分,委员会可自行决定要求对申请人的执照资格进行口头审查。

15.3　本条中的任何内容都不得解释为剥夺申请人根据其他法律规定提出上诉的权利。

第 32 - 3 - 16 条　非执业执照

16.1　任何未积极从事针灸实践的针灸师,如果希望获得的《法典》第 30 - 36 - 16 条规定的非执业执照,或希望将非执业执照恢复为执业状态,应按照委员会提供的表格向委员会提交申请(执业-非执业执照申请)。申请人无须将他或她的执照或执照副本随申请一起提交给委员会。

16.2　为了将非执业执照恢复到执业状态,持证人应在申请恢复执业状态之前的两年内完成至少四十八学时的经批准的继续教育,并遵守本章第九节《继续教育要求》的规定。如果执照处于非执业状态不超过一年,至少需要二十四学时的继续教育。

16.3　持证人的执照处于非执业状态时,委员会依然有权根据法律规定给予持证人纪律处分,或维持其纪律处分,或根据此类规定下达吊销或撤销其执照的命令,或给予其他纪律处分。

第四节　针灸委员会费用

第32-4-1条　总则

1.1　范围:本节规定了与委员会相关的费用。

1.2　权限:《西弗吉尼亚州法典》第30-36-7条和第30-36-8条。

1.3　提交日期:2020年4月20日。

1.4　生效日期:2020年4月30日。

失效条款:本节将于2030年4月30日到期后终止,不再具有任何效力。

第32-4-2条　申请

本规则规定适用于所有申请人、执业针灸师、见习针灸师、针灸学员和继续教育讲师。

第32-4-3条　费用

3.1　申请费:不可退还的申请费为七十五美元。

3.2　执照费:两年期的初始执照费为四百二十五美元。

3.3　续期费:两年期的续期费为四百二十五美元。

3.4　非执业执照:两年期的非执业执照费用为三百二十五美元。

3.5　逾期费:逾期申请的逾期费为五十美元。

3.6　复制执照:复制或更换挂墙执照的费用为二十五美元。复制或更换续期收据或口袋执照的费用为十美元。

3.7　背书费:背书信的费用为十美元。

3.8　耳穴戒毒证书费:两年期的耳穴戒毒证书费用为六十美元。耳穴戒毒疗法授权证书的有效期为两年,从颁发之日的月底算起。

3.9　耳穴戒毒证书续期费:两年期的耳穴戒毒证书续期费为五十美元。新的耳穴疗法授权证书的有效期为两年,从颁发之日的月底算起。

3.10　尽管本费用表中规定了费用,申请人仍可根据本章第十五节的规定寻求豁免初始执照费。

第32-4-4条　针灸辅导

针灸辅导讲师和学员应当在完成经批准的年度针灸培训后的三十日内支付每年一百美元的注册续期费。

第 32 - 4 - 5 条　继续教育提供者

每个继续教育提供者的批准年费为五十美元。

第 32 - 4 - 6 条　到期执照的续期

失效或到期的执照可在到期后三年内随时续期。持证人应支付所有应计未付的续期费用,加上申请续期的逾期费。

第五节　执业针灸师的广告

第 32 - 5 - 1 条　总则

1.1　范围:本规则为针灸广告制定了标准。

1.2　权限:西弗吉尼亚州第 30 - 36 - 7 条和第 30 - 36 - 14 条(f)款。

1.3　提交日期:1999 年 5 月 21 日。

1.4　生效日期:1999 年 5 月 21 日。

第 32 - 5 - 2 条　申请和执行

本立法规则适用于所有执业针灸师、见习针灸师和针灸学员。本节规则由委员会执行。

第 32 - 5 - 3 条　认可的头衔

在西弗吉尼亚州执业的针灸师可使用包括但不限于以下学术和专业授予的头衔:

3.1　L.Ac.和 Lic.Ac:执业针灸师。

3.2　O.M.D.:东方医学医生。

3.3　MSOMed.:东方医学理学硕士。

3.4　D.Ac.:针灸师。

3.5　C.A.:认证针灸师。

3.6　D.O.M.:东方医学博士。

3.7　A.P.:针灸医师。

第 32 - 5 - 4 条　广告

获得委员会许可的执业针灸师可在委员会依法典第 30 - 36 - 2 条授权的执业范围内,向公众宣传任何针灸服务。广告不得推广过度或不必要的针灸服务。

第 32 - 5 - 5 条　医生头衔的使用

5.1　当针灸师拥有经认可、批准或授权的针灸、东方医学或生物科学教育机构授予的博士学位时,他或她可以使用“医生”的头衔或“Dr”的缩写。本款授权的针灸师使用“医生”头衔或缩写“Dr”,而没有进一步说明授权使用的执照、证书或学位的类型,属违反职业道德的行为。

5.2　针灸医生应以书面和口头方式向其患者明确解释,他或她不是获得执业内科医师或外科医生执照的医生,除非他或她获得依《法典》第 30 - 3 - 1 条及其后各条和第 30 - 14 - 1 条及其后各条的规定获得执照。

第六节　执业针灸师的针灸实践标准

第 32 - 6 - 1 条　总则

1.1　范围:本规则确立了本州针灸实践的最低标准。

1.2　权限：西弗吉尼亚州第 30-36-7 条。

1.3　提交日期：1999 年 5 月 21 日。

1.4　生效日期：1999 年 5 月 21 日。

第 32-6-2 条　申请

本立法规则适用于所有执业针灸师、见习针灸师和针灸学员。

第 32-6-3 条　定义

3.1　洁针技术：由 CCAOM 管理的标准协议测试。

3.2　CCAOM：针灸和东方医学学院委员会。

3.3　FDA：联邦食品和药品管理局。

3.4　OSHA：联邦职业安全与健康管理局。

第 32-6-4 条　办公条件

4.1　每个针灸办公室、诊所、治疗中心或机构应始终保持清洁卫生，并应为男性和女性患者提供无障碍洗手间。

4.2　委员会或其代表可在正常营业时间进行事先通知或无事先通知的办公室检查，以确保卫生条件得到保持。委员会或其代表可以检查治疗区和非治疗区。患者档案和记录应由委员会或其官方代表授权检查。

第 32-6-5 条　一次性针头；消毒设备

5.1　一次性针头。所有针灸诊所、诊所、治疗中心和机构应仅使用预消毒的一次性针头。医师应根据"洁针技术"和 CCAOM 制定的执业标准使用预先消毒的一次性针头。

5.2　灭菌设备。所有针灸办公室、诊所、治疗中心和机构应配备消毒设备，对患者正常和常规治疗中使用的非针类设备进行消毒，或者应与当地医院或医疗服务机构签订合同，对非针类设备进行运输和消毒。劳工部检查员应至少每两年检查一次灭菌设备。

第 32-6-6 条　治疗程序

执业针灸师在治疗过程中应遵循 FDA 和 CCAOM 的标准方案，并遵循以下程序：

6.1　洗手。针灸师在检查患者或操作针灸针和其他器械之前以及在治疗不同患者的间隙，应立即用肥皂和温水用力搓手。

6.2　器械灭菌。所有非针类器械在使用前应进行完全灭菌（破坏所有微生物）。所有装有无菌针头的针盘也应处于无菌状态。每次对非针类器械进行灭菌时，针灸师应使用指示胶带或指示卡，指示灭菌过程已完成。

6.3　针灸针。医生只能使用预包装、预消毒的一次性针头进行针灸治疗。针头不得在同一患者身上重复使用，即使是在同一治疗过程中。

6.4　穴位。在插入针头之前，医师应使用适当的消毒剂清洁患者身体上要插入针头的部位。

6.5　皮下断针。如刺入患者皮下的针灸针断裂，提供治疗的针灸师应立即咨询医师。针灸师不得切断或穿透组织取针。

6.6　并发症的医疗处理。当需要立即治疗时，针灸师应立即将针灸治疗引起的任何并发症（包括但不限于血肿、腹膜炎或气胸）转介给西医、整骨医生或足科医生。

6.7　点刺（皮下注水法）。医师应使用无菌一次性注射器和无菌溶液进行点刺注射。

6.8　针头处理。针灸医师应将所有针灸针,穿刺针和器械丢弃到坚硬的生物危害容器中。针灸医师应以下列两种方式之一对针头进行分类丢弃:

6.8.1　针头应进行消毒,并丢弃在密闭容器中;或

6.8.2　应将其置于标有"危险废物"的密闭不易碎容器中,并按照符合 OSHA 有害生物废料法规的方式进行处理。

第 32－6－7 条　知情同意

医师应根据任何治疗的需要,以书面和口头形式告知患者治疗计划中可能出现的任何并发症。

第 32－6－8 条　诊室外的治疗

8.1　在诊室外提供针灸治疗的医师应携带所需的无菌针头和其他器械,置于无菌密闭容器中。

8.2　医师在其诊室外提供治疗时,应遵守适用于治疗的所有实践标准。

第 32－6－9 条　针灸病历的内容与留存

9.1　针灸师应保存书面医疗记录,证明每位患者的治疗过程。这些记录应至少包括每名患者的下列内容:

9.1.1　患者的病史。

9.1.2　针灸与东方医学诊断。

9.1.3　诊断测试和成像程序及实验室检查结果。

9.1.4　每次就诊时使用的穴位和实施的任何治疗程序。

9.1.5　针灸医师的处方和建议。

9.1.6　包含病程记录的患者治疗计划。

9.2　针灸医师应保存所有病历资料,保存期为自最后一次记录之日起五年。

第 32－6－10 条　财务责任

10.1　财务责任。作为颁发执照或执照续期的先决条件,每个针灸师应投保医疗事故保险或职业责任保险,并向委员会提供其财务责任的证明。每名持证人应享有下列权利之一:

10.1.1　专业责任保险的每次索赔金额不低于一万美元,授权保险公司的最低年度赔偿金额不低于三万美元。

10.1.2　每项索赔金额不低于一万美元的未到期不可撤销信用证,最低总可用信用证金额不低于三万美元。当最终判决或结算是由于提供或未能提供针灸服务而提出的索赔时,应在提交指明责任和赔偿损失的最终判决时,或在提交由协议各方签署的和解协议时,向作为受益人的针灸师支付该信用证,该信用证不得转让。信用证应由根据《西弗吉尼亚州法典》组建的任何银行或储蓄协会签发。

10.1.3　每次索赔的履约保证金额不少于一万美元,最低年度总额不少于三万美元,由西弗吉尼亚州具备营业执照的公司出具。

10.2　豁免。在向委员会提出申请后,满足下列条件的持证人可免于遵守本条的要求:

10.2.1　任何专门作为西弗吉尼亚州联邦政府或其机构或分支机构的官员、雇员或代理人执业的针灸师。为本节之目的,西弗吉尼亚州、其代理机构或其分支机构的代理人是指有

资格享受西弗吉尼亚州提供的任何计划保险的人。

10.2.2　持有非执业执照且不在本州执业的任何持证人。任何申请重新激活执照的持证人应满足下列条件之一：表明其持有长尾保险，该保险在1998年1月1日或在西弗吉尼亚州的初始许可日期后（以较晚者为准），以及在执照进入非执业状态之日前，为发生的事故提供了责任保险；或者该持证人应提交一份宣誓书，声明其在申请重新激活时没有未解决的医疗事故判决或和解。

10.2.3　仅在认证学校履行其教学职责的任何持证人。持证人可从事针灸实践，前提是该实践是其履行学校教学岗位相关职责的伴随工作和必要部分。

10.2.4　任何依据《法典》第30-36-1条及其后各条持有西弗吉尼亚州现行执照，且不在西弗吉尼亚州执业的持证人，如该人在本州开始或恢复执业，他或她应将其执业活动告知委员会，并履行获得保险的义务。

10.2.5　任何能够向委员会证明他或她在西弗吉尼亚州没有渎职行为的持证人。

第七节　针灸师的纪律处分和投诉程序

第32-7-1条　总则

1.1　范围：本规则为委员会的纪律处分和投诉程序设立了适当的程序。依据《法典》第30-36-18条，委员会负有以上职责。

1.2　权限：《西弗吉尼亚州法典》第30-1-8条(a)款和第30-36-1条。

1.3　提交日期：2008年4月16日。

1.4　生效日期：2008年4月16日。

第32-7-2条　申请和强制执行

本立法规则适用于所有执业针灸师、见习针灸师和针灸学员。

第32-7-3条　定义

3.1　"委员会"系指西弗吉尼亚州针灸委员会。

3.2　"持证人"系指持有针灸委员会颁发的针灸和东方医学执照的针灸师。

3.3　"执照"系指由委员会颁发的执照。

3.4　"针灸与东方医学的实践"系指《西弗吉尼亚州法典》第30-36-2条定义的针灸实践，包括执业针灸师、见习针灸师和针灸学员。

3.5　"虚假和欺骗性广告"系指一项声明，包括谎报事实，因未能披露重要事实，可能导致误导或欺骗，意图或可能制造虚假或不合理的有利结果的预期，或包含表达或暗示，有较大可能导致一个谨慎的普通人误解或被欺骗。

3.6　"裁决性听证"系指由委员会或指定的听证官进行的正式行政听证，以确定对持证人提出的投诉的真实性和有效性。

3.7　"察看期"系指委员会依法对持证人施加一段时间内的条件和要求。

第32-7-4条　拒绝执照申请、将持证人列入察看期、限制持证人、给予纪律处分、吊销或撤销执照的原因

4.1　委员会可拒绝执照申请，将持证人列入察看期，吊销执照，限制持证人，或撤销委

员会颁发的任何执照,只要有充分证据证明持证人存在下列行为:

4.1.1 故意制作、出示或使其制作或出示与执照申请有关的任何虚假、欺诈或伪造的声明、书面文件、证书、文凭或其他材料。

4.1.2 曾经或正在涉及与执照考试有关的欺诈、伪造、欺骗、串通或串谋。

4.1.3 对管制药品上瘾。

4.1.4 成为一个长期或持续的酗酒者。

4.1.5 从事有可能欺骗、欺诈或伤害公众或公众成员的不光彩、不道德或违反职业道德的行为。

4.1.6 故意违反保密通信。

4.1.7 在任何其他州、准州、司法管辖区或外国的针灸或东方医学执照被撤销、吊销或限制,或被采取其他行动,或受到其发证机构的任何其他纪律处分,或不予为其颁发执照的。

4.1.8 曾经或当前因疾病、酗酒、过度使用酒精、药物、化学品或任何其他物质,或因任何身体或精神异常,无法利用合理技能安全从事针灸或东方医学实践。

4.1.9 缺乏利用合理技能安全从事针灸或东方医学实践的专业能力。如针灸师多次表现出未能适当治疗患者的行为,委员会可对此予以考虑,并可要求针灸师参加由委员会成员,其代理人或指定人员组织的书面或口头的调查或考试,以便确定持证人的专业资质。

4.1.10 从事了违反职业道德的行为,包括但不限于任何偏离或不符合普遍认同的东方医学执业标准,或东方医学职业道德,或委员会规则、执业针灸师道德规范、委员会 32CSR10 规则列出的违反职业道德的行为。不论患者是否因其行为而受到伤害,或是否有违反诚实、正义或良好道德的行为,不论该行为是在他或她的执业过程中还是在其他过程中发生的,也不论该行为是在本州境内还是境外发生的。

4.1.11 在任何司法管辖区内被判有罪,而该罪直接与针灸或东方医学的实践或与针灸或东方医学的能力有关。为本节之目的,不抗辩答辩将视为定罪。

4.1.12 以本人以外的名字宣传、从事针灸实践或试图从事针灸实践。

4.1.13 持证人知悉任何人员违反本规则或《西弗吉尼亚州针灸实践法》条款,而未能向委员会报告。

4.1.14 帮助、协助、怂恿或建议任何无证人员从事违反本规则或《西弗吉尼亚州针灸实践法》的东方医学实践。

4.1.15 未能履行针灸师所承担的任何法定或法律义务。

4.1.16 作出或提交一份持证人明知是虚假的报告,故意或因疏忽未能提交州或联邦法律要求的报告或记录,故意妨碍或阻碍提交报告或诱使他人这样做。报告或记录仅包括以执业针灸师身份签署的报告或记录。

4.1.17 直接或间接地向针灸师、组织、机构或个人支付或收取任何佣金、奖金、回扣或回赠,或以任何形式参与任何费用分成,而将患者转介至医疗保健产品和服务提供单位,包括但不限于医院、疗养院、临床实验室、门诊手术中心或药房。本项规定不得解释为阻止针灸师收取专业咨询服务费。

4.1.18 在患者-医师关系中施加影响,目的是让患者发生性行为。

4.1.19　在东方医学实践中作出欺骗性、不真实或欺诈性的陈述，或在东方医学实践中使用欺骗性的伎俩，不符合东方医学界普遍流行的治疗标准。

4.1.20　通过使用欺诈、恐吓、不当影响，或通过过度接触或无理的行为，亲自或通过代理人来招揽患者。招揽系指直接或含蓄地要求接收方立即回应的任何讯息。

4.1.21　未能保存证明患者治疗过程的书面记录，包括但不限于患者病史、检查结果、检测结果以及治疗（如有）。

4.1.22　通过向患者或客户施加影响并实施盘剥，为自身或第三方谋取经济利益。其行为方式包括但不限于，推广或销售服务、商品、电器用具或药品，或者推广或宣传药店的处方。为本分部之目的，不适当地或过量或以不适当剂量开处方、配药、给药、混合或以其他方式配制药物，包括所有管制和非管制药品。无论涉案人出于何种意图，此种行为不符合患者的最佳利益，也不是针灸师或东方医学医师实践过程的行为。

4.1.23　玩忽职守，或其从事针灸或东方医学实践过程中的护理、技能或治疗水平未能达到相同或相似专业的理性、谨慎的东方医学医师认为在类似条件和情况下可接受的水平。

4.1.24　在未事先得患者充分知情和书面同意的情况下，实施根据学界通行的东方医学实践标准构成人体试验的任何程序或处方。

4.1.25　从事或提供超出《西弗吉尼亚州针灸实践法》允许范围的针灸实践，或接受并履行持证人知悉或有理由知悉他或她没有能力履行的专业职责。

4.1.26　将专业责任委托给持证人知悉或有理由知悉的，缺乏培训、经验或执照而不具备资格履行责任的人。

4.1.27　违反或试图违反与针灸实践有关的任何司法管辖区的任何法律或规则。

4.1.28　违反或未能遵守委员会的合法命令，或违反根据委员会启动的任何程序作出的任何法院命令。

4.1.29　提供、采取或同意通过秘密方法、手术、疗法或药物治愈或治疗疾病；或已采用秘密方法、手段和手术治疗多人的情形下，在委员会问询时拒绝透露相关情况。

4.1.30　从事虚假或者欺骗性广告的。"虚假或欺骗性广告"系指一项声明，包括谎报事实，因未能披露重要事实可能导致误导或欺诈，意图或可能制造虚假或不合理的有利结果的预期，或包含表达或暗示，有较大可能导致一个谨慎的普通人误解或被欺骗；或

4.1.31　从事不符合公众利益的广告活动。不符合公众利益的广告包括：

4.1.31.a　造成恐吓或过度压力效果的广告。

4.1.31.b　使用客户评价的广告。

4.1.31.c　虚假、欺骗性、误导性、夸张或浮夸的广告。

4.1.31.d　承诺患者满意或治愈疾病的广告。

4.1.31.e　以欺骗公众为目的提供免费服务或折扣的广告。本项不适用于包含议价提议的广告，也不适用于与患者免费护理的既定政策或计划相结合的广告。

4.1.31.f　声称持证人职业优势的广告，但是无法证明。

4.2　为第4.1条之目的，被宣布为构成可能欺骗、欺诈或损害公众或其任何成员的不光彩、不道德或违反职业道德的行为，包括但不限于：

4.2.1 处方或分发《西弗吉尼亚州法典》第60A－1－101(d)中定义的任何"管制药品",但按照东方针灸医学理论原则执行的《西弗吉尼亚州法典》第30－36－2中定义的除外。

4.2.2 以任何方式公布或发表极不可能或夸张的陈述,而该陈述有欺骗或欺诈公众或其成员的倾向,包括但不限于:

4.2.2.a 声称患者或客户能够通过持证人知之甚少或没有治疗价值的任何方法、手术、疗法或药物来治疗或治愈明显无法治愈的病症或者体弱的任何陈述。

4.2.2.b 代表、宣称或表明自己有能力并愿意通过系统的或学校的实践方法治疗病症或体弱,但以下情况除外:

4.2.2.b.1 持有委员会认可的学校的学位或文凭。

4.2.2.b.2 他或她声称是自学成才的。

4.2.3 在针灸实践过程中发生的严重过失行为或一系列过失行为,在相关情况下会被视为严重不称职、严重无知、重大过失或渎职,包括执行任何不必要的服务或程序。

4.2.4 旨在使针灸或东方医学行业名誉扫地的行为,包括但不限于任何偏离或不符合本州普遍接受的东方医学实践标准的行为。

4.2.5 在持证人宣传免费服务、免费检查或免费治疗的情况下,在患者首次就诊后四十八小时内收取任何类型服务的任何费用。

4.2.6 与根据《西弗吉尼亚州法典》第30章获得执照的任何类别的卫生保健从业者签订任何监督和/或合作协议,但不符合与之相关的实践标准。

4.2.7 收取过高或不合理的费用。在确定费用的合理性时,应考虑的指导因素包括:

4.2.7.a 所需时间和精力。

4.2.7.b 手术或治疗的新颖性和难度。

4.2.7.c 正确执行该手术或治疗所需的技能。

4.2.7.d 患者或其病情所导致的任何要求或条件。

4.2.7.e 与患者的专业关系的性质和时间长度。

4.2.7.f 持证人的经验、信誉和能力。

4.2.7.g 提供服务所处环境的性质。

4.2.8 在任何情况下,如发现除根据本条第4.3款的规定采取的任何行动外,已收取了过多的、不合理的费用,委员会可要求持证人减少或退还该费用。

4.3 当委员会发现任何申请人没有资格获得执照,或发现任何持证人应根据《西弗吉尼亚州针灸实践法》或委员会的规则受到纪律处分时,委员会可对任何人或多人采取以下行动:

4.3.1 拒绝向申请人颁发执照。

4.3.2 公开申斥。

4.3.3 吊销或限制任何执照一定期限,该期限不超过五年。

4.3.4 要求任何持证人参加委员会规定的教育计划。

4.3.5 撤销任何执照。

4.3.6 要求持证人接受医生或其他专业人员的护理、咨询或治疗。

4.3.7　要求其在其他医师的指导或监督下执业。

4.3.8　要求持证人提供一段时间的免费公共或慈善服务。

4.3.9　除上述行动外，或结合上述行动，委员会可作出不利于持证人或申请人的判决，但保留判决或处罚的实施；或者，委员会可作出判决和处罚，但暂停处罚的执行，并将针灸师列入察看期，如针灸师不遵守委员会规定的任何条款，可取消察看期。委员会可自行决定，根据《西弗吉尼亚州针灸实践法》《西弗吉尼亚州法典》第30－36－1条及其后各条，恢复并重新颁发执照。作为条件，委员会可以实施本规则或《西弗吉尼亚州针灸实践法》中规定的任何纪律处分或补救措施。

4.4　委员会有权将持证人列入察看期，并在察看期向持证人附加不同的限制条件。在得出执业针灸医师应被列入察看期的结论后，委员会可对任何人或多人施加以下限制条件：

4.4.1　委员会可委任一名或多名委员会成员，负责定期提交察看期持证人的面谈报告。该类面谈可按照委员会的决定定期进行，指定的委员会成员届时将在委员会定期会议上向委员会报告持证人的进展。

4.4.2　委员会可要求察看期持证人按委员会确定的间隔时间赴委员会出庭，该执照持有人可报告其进展。在察看期持证人出庭期间，委员会可向察看期持证人提出问题，以观察其行为和进展。

4.4.3　委员会可选择一名医生或要求察看期持证人选择一名将获得委员会批准的医生，该医生应按委员会的指示定期提交有关察看期持证人的进展报告。

4.4.4　委员会可任命一名医疗顾问，其职责是与察看期持证人进行面谈。然后，察看期持证人应按委员会规定的时间定期向指定的医疗顾问报告，医疗顾问应按委员会规定的时间间隔向委员会报告。

4.4.5　在酗酒和/或滥用药物的情况下，作为察看期的条件，委员会可要求察看期持证人定期提交血液样本和/或尿液药物筛选样本。

4.4.6　委员会可要求察看期持证人授权其私人医生向委员会提交察看期持证人的病历，包括私人医生在其察看期内可获得的过去的病史和所有新病历，以供审查。

4.4.7　委员会可要求察看期持证人报告其可能使用的所有药物，并按委员会规定的间隔时间向委员会报告。

4.4.8　委员会可要求察看期持证人在察看期终止前定期出席委员会会议，并向委员会提供其可能要求的信息；委员会可在其认为必要的情况下利用传票、书面文件传票及其调查人员，收集事实和证据，以确定察看期持证人是否遵守察看期条款。

4.4.9　在有指示的情况下，委员会可对最初被列入察看期的持证人施加额外的察看期、限制或撤销察看条件。察看期自启动之日起不得超过五年。

第32－7－5条　投诉的处理方式

5.1　任何个人、医疗同行评审委员会、事务所、公司、委员会成员或公职人员均可向委员会投诉，指控针灸师违反《法典》第30－36－1条及其后各条或委员会规则。委员会可为此提供表格，但投诉可以任何书面形式提出。除了描述要投诉的违规行为外，投诉还应包括以下内容：

5.1.1 被投诉人员的姓名和地址。

5.1.2 医疗或其他事件发生日期。

5.1.3 在所述事件发生后可能治疗过的患者的姓名。

5.1.4 在所述事件发生后或发生期间,患者住院或就诊的任何医疗机构的名称。

5.2 委员会可制定投诉表格,并按照要求提供给投诉人。

5.3 任何投诉信息应由委员会发送给被投诉的针灸医师,以取得其书面意见,该针灸医师将在二十日内提交书面答复,或放弃书面答复的权利。

第 32－7－6 条　申诉

6.1 任何执照申请被委员会拒绝的申请人,可根据争议案件听证程序,《西弗吉尼亚州法典》第 29A－5－1 条及其后各条和委员会规则,可在三十日内对该项命令提出申诉:但委员会在对申请人的知识或能力进行考核后,对考核是否公平或者申请人是否通过考核有争议而拒绝颁发执照或证书的,该申请人不得申诉。

6.2 任何持证人在本州实施针灸和东方医学服务,委员会发布命令拒绝其执照申请、吊销、限制或撤销执照的,可根据争议案件听证程序,《西弗吉尼亚州法典》第 29A－5－1 条及其后各条以及委员会规则,在三十日内对该项命令提出申诉。

第八节　有争议案件的听证程序

第 32－8－1 条　总则

1.1 范围:本规则规定了委员会对争议案件听证的裁决程序。

1.2 权限:《西弗吉尼亚州法典》第 30－36－1 条,第 30－1－1 条,第 29A－5－1 条及其后各条。

1.3 申请日期: 2007 年 7 月 17 日。

1.4 生效日期: 2007 年 9 月 1 日。

第 32－8－2 条　定义

除上下文另有规定外,本节规则中下列术语具有如下含义:

2.1 "委员会"系指西弗吉尼亚州针灸委员会。

2.2 "申请方"系指被委员会拒绝颁发针灸和东方医学执照并因此申请委员会就该拒绝命令举行听证会的个人。

2.3 "被控方"系指持有委员会颁发的针灸和东方医学执照,并已根据本节第 3.4 款所述被委员会指控的个人。

2.4 "持证人"系指持有委员会颁发的针灸和东方医学执照的针灸师,或持有教育培训执照的"学员"。

2.5 "执照"系指委员会根据《西弗吉尼亚州法典》第 30－36－1 条颁发的执照。

2.6 "针灸和东方医学实践"系指美国《西弗吉尼亚州法典》第 30－36－1 条及其后各条定义的针灸和东方医学实践。并包括执业针灸师、见习针灸师及针灸学员。

第 32－8－3 条　听证程序

3.1 任何人被委员会吊销、限制或撤销执照/培训执照的,认为该命令违反了《西弗吉尼亚州法典》第 30 - 1 - 1 条及第 30 - 36 - 1 条或其他规定,有权对该命令举行听证。

3.2 任何人希望就本条第 3.1 款所述理由举行听证的,必须向委员会提出书面申请。

3.3 委员会主席或其授权指定人员收到此类听证申请的,应在收到书面申请后四十五日内安排听证,但经双方同意延期的除外。

3.4 当有合理根据相信任何执业针灸师、见习针灸师及针灸学员存在相关行为或情形,导致其执照应根据《西弗吉尼亚州法典》第 30 - 36 - 1 条及其后各条或委员会立法规则的一个或多个原因被吊销、撤销或以其他方式处罚时,委员会可对其提出指控。指控可基于委员会收到的经核实的书面投诉信息,以及委员会在调查该等投诉时所收集的补充信息。指控也可仅基于委员会进行调查活动所获信息。

3.5 根据本条第 3.4 款所述对持证人或学员提出的指控,须在以委员会的名义发出的投诉及听证通知中载明,该委员会是本州监管针灸及东方医学实践的机构。该投诉及听证通知应指定委员会为"投诉人",并应指定参与听证程序的执业针灸师、见习针灸师及针灸学员为"答辩人";应列出每项违法行为的实质内容,并应充分详细地告知答辩人被投诉行为或情形的性质、时间和地点;应写明开庭的日期、时间和地点;并应附有委员会委任听证官的意向陈述书。

3.6 在收到本条第 3.1 和 3.2 款所述的听证要求后,主席或其指定人员应向申请方提供以委员会的名义发出的投诉和听证会通知,该委员会是本州监管针灸和东方医学实践的机构。该投诉及听证通知应指定提出申请的一方为"投诉人",并应指定委员会为"答辩人";应列明委员会拒绝向申请方提供执照的每一理由的实质内容,且应充分详细地告知申请方其中有争议的行为或情形的性质、时间及地点;应写明开庭的日期、时间和地点;并应附有委员会委任听证官的意向陈述书。

3.7 委员会可在其认为适当的情况下,修改投诉及听证通知中所载的指控。

3.8 投诉和听证通知应至少在听证日期前三十日送达申请方或被控方。

3.9 在不迟于听证日期前二十日收到委员会的书面动议后,委员会应在听证日期前至少十五日向申请方或被控方或其律师提供更明确的陈述,说明被控的事项或拒绝颁发执照的理由。

3.10 听证会应按下述方式进行:

3.10.1 出席听证会的任何一方均有权委托一名在西弗吉尼亚州具有合法执业资格的律师代理。

3.10.2 委员会可由西弗吉尼亚州总检察长办公室代表。

3.10.3 不相关的、不重要的或者过分重复的证据应予以排除。此外,还应遵循本州巡回法院在民事案件中适用的证据规则。但是,如需确定根据上述规则无法合理证明的事实,则根据上述规则不予采纳的证据可以被采纳,前提是该证据属于理性谨慎的人在处理其事务时通常信赖的一类证据,根据法规排除的情况除外。

3.10.4 应遵守本州法律所承认的特权规则。

3.10.5 对证据的异议,应记入笔录。听证的任何一方可以就笔录中排除的证据或者其他证据作出证明。

3.10.6 听证当事人可以带证人出庭作证;可由本人、律师或双方同时进行听证;可出示委员会或其指定的听证官认为适当的其他证据以支持其立场;在适当情况下,可以盘问委员会为支持指控或为拒绝颁发执照或教育培训执照的决定进行辩护而传唤的证人。

3.10.7 听证须在委员会指定的时间和地点举行,至少三十日内书面通知被控方或申请方和/或其律师,否则不得进行听证;或者,如未能找到他或她,可在他或她通常居住的地方将该通知送交其妻子或丈夫,或其年满十六岁的家庭成员,并提供有关通知的目的;或者,如找不到任何这样的人,可在该住所前张贴该通知;或者,如果他或她不在本州居住,该通知可由本州报纸连续三个星期每周出版一次;或通过挂号信或挂号邮件送达该通知。

3.10.8 听证应向社会公开。

3.10.9 委员会成员及其官员、代理人和雇员有权在听证会上就材料和相关事宜作证;但在听证会上作证的委员会成员不得参与委员会就其作证的案件进行的审议或作出的决定。

3.10.10 听证可由一名或多名委员会成员或委员会指定的听证官举行。

3.10.11 听证的记录,包括投诉(如适用)、听证通知书、所有诉状、动议、裁定、规定、证物、文件证据、证据证词及听证速记报告,均须记录在案,并在委员会的档案内保存副本。依申请,可向任何一方提供一份副本,费用由其承担。

3.10.12 证明文件可以副本或摘要的形式收录,也可以通过引用的方式合并收录。

3.10.13 在根据本条第 3.4 和 3.5 款向持证人提出指控后,应委员会的要求举行了听证,则委员会应负有举证责任,并应首先提出证据和/或证词,以支持该指控。

3.10.14 如果根据本条第 3.1、3.2、3.3 和 3.6 款的规定举行了听证,则申请方负有举证责任,因此应首先出示其证据。委员会可要求申请进行听证的人员就听证费用提供担保。如申请听证的人员在实质上未能取得胜诉,委员会可评估有关事实,并可在民事诉讼中通过其他适当的方法收集有关事实。

3.10.15 在委员会根据本条第 3.10.13 款提交证据后,答辩人或被控方有权在答辩中提交证据。

3.10.16 在要求申请方根据本条第 3.10.14 款提交证据的程序结束后,委员会有权在答辩中提交证据。

3.10.17 委员会可传唤证人出庭作证,支持其拒绝颁发执照的决定或支持对持证人提出的指控;可以提交其他证据来支持其立场;并且,可以盘问申请方或被控方为支持其立场而传唤的证人。

3.10.18 各方均有权进行开场和结案陈词,每次陈述不得超过十分钟。

3.10.19 委员会因对持证人的指控而举行的听证,可由委员会或其指定人员在向各方发出适当通知的情况下,继续举行听证或延期至较晚的日期或不同的地点。

3.10.20 在提出正当理由后,可批准继续听证的动议。延期的动议必须以书面形式提出,并于听证日期前七日内送交委员会办公室。在确定是否存在正当理由时,将考虑申请继续听证程序的一方在没有继续听证的情况下有效进行听证的能力。在听证之日起七日内提出的延期动议应被驳回,除非该动议的理由不能较早查明。在听证日期前提出的延期听证的动议,可由委员会的执行秘书或助理执行秘书或指定的听证官裁定。所有其他申请继续进行听证的动议,须由委员会成员或主持听证的听证官裁定。

3.10.21　除延期动议及在听证期间提出的动议外,与提交委员会审理的案件有关的所有动议均须以书面形式提出,并须在听证日期至少十日前送交听证委员会办公室。审前动议应在审前会议上或作证开始前的听证会上听取。委员会成员或在听证中主持听证的听证官须听取另一方的动议及回应,并须就该动议作出相应裁决。

第32－8－4条　证词和证据的抄录

4.1　所有证词、证据、辩论以及证词、证据可采性的裁定,均应以速记笔录、速记文字或者机械方式加以记录。

4.2　所有录得的材料都要抄录。委员会应负责组织对证词、证据的抄录。

4.3　在委员会或任何一方提出动议,指出任何听证记录的任何部分有错误或遗漏时,委员会或其指定的听证官须解决有关记录是否真正揭示听证所发生的情况的所有分歧,并须对记录作出适当的更正和/或修订,以使其符合事实。

4.4　在就任何执照或执照纪律事项的决定进行表决前至少十日,须向委员会所有成员提供一份听证记录,以供审阅。

第32－8－5条　提交拟议的事实调查结果和法律结论

5.1　任何一方均可按委员会或其正式委任的听证官指定的时间和方式提交事实调查结果的建议和法律结论。

第32－8－6条　听证官

6.1　委员会可任命一名听证官,其有权传唤证人和调取文件、主持宣誓和证词、审查证人宣誓、裁决证据事项、在当事人同意的情况下为解决或简化问题举行会议、安排编制听证会记录,以便委员会能够履行其职能,并按照第24－3－3.10款的规定举行听证会。

6.2　由委员会委任的听证官无权授予、吊销、撤销或以其他方式处罚任何执照。

6.3　听证官须拟备事实调查结果的建议及法律结论,以提交委员会。委员会可通过、修改或拒绝接受有关事实的调查结果和法律结论。

第32－8－7条　会议;非正式处理案件

7.1　在听证前或听证后的任何时间,委员会、其指定人员或其正式指定的听证官可为下列目的举行会议:

7.1.1　处理程序请求、审前动议或类似事项。

7.1.2　经当事人同意简化或解决问题;或

7.1.3　以规定或协议方式约定案件的非正式处理。

7.2　委员会或其委任的听证官可自行动议或在当事人的申请下,安排举行该等会议。

7.3　委员会也可就案件的非正式处理提出或考虑规定或协议,并可在不举行会议的情况下订立这些规定和/或协议。

第32－8－8条　口供

8.1　与本州巡回法院的民事诉讼一样,口供可被接受和宣读,也可作为证据。

第32－8－9条　传票

9.1　委员会或其执行秘书,以及由委员会委任的听证官,可发出传票,要求证人出庭作证和出示文件。该传票应根据《西弗吉尼亚州法典》第29A－5－1(b)款发出。

9.2　一方当事人根据本条第9.1款规定发出传票或书面文件传票的,应在安排的听证日期前至少十日提交至委员会。申请发出传票或书面文件传票的一方当事人应确保传票按照《西弗吉尼亚州法典》第29A－5－1(b)款的规定送达。

第32－8－10条　命令

10.1　根据本节举行听证会后,委员会的任何最终命令应根据《西弗吉尼亚州法典》第29A－5－3条和30－1－8(d)款的规定作出。该等裁定应在妥善处理案件所需的所有文件和材料(包括笔录)提交后的四十五日内作出,并应包含事实调查结果和法律结论。

10.2　事实调查结果和法律结论必须经投票或定期会议上的多数通过,才能进入最终命令程序。经委员会多数成员批准的最终裁定副本,须在委员会批准后五日内,以直接送达或以挂号信或挂号邮件送达申请方和被控方和/或其律师(如有)。

第32－8－11条　申诉

11.1　对根据本节作出的任何最终命令的申诉,应符合《西弗吉尼亚州法典》第30－1－9条的规定。

第32－8－12条　可分割性

12.1　如果本规则的任何条款或其对任何人或情形的适用性被认定无效,此无效性不应影响本节的条款或适用性,而本节的条款或适用性可在除去无效条款或不适用情形的情况下仍然有效,为此,本节的各条款被宣布为可分割的。

第九节　继续教育要求

第32－9－1条　总则

1.1　范围:根据《西弗吉尼亚州法典》第30－36－14(d)款规定,本节规定了对执照续期的继续教育要求。

1.2　权限:《西弗吉尼亚州法典》第30－36－7(a)和30－36－14(c)款。

1.3　申请日期:2008年4月16日。

1.4　生效日期:2008年4月16日。

第32－9－2条　申请

本立法规则适用于续期执照的持证人和继续教育课程讲师。

第32－9－3条　定义

3.1　获批的继续教育提供者。获得委员会批准的,在西弗吉尼亚州提供继续教育的人员或组织。

3.2　课程。一段系统的学习经历,时长不少于一学时,旨在习得与针灸实践相关的知识、技能和信息。

3.3　学时。在一门课程中花费至少五十分钟时间参与有组织的学习。

第32－9－4条　继续教育提供者的标准

4.1　为成为经批准的继续教育提供者,其应向委员会提交一份由委员会提供的表格的申请,并附委员会32CSR4规则所要求的费用。提交委员会的所有继续教育提供者申请和文件均应采用英文打印稿。

4.2　对继续教育提供者的批准自委员会签发之日起一年到期，并可在提交所需的申请和费用后续期。

4.3　根据《西弗吉尼亚州法典》第30－36－10条，经委员会批准的针灸学校和学院视为获批的继续教育提供者。

第32－9－5条　获批的继续教育提供者

5.1　为本规则之目的，只有在个人或组织提交了继续教育培训机构申请表、缴纳了适当的费用并获得了提供者编号后，提供者才能使用"获批的继续教育提供者"这一名称。以下组织或其继受机构提供的计划将视为"获批"：

5.1.1　西弗吉尼亚东方医学协会（WVAOM）。

5.1.2　美国针灸和东方医学协会（AAAOM）。

5.1.3　针灸和东方医学学院委员会（CCAOM）。

5.1.4　美国医学针灸学会（AAMA）。

5.1.5　全国针灸师协会。

5.1.6　国家针灸戒毒协会。

5.1.7　经认可的学校或学院。

5.2　委员会应只向一个人或组织分配一个提供者编号。当两个或两个以上获批的继续教育提供者共同主办课程时，只能由一个提供者的编号标识该课程，该提供者应负责记录保存、广告宣传、证书颁发和确定讲师资格。

5.3　获批的提供者须在指定地点将下列记录保存四年：

5.3.1　每门获批课程的课程大纲。

5.3.2　每门获批课程的时间及地点。

5.3.3　课程讲师的个人简历。

5.3.4　每门获批课程的出勤记录（包括参加该课程的针灸师姓名、签字及执照号）以及给该课程学员颁发证书的记录。

5.3.5　每门获批课程的学员评价表。

5.4　在完成获批课程后十日内，提供者应向委员会提交下列文件：

5.4.1　出席获批课程的执业针灸师姓名、签名及执照号。

5.4.2　获批课程的参与者评价表。

5.5　在一门获批课程结束后六十日内，获批的提供者应向每位已完成课程的参与者颁发结业证书，其中包括以下信息：

5.5.1　提供者的名称和号码。

5.5.2　课程名称。

5.5.3　参与者姓名及针灸执照号码（如适用）。

5.5.4　课程的日期和地点。

5.5.5　完成的继续教育学时数。

5.5.6　要求针灸师自课程完成之日起将证书保留至少四年的声明。

5.6   获批的提供者对已获批课程的日期或地点做出任何更改,须通知委员会。如果新的日期在提交课程申请后四十五日内,则获批的提供者不得将课程的日期更改为课程获批之前的日期。

5.7   对获批课程的内容或讲师的任何更改都需要事先得到委员会的批准。对获批课程的内容或讲师的更改请求,应在课程开始前至少十日送交委员会。

5.8   获批的提供者应在三十日内通知委员会其组织结构或继续教育课程负责人的任何变化,包括姓名、地址或电话号码的变化。

5.9   继续教育提供者的批准不可转让。

5.10   委员会可在合理的工作时间内对经批准的提供者的记录、课程、讲师和有关活动进行审计。

第 32-9-6 条   继续教育课程的批准

6.1   只有获批的提供者才能提供继续教育课程。

6.2   继续教育所有课程的内容应与针灸实践有关,并应:

6.2.1   与针灸实践所需的知识和/或技术技能有关;或

6.2.2   与直接和/或间接的患者护理有关。也可涵盖针灸服务管理或医德课程。

6.3   每门课程应包括一种方法,供课程参与者评估以下内容:

6.3.1   该课程达到其所述教学目标的程度。

6.3.2   讲师对该课程了解的充分程度。

6.3.3   相应教学方法的运用程度。

6.3.4   课程资料的适用性或实用性。

6.3.5   其他相关意见。

第 32-9-7 条   继续教育学分课程的内容

7.1   续期执照时,需参加至少四十八学时以下类型的继续教育或继续医学教育。

7.2   在每两年的续期周期内,持证人须获得获批的提供者提供的至少二十四学时的针灸或东方医学指导。

7.3   在每两年的续期周期内,持证人可接受不超过二十四学时的由以下组织或其继受机构主办或认证的西方临床科学、医疗实践、医学伦理学或医学研究的教学:

7.3.1   世界卫生组织(WHO)。

7.3.2   国家卫生研究院(NIH)。

7.3.3   美国医学协会(AMA)。

7.3.4   美国骨科协会(AOA)。

7.3.5   美国护士协会(ANA)。

7.3.6   当地医院;或

7.3.7   地方学院,并且。

7.4   在每个续期周期内,持证人可接受不超过十二学时的认证课程培训,以协助持证人履行其专业管理职责,包括但不限于:

7.4.1   办公室、医院或行政管理。

7.4.2　语言训练，如以汉语或英语作为外语；或

7.4.3　教育方法。

7.5　针灸师可以在任何其他事先得到委员会自行批准的计划中获得学分。

第32-9-8条　申请课程批准

8.1　为获得课程批准，获批的提供者应在委员会提供的表格或类似格式文件上以英文向委员会提交课程批准申请。申请应包含下列信息：

8.1.1　提供者的姓名、号码、地址、电话号码和联系人。

8.1.2　课程名称、日期、地点和继续教育学时数。

8.1.3　教学的类型和方法以及要达到的教育目标。

8.1.4　课程大纲，课程说明，以及讲师的信息和资格。

8.1.5　所有拟议的公共广告，供经批准的提供者用于宣传课程。如果提供者使用的公共广告是在课程获得批准后制作的，且未随课程申请一起提供给委员会，提供者应在该广告发布后十日内向委员会邮寄该广告的副本。

8.2　获批的提供者应就提供继续教育学分的每一门课程获得委员会批准。如果要重复先前批准的课程，提供者应就该课程的后续管理向委员会申请批准。

8.3　获批的提供者应在课程首次开设前至少四十五日向委员会提交所有课程批准申请。

第32-9-9条　讲师

9.1　各获批的提供者有责任聘用合格的讲师。

9.2　教授获批继续教育课程的讲师，须至少具备以下资格：

9.2.1　针灸讲师应（A）持有现行有效的针灸执照，或根据《西弗吉尼亚州法典》第30-36-9(b)款获授权担任客座针灸师，且未受委员会的任何纪律处分或察看处分，（B）对课程主题有充分了解、熟悉前沿知识并熟练掌握技能，可通过以下方式证明：

1. 持有学院或大学学士学位或更高学位，以及具备相关经验的书面证明；或

2. 在该课程开始前的两年内，有教授类似课程内容的经验。

3. 最近两年内在其所任教的专业领域有不少于一年的工作经验。

9.2.2　非针灸讲师，须：

1. 在其专业领域获得现行执照或证书（如合适）。

2. 出示专业培训的书面证明，包括但不限于特定学科领域的培训证书或高级学位。

3. 过去两年内，在其所任教的专业领域有不少于一年的教学经验。

第32-9-10条　广告

10.1　获批的提供者传播的信息应真实，无误导性，并包括以下内容：

10.1.1　对课程内容和/或目标的清晰、简明的描述。

10.1.2　课程的日期和地点。

10.1.3　提供者的姓名和电话号码。

10.1.4　声明"这门课程已获西弗吉尼亚州针灸委员会批准，提供者编号_____，共_____学时的继续教育"。

10.1.5　提供者针对缺勤、取消课程情况的退款政策。

10.2　提供者在收到委员会的书面确认前,不得声称其课程已获委员会批准。如果提供者正在等待委员会的批准决定,可在广告中表明其课程处于待批准状态。如提供者表明其课程处在待批准状态,而委员会随后拒绝批准该课程,则提供者应承担全部责任。

第 32-9-11 条　拒绝、撤回和申诉

11.1　委员会可以撤回对提供者的批准,或拒绝其申请,理由包括但不限于:

11.1.1　与提供者的活动有重大关系的定罪;或

11.1.2　未遵守《西弗吉尼亚州法典》第 30-36-1 及其后各条的任何规定。

11.2　在需提交至委员会的信息中,如提供者或申请人对事实做出重大谎报,即构成撤回批准或否决申请的理由。

11.3　在向提供者发出书面通知说明撤销理由,并给予其合理机会向委员会或委员会指定人员陈词后,委员会可撤销对提供者或课程的批准。

11.4　如委员会驳回提供者或课程申请,申请人可向委员会递交上诉书说明上诉理由:上诉书须在委员会驳回申请通知发出后十日内由委员会备案。该上诉须由委员会或其指定人员进一步商议。如委员会或其指定人员在上诉提出日期之后对该上诉予以考虑,可准予追溯批准。

第 32-9-12 条　对不遵守规定的行为实施处罚

12.1　在执照续期时,每名针灸师证人应签署一份声明,说明其是否遵从了继续教育规定,该声明须遵循虚假宣誓相关的法律条款。持证人须提交有关文件的影印本及获批的续期申请表。

12.2　委员会可每年对按照继续教育要求报告的针灸师进行一次随机审查。任何针灸师每两年不得接受一次以上的审查。

12.3　任何针灸师虚报所需继续教育的完成情况,构成违反职业道德的行为。

12.4　被选中接受审查的针灸师应提交其参加和完成的继续教育课程的原始文件或记录。

12.5　每位针灸师应将其参加过的所有继续教育计划的记录保留至少四年,记录中应注明提供者的名称、课程或计划名称、课程日期、课程地点以及已获得的继续教育学分。

12.6　获批的继续教育课程的讲师每年最多可获得两学时的继续教育学分。讲师只有在担任获批课程的讲师时,才可以申请学分。此外,在委员会批准的继续教育课程中,每完成一个学时应累积一个学分。以小组成员的身份参加获批课程的专题演讲,没有资格获得继续教育学分。

第十节　执业针灸师道德规范

第 32-10-1 条　总则

1.1　范围:本规则在本州确立了针灸和东方医学的道德规范。

1.2　权限:《西弗吉尼亚州法典》第 30-36-7(a) 和 30-36-7(b) 款。

1.3　申请日期:1999 年 5 月 21 日。

1.4 生效日期：1999年5月21日。

第32－10－2条 申请

本立法规则适用于本州所有执业针灸师、见习针灸师和针灸学员。

第32－10－3条 道德规范

执业医师应在每个针灸师办公室、诊所或治疗中心张贴本条规定：

3.1 针灸医师的主要目的是恢复、维持和增进人体健康。

3.2 针灸医师根据自己的能力和判断，遵循东方医学的原则，通过提供个性化的医疗服务来恢复、维持和增进健康。

3.3 任何情况下，针灸医师首先应努力做到不伤害患者，并以最小的风险提供最有效的医疗服务（不论任何情况，切勿伤害患者）。

3.4 针灸医师应认识、尊重和促进每个患者身体内在的自愈能力（尊重自然的痊愈力量）。

3.5 针灸医师应努力识别和消除病因，而不是仅仅消除或抑制症状（对病因进行识别和治疗）。

3.6 针灸医师应教育患者，激发患者的合理希望，鼓励其对自身健康负责（承担教师职责）。

3.7 针灸医师进行治疗时，应考虑所有个人健康因素及其影响（重视整体）。

3.8 为促进公众健康，针灸师应重视卫生健康领域，从而为个人、社会乃至全世界预防疾病（健康促进、最佳预防）。

3.9 针灸医师应承认每个人的价值和尊严，因此，不应基于民族、种族、性别或性取向而拒绝提供治疗。

3.10 针灸医师应保障患者的隐私权，只有在患者授权或法律授权的情况下才可披露机密信息。

3.11 当任何人不称职或不道德的做法对医疗质量和安全产生不利影响时，针灸医师应明智地保护患者和公众。

3.12 针灸医师应保持东方医学执业能力，并通过评估个人优势、局限性和有效性，提高专业知识，努力实现卓越的专业能力。

3.13 针灸医师应以诚实、正直和对个人的判断和行为负责的态度进行其执业和专业活动。

3.14 针灸医师应努力参与专业活动，以提高东方医学的医疗水平、知识体系和公众意识。

3.15 针灸医师应尊重所有有道德、有资格的卫生保健从业者，并与其他卫生保健从业者合作，促进个人、公众乃至全球社会的健康。

3.16 针灸医师应努力体现个人的健康、道德品质和作为卫生保健专业人员的可信度。

第32－10－4条 在诊室销售东方药物的相关道德规范

4.1 在针灸师诊室销售药物应以满足患者的需要为基础。盈利总是被视为次要考虑因素。本条为州和国家针灸医师协会道德规范的延伸。

4.2 尽管药物零售可解释为医生的利益冲突;但只要潜在的意图仍是患者的最佳利益,而不是盈利,而且医生认为不存在成分和质量适用于该患者的其他药物,这仍然是一个合法可行的服务。

4.3 执业针灸师可处方的东方药物包括但不限于:

4.3.1 草药,单独的草药和配方。

4.3.2 腺体制剂。

4.3.3 矿物药。

4.3.4 维生素。

4.3.5 中成药。

4.4 持证人应遵守美国食品药品监督管理局(U.S.Food and Drug Administration)有关非处方药、草药和药品销售的规定。

第十一节 教 育 要 求

第 32－11－1 条 总则

1.1 范围:规定了从针灸或东方医学学校或学院毕业的针灸执照申请人的教育要求。

1.2 权限:《西弗吉尼亚州法典》第 30－36－7 条。

1.3 申请日期:1999 年 5 月 21 日。

1.4 生效日期:1999 年 5 月 21 日。

第 32－11－2 条 申请

本立法规则适用于从针灸或东方医学学校或学院毕业的执照申请人。

第 32－11－3 条 定义

3.1 获批的学校或学院。获得国家针灸和东方医学学校和学院认证委员会(NACSSAOM)认可或者作为其候选认可机构。

3.2 NACSSAOM。国家针灸和东方医学学校和学院认证委员会。

第 32－11－4 条 批准针灸培训计划的一般标准

4.1 东方医学理论培训的总时数应包括至少一千八百学时,临床指导的总时数应包括至少三百学时。课程学习应至少延长四个学年,或八个学期,或十二个季度或九个三学期制学期,或三十六个月。

4.2 录取考生应已顺利完成经批准的高中课程或通过同等学力的标准考试。

4.3 培训课程应设在西弗吉尼亚州州立大学或学院,或经委员会批准的机构,如果培训计划位于西弗吉尼亚州以外,则应在经相关政府认证机构或美国教育部认可的认证机构批准的机构中进行。

4.4 该培训计划须制定评估机制,以确定其理论及临床培训计划的有效性。

4.5 课程学习应包含学分。

4.6 培训计划临床部分的导师应是执业针灸师或其他经授权可从事针灸实践的执业医师。

4.7 所有讲师应凭借其教育、培训和经验,有能力教授其指定课程。

4.8 每门获批的培训课程应获得美国教育部批准的机构对学校和学院的认可或批准，否则经委员会批准的培训课程将自动失效。

第 32-11-5 条　批准针灸培训的具体课程要求

5.1 为了得到委员会的批准，根据规定第 30-36-1081B 条，针灸培训课程应符合以下课程标准：

5.1.1 普通生物学：八个学期。

5.1.2 化学：包括有机和生物化学，八个学期。

5.1.3 普通物理学：包括生物物理学的一般考察，八个学期。

5.1.4 普通心理学：包括咨询技巧，八个学期。

5.1.5 解剖：显微解剖学、大体解剖学和神经解剖学的考察，四个学期。

5.1.6 生理学：包括神经生理学，内分泌学和神经化学在内的基本生理学考察，四个学期。

5.1.7 病理学：对疾病性质的考察，包括微生物学、免疫学、精神病理学和流行病学，四个学期。

5.1.8 营养和维生素，顺势疗法和草药学，四个学期。

5.1.9 医学史：医学史考察，包括跨文化治疗实践，三个学期。

5.1.10 医学术语：英语医学术语基础，三个学期。

5.1.11 临床科学：内科综述、药理学、神经学、外科、产科/妇科、泌尿学、放射学、营养和公共卫生，八个学期。

5.1.12 临床医学——医学、整骨疗法、牙科、心理学、护理学、整脊疗法、足科和顺势疗法的临床实践概述，让针灸医师熟悉其他卫生保健从业者的实践经验，八个学期。

5.1.13 西药学，八个学期。

5.1.14 心肺复苏（CPR），八个面授学时。

5.1.15 东方传统医学：对其传统诊断和治疗方法的理论与实践考察，八个学期。

5.1.16 针灸解剖学与生理学：针灸学基础。包括经络系统，经外奇穴，以及耳针疗法，八个学期。

5.1.17 针灸技术：针刺技术，艾灸和电针的指导，包括预防措施（如针头灭菌）、禁忌证和并发症，八个学期。

5.1.18 指压技术：指导使用手工按压治疗，八个学期。

5.1.19 呼吸技巧：气功入门课程，四个学期。

5.1.20 传统东方功法：太极拳入门课程，四个学期。

5.1.21 传统东方草药学，包括植物学：部分学时应在临床环境中进行，十二个学期，加上一百个临床学时。

5.1.22 实践管理：保持专业实践的法律和道德方面的指导，包括记录保存、专业责任、患者账户和转诊程序，三个学期。

5.1.23 与针灸实践相关的伦理学，两个学期。

5.2 课程应包括充分的临床指导，其中 75% 应在由课程培训方经营的诊所进行。在以

下适当情形下,可直接接触患者:

5.2.1　实践观察:对针灸临床实践进行监督观察,并进行病例报告和讨论,五十个临床学时。

5.2.2　诊断和评估:中西医结合的诊断方法在患者评价中的应用,五十个临床学时。

5.2.3　指导实践:对患者进行临床针灸治疗,五十个临床学时。

5.3　在诊断、评估和临床实践的最初一百学时内导师在患者诊断和治疗过程中应始终在场。在随后一百学时内,导师应在患者接受针灸治疗时始终在场。

5.4　此后,在进行临床指导期间,导师应在患者接受治疗的地点附近。学生也应在每次治疗前和治疗后,请教导师。

第 32‐11‐6 条　培训课程的评估

6.1　本州的每个培训计划都应建立一种机制,评估并授予学生先前课程学习和经验的转学分,以获得本规则第 32‐11‐5 条所要求的课程学习和临床教学的同等学分。培训课程评估和授予转学分的政策和程序应以书面形式提出,并提交委员会。政策和程序应包括以下所有内容:

6.2　学分只能根据学生实际完成的课程学习或直接相关的经验授予。本规则中,"经验"系指学生直接参与本条要求的课程领域的学术相关学习,包括综合的现场和临床实习、学徒制、辅导计划和合作教育计划。

6.3　若申请人的课程学习及临床教学在未获委员会批准的针灸学校完成,则对申请人的评估应包括学校在可授予转学分的学科领域组织的考试。

6.4　先前的教育和经验可获得的学分应相当于在培训方案中完成同一科目的一般学生可获得的学分,并应符合培训计划的课程标准和毕业要求。

6.5　在委员会批准的另一所针灸学校或学院顺利完成课程学习和临床教学,可获得转学分。

6.6　在美国教育部认可的认证机构批准的学校顺利完成的生物学、化学、物理、心理学、解剖学、生理学、病理学、营养和维生素、医学史、医学术语、临床科学、临床医学、西方药理学、心肺复苏、实践管理和伦理等课程,最高可获得高达 100% 的转学分。

6.7　在传统东方医学、针灸解剖学和生理学、针灸技术、穴位按摩、呼吸技巧、传统东方功法等方面的临床课程学习和教学中获得学分,或在未获委员会批准的学校顺利完成的传统东方草药学,可由委员会批准的学校授予学分,但要求这些学科领域的学时至少有 50% 是在委员会批准的学校顺利完成的。

6.8　培训计划中评估及授予学生转学分的完整记录,应归入学生的学业档案,并作为该学生成绩单的正式部分,根据学生要求提交委员会存档。

6.9　所有学生入学时,应收到培训计划关于评估及授予转学分相关政策及程序的副本。

第 32‐11‐7 条　批准所需的文件

寻求批准针灸培训计划的教育机构或方案应向委员会提供任何必要的文件和其他证据,以便委员会确定所提供培训的实际性质和范围,包括但不限于:目录,课程描述,课程计划和学习简报。

第 32－11－8 条　吊销或撤销批准

委员会可因任何未能遵守《西弗吉尼亚州法典》第 30－36－1 条及其后各条或本节规则的行为而拒绝、吊销或撤销对任何针灸培训计划的批准，或将其列入察看期。

第 32－11－9 条　学校监控；记录；报告

9.1　每一所经批准的西弗吉尼亚州针灸学校，应在该学校财政年度结束后六十日内向委员会提交一份当前的课程目录，并附上信函概述下列内容：

9.1.1　增加或删除的课程或相较前一年的课程任何重大变化。

9.1.2　教师、行政或主管部门的变化。

9.1.3　学校设施的重大变化。

9.1.4　一份关于学校财务状况的声明，使委员会能够评估学校是否有足够的资源来确保其有能力进行入学学生的培训计划。

9.2　如果委员会认为有必要，委员会的代表应到学校实地考察，审查和评估学校的状况。学校应向委员会偿还进行审查和评估所产生的直接费用。

9.3　所有学生记录须以英文备存。

9.4　各获批针灸学校应在三十日内，向委员会报告其设施或诊所及本规则规定的课程设置的重大变化。

第十二节　辅导教育要求

第 32－12－1 条　总则

1.1　范围：本条规定了针灸执照申请人完成辅导或学徒计划的教育要求。

1.2　权限：《西弗吉尼亚州法典》第 30－36－7 条。

1.3　申请日期：1999 年 5 月 21 日。

1.4　生效日期：1999 年 5 月 21 日。

第 32－12－2 条　申请

本立法规则适用于申请执照和申请辅导计划。

第 32－12－3 条　定义

3.1　针灸辅导。一项针灸学徒计划，该计划由委员会根据本法典批准，在顺利完成后应符合《西弗吉尼亚州法典》第 30－35－10(3) 款关于针灸执照的要求。

3.2　针灸导师。一名执业针灸师，经委员会批准，向在委员会注册的学员提供针灸辅导。

3.3　学员。经委员会注册，在针灸导师的指导下参加针灸辅导的人。

第 32－12－4 条　事先批准作为针灸学员执业

在针灸辅导中从事针灸实践的人员应取得委员会的事先批准。

第 32－12－5 条　事先批准辅导一名针灸学员

针灸师应事先获得委员会的批准，才能在针灸辅导中指导任何针灸学员。

第 32－12－6 条　申请存档：预培训学分

6.1　针灸学员申请人应使用委员会提供的表格提交批准，并附上 32CRS4 规定的申请费。

6.2　针灸导师申请人应使用委员会提供的表格提交批准，并附上任何必要的文件，包括培训协议和 32CRS4 规定的申请费。

6.3 具有符合委员会标准的预培训和经验的针灸学员可根据先前的培训和经验减少所需的理论和临床培训时间。应将预培训和经验的证明连同学员注册申请提交委员会审查。

第 32－12－7 条 批准针灸辅导的要求

7.1 针灸导师和针灸学员应制定一份书面培训协议,其中包括针灸辅导的必要内容。该协议应为学员提供结构化的学习经历,包括独立进行针灸实践所需的所有基本技能和知识,并应为学员参加委员会的针灸执照考试做好准备。

7.2 培训协议应明确针灸辅导是否为就业性质。就业可以是全职或兼职。

7.3 针灸辅导须提供正规临床培训及补充的理论及教学指导。在《西弗吉尼亚州法典》第 30－36－10 条中要求的培训来自经批准的针灸学校或其他中学后教育机构,该机构是由美国教育部授权的区域认证机构认证或批准的。

7.4 该临床培训须至少达到三百学时,包含下列课程:

7.4.1 实践观察。

7.4.2 病史及体格检查。

7.4.3 治疗计划。

7.4.4 患者准备工作。

7.4.5 灭菌设备的灭菌,使用和维护。

7.4.6 艾灸。

7.4.7 电针(交流和直流电压)。

7.4.8 体针和耳针。

7.4.9 急救治疗,包括心肺复苏。

7.4.10 对患者进行治疗前后的指导。

7.4.11 禁忌证及注意事项。

7.5 针灸辅导的理论及教学训练须至少达到二千七百学时(约二百七十学期学分),包含下列课程:

7.5.1 传统东方医学:对传统诊疗方法的理论与实践综述的研究。

7.5.2 针灸解剖学和生理学:针灸基础,包括经络系统,经外奇穴,以及耳针疗法。

7.5.3 针灸技术:指导使用针刺技术、艾灸、电针,包括预防措施(如针头灭菌)、禁忌证和并发症。

7.5.4 临床医学:医学、整骨疗法、牙科、心理学、护理学、整脊疗法、足科和顺势疗法的临床实践概述,让针灸医师熟悉其他卫生保健从业者的实践经验。

7.5.5 医学史:对医学史的研究,包括跨文化治疗实践。

7.5.6 医学术语:英语医学术语基础。

7.5.7 普通科学:对一般生物学、化学和物理学的研究。

7.5.8 解剖:对显微、大体解剖学和神经解剖学的研究。

7.5.9 生理学:对基础生理学的研究,包括神经生理学,内分泌学和神经化学。

7.5.10　病理学：对疾病性质的研究,包括微生物学、免疫学、精神病理学以及流行病学。

7.5.11　临床科学：内科、药理学、神经学、外科、产科/妇科、泌尿学、放射学、营养和公共卫生综述。

7.6　学员须以不危害患者健康和幸福的方式提供针灸服务。学员应告知患者,针灸服务将由该学员提供。每次治疗中,须告知患者学员将在针灸导师的监督下进行针灸治疗,且患者在治疗前已通过书面形式同意学员对其进行针灸治疗。上述规定也适用于学员协助针灸导师提供针灸服务的情况。

7.7　针灸辅导培训计划应在导师和学员签署的书面协议中加以说明,该书面协议应包括但不限于培训计划、培训时长、提供理论及教学培训的方法,以及学员提供针灸服务的培训指南。在申请审批时须提交该书面协议的复印件。

第 32‐12‐8 条　针灸导师的责任

针灸导师须承担以下职责：

8.1　导师须按本规则规定,随时负责并监督学员的工作。

8.2　导师只应分配学员其有能力进行安全有效治疗的患者。导师应在学员提供服务时,对其进行持续的指导和即时的监督,并应在插针和拔针期间保持近距离。

8.3　导师须确保必要时获得患者知情同意。

8.4　导师须确保提交的培训计划目标由学员提供并实现。

8.5　导师须确保学员符合执业标准。

8.6　导师须按委员会提供的表格,按季度向委员会提交进度报告,该报告应列出对学员进行理论、教学和临床培训的日程安排。

8.7　导师须确保学员在提供服务或以其他方式从事专业活动过程中,始终明确其"针灸学员"的身份;并佩戴第 1399.427 条规定的身份徽章。

8.8　导师不得允许学员单独计费。

8.9　导师应遵守《西弗吉尼亚州法典》第 30‐36‐1 条及其后各条,有关支付给雇员或学徒的工资、报酬、最长工作时间和工作环境的适用法律和规则。学员如需加班,不得干扰或影响其培训计划,也不得损害学员或患者的健康及安全。

第 32‐12‐9 条　学员的责任

9.1　辅导计划学员不得在没有按照规定受到监督的情况下自主提供针灸服务,也不得提供其未受训练或不能胜任的任何服务。

9.2　针灸辅导的学员须达到向委员会呈交的培训计划中的教学目标,包括所需的理论训练。

9.3　学员须遵守 32CRS6 规定的针灸执业标准。

9.4　针灸辅导的学员在提供服务或以其他方式从事专业活动时,须表明其学员身份,并应在外衣上佩戴身份徽章,该徽章须清楚显示学员姓名及"针灸学员"的身份。

9.5　如果导师没有向委员会报告针灸辅导的延迟、中断或终止状况,应由辅导学员向委员会报告。

第 32－12－10 条　终止或更改培训计划

10.1　无论任何原因导致针灸辅导终止,导师均应在十日内以书面形式告知委员会。委员会收到通知时,委员会应取消导师和学员的注册信息。如导师或学员其后参加针灸辅导,应向委员会重新提交注册申请。

10.2　如针灸辅导的培训计划有实质性修改,须向委员会提交修改报告。提交此报告不收取任何费用。

10.3　如导师不能完成培训,委员会可酌情制定计划,允许学员完成培训课程。委员会可指派一名新的针灸导师。

第 32－12－11 条　资格审查及口试申请

完成辅导计划后,学员可申请执照。

第 32－12－12 条　拒绝、吊销或撤销导师的注册

针灸辅导中,委员会可基于下列原因,拒绝、授予(在符合相关条款及条件的前提下)、吊销、撤销导师的注册,或将其列入察看状态:

(a)未能遵守《西弗吉尼亚州法典》第 30－36－1 条及其后各条或本节的规定。

(b)违反 32CRS5 实践标准。

(c)导师是纪律处分的对象,或已受到纪律处分的指控。

(d)通过欺诈、谎报或向委员会提供关于针灸辅导的虚假或误导性信息的方式注册为导师。

(e)导师或学员未遵守患者知情同意的条例;或

(f)学员在针灸辅导中提供违反本规则的针灸服务,无论针灸导师是否知悉。

第 32－12－13 条　拒绝、吊销或撤销学员的注册

针灸辅导中,委员会可基于下列原因,拒绝、颁发(在符合相关条款及条件的前提下)、吊销、撤销学员的注册,或将其列入察看状态:

(a)未能按本细则规定批准注册学员的。

(b)违反《西弗吉尼亚州法典》第 30－36－1 及其后各条,或委员会规则 32CRS1 及其后各条。

(c)通过欺诈、谎报或向委员会提供关于针灸辅导的虚假或误导性信息的方式注册为学员。

(d)未遵守患者知情同意的条例。

(e)在获批的针灸辅导以外提供针灸服务。

(f)未表明针灸学员身份,或在提供针灸服务时未佩戴身份徽章。

(g)在针灸导师的指导下提供针灸服务,而该导师未获委员会批准,或已被吊销导师注册。

第十三节　专业有限责任公司的成立及批准

第 32－13－1 条　总则

1.1　范围:本立法规则规定了针灸师专业有限责任公司的成立和批准程序。

1.2　权限：《西弗吉尼亚州法典》第 31B－13－1304 条。

1.3　申请日期：1999 年 5 月 21 日。

1.4　生效日期：1999 年 5 月 21 日。

第 32－13－2 条　定义

2.1　委员会：西弗吉尼亚州针灸委员会,根据《西弗吉尼亚州法典》第 30－36－1 条及其后各条成立。

2.2　专业有限责任公司：根据《西弗吉尼亚州法典》第 31B－13－1 条及其后各条成立的以提供专业服务为目的的有限责任公司。

2.3　专业服务：根据《西弗吉尼亚州法典》第 30－36－1 条及其后各条规定由针灸师提供的服务。

第 32－13－3 条　针灸师专业有限责任公司的成立和批准程序费用

3.1　在本州持有针灸执照的针灸师,希望以有限责任公司的形式提供针灸和东方医疗服务的,应遵守《西弗吉尼亚州法典》第 31B－13－1301 条及其后各条的规定。任何专业有限责任公司的成员不得提供该公司的专业服务,正式获得执照或依法授权提供专业服务的人员除外。

3.2　专业有限责任公司的名称应包含"专业有限责任公司"或缩写"P.L.L.C."或"Professional L.L.C."

3.3　每家专业有限责任公司应在成立时,以及每年 7 月第一日之前向委员会提交其两名或两名以上成员的姓名、该专业有限责任公司持有至少一百万美元专业责任保险的书面文件,以及一百美元的初始备案费和一百美元的年度续期费。

3.3.a　如果专业有限责任公司通过下列方式,提供一百万美元专门指定的隔离基金,用于执行对公司成员或其向公司的患者或客户提供的任何专业或非专业服务的判决,则满足持有一百万美元专业责任保险的要求：

3.3.a.1　以信托方式,或以现金、银行存单或美国国债的银行托管方式存入;或

3.3.a.2　银行信用证或保险公司债券。

3.4　每一家有限责任公司应向委员会提交一份年度报告副本,该报告必须根据《西弗吉尼亚州法典》第 31B－2－211 条提交州务卿。年度报告副本以及向州务卿提交备案的任何更正后的年度报告副本,应在每年 7 月 1 日或之前向委员会提交。

3.5　符合本规则所有规定的专业有限责任公司,均应由委员会批准并始终由委员会批准。

3.6　如任何持证人不再是专业有限责任公司的成员,该公司应在二十日内书面通知委员会,告知该持证人已不再是专业有限责任公司的成员。持证人不再是专业有限责任公司成员的事实不影响委员会对该专业有限责任公司的批准,但前提是委员会认定该专业有限责任公司仍遵守本规则的所有规定。

第 32－13－4 条　违规通知,停止提供专业服务

4.1　如委员会认定专业有限责任公司并未遵守本规则的所有规定,并应停止在本州提供专业服务,委员会应书面通知该专业有限责任公司。该专业有限责任公司接到书面通知后,应停止在本州提供专业服务。

第 32－13－5 条 医师-患者关系

5.1 本规则条款不得解释为改变或影响医师-患者关系。

第十四节 耳穴戒毒疗法证书

第 32－14－1 条 总则

1.1 范围：本规则根据《西弗吉尼亚州法典》第 30－36－10 条规定了耳穴针灸证书持有人的申请、证书、资格和期限。

1.2 权限：《西弗吉尼亚州法典》第 30－36－7(d)款和第 30－36－10 条。

1.3 申请日期：2020 年 4 月 20 日。

1.4 生效日期：2020 年 4 月 30 日。

1.5 失效条款：本节将于 2030 年 4 月 30 日到期时终止，不再具有任何效力。

第 32－14－2 条 申请

本立法规则适用于耳穴戒毒证书持有人的申请、证书颁发、续期、资格和期限等。

第 32－14－3 条 定义

3.1 耳穴戒毒疗法。指经委员会批准或国家针灸戒毒协会（NADA）规定的治疗药物滥用、酗酒、化学依赖、戒毒、行为治疗或创伤恢复的疗法。经证明这些人已顺利完成了实施耳穴戒毒疗法所需的学习课程。

3.2 证书持有人。系指经委员会授权接受耳穴戒毒训练并符合耳穴戒毒治疗师或专家资格的人。

3.3 国家针灸戒毒协会（NADA）协议。系指国家针灸戒毒协会关于耳穴戒毒疗法的协议。

第 32－14－4 条 证书持有人的申请、期限及续期

4.1 如欲取得耳穴戒毒治疗师或耳穴戒毒专家的证书，应以委员会规定的格式向委员会提出申请，并根据《西弗吉尼亚州法典》第 32 章第 4 节，按照委员会规则支付相应的委员会费用。

4.2 实施耳穴戒毒疗法的授权证书有效期为两年，从委员会颁发之日的月底起算。此类初步批准应以书面形式告知本节第 5.1.2 款所列的相关专业委员会。

4.3 实施耳针疗法的证书应按照要求并缴纳适当的费用，以委员会规定的格式向委员会申请续期。

第 32－14－5 条 证书获取要求

5.1 为取得耳穴戒毒专家证书，申请人应：

5.1.1 年满十八岁。

5.1.2 被授权在本州从事下列任何一项：

5.1.2.a 医师助理，根据本法典第 30－3E－1 条及其后各条。

5.1.2.b 牙医，根据本法典第 30－4－1 条及其后各条。

5.1.2.c 注册专业护士，根据本法典第 30－7－1 条及其后各条。

5.1.2.d 经验护士，根据本法典第 30－7A－1 条及其后各条。

5.1.2.e 心理学家,根据本法典第30－21－1条及其后。

5.1.2.f 职业治疗师,根据本法典第30－28－1条及其后各条。

5.1.2.g 社会工作者,根据本法典第30－30－1条及其后各条。

5.1.2.h 专业顾问,根据本法典第30－31－1条及其后各条。

5.1.2.i 紧急医疗服务提供者,根据本法典第16－4C－1条及其后各条;或者

5.1.2.j 根据本法典第15A－1－1条及其后各条,提供矫正医疗服务。

5.1.3 提供顺利完成委员会批准的耳针计划的证据。

5.1.4 按委员会规定提交完整的申请。

5.1.5 提交立法规则规定的适当费用。

5.2 证书可根据本规则的规定续期。

5.3 证书持有人应根据《西弗吉尼亚州法典》第30－36－10条和本条第5.1.2款的要求维持和保持其专业能力和有效授权。

第32－14－6条 拒绝颁发、限制、处分、吊销或撤销耳穴证书或将其列入察看期的原因

6.1 委员会可拒绝证书申请,将证书持有人列入察看期,吊销证书,限制证书,或撤销委员会颁发的任何证书,但须有充分证据能够证明该证书持有人:

6.1.1 在申请证书时故意作出、提供或导致作出或提供任何虚假、欺诈或伪造的陈述、文书、证书、文凭或其他材料。

6.1.2 曾经或正在涉及与认证申请有关的欺诈、伪造、欺骗、串通或共谋。

6.1.3 对管制药品上瘾。

6.1.4 成为一个长期或持续的酗酒者。

6.1.5 从事有可能欺骗、欺诈或伤害公众或公众成员的不光彩、不道德或违反职业道德的行为。

6.1.6 故意违反保密通信。

6.1.7 根据《西弗吉尼亚州法典》第30－36－10条和本规则第5.1.2款,在本州或任何其他州、准州、司法管辖区或外国撤销、吊销或限制其执照,或以其他方式对其采取行动,或受到执照或管理部门的任何其他纪律处分,或被剥夺在本州或任何其他州、准州、司法管辖区或外国的执照或授权。

6.1.8 表现出缺乏为患者提供耳穴治疗的专业能力,无法保障合理的技能和安全。在这方面,委员会可考虑持证人多次表现出未能妥善治疗患者的行为,并可要求证书持有人在委员会认为有必要确定其专业资格时,接受委员会成员、其代理人或指定人员的书面或口头询问或检查。

6.1.9 根据国家针灸戒毒协会关于耳穴戒毒疗法的指南制定的准则,从事违反职业道德的行为,包括但不限于任何偏离或不符合可接受的实践标准的行为,无论患者是否受到该行为的伤害,或实施了任何违反诚实、正义或良好道德的行为,无论该行为是在其实践过程中还是在其他方面实施,也无论是否在本国境内实施。

6.1.10 证书持有人在任何司法管辖区被判犯有与耳穴戒毒疗法实践直接有关的罪行,

或与根据《西弗吉尼亚州法典》第30-36-10条和本规则第5.1.2款所述的专业授权或其他授权有关的罪行。为本规则之目的,放弃答辩将视为有罪。

6.1.11 关于初步证明,在任何司法管辖区被判有罪且尚未撤销,并与耳穴戒毒疗法实践或根据《西弗吉尼亚州法典》第30-36-10条和本节第5.1.2款所述的专业授权或其他授权有合理关系。为本规则之目的,不抗辩答辩将视为有罪;在确定定罪是否与耳穴戒毒疗法实践或根据《西弗吉尼亚州法典》第30-36-10条和本规则第5.1.2款所述的专业授权或其他授权有合理关系时,委员会至少应考虑:

6.1.11.a 其被判罪行的性质和严重性。

6.1.11.b 自犯罪发生以来的时间。

6.1.11.c 该罪行与履行职业或专业责任所需的能力和健康状况的关系。

6.1.11.d 其进行康复或治疗的任何证据;尽管有任何其他相反的法律规定,如果申请人因先前的刑事定罪而被取消认证资格,委员会应允许其随后按照《西弗吉尼亚州法典》第30-1-24条的规定提出申请。

6.1.12 以本人以外的名字宣传、从事针灸实践或试图从事针灸实践。

6.1.13 未能向委员会报告证书持有人知悉的违反本规则或违反第30-1-1条及其后各条所述的任何职业行为准则。

6.1.14 未能履行证书持有人的任何法定或法律义务。

6.1.15 制作或提交一份证书持有人明知是虚假的报告,故意或过失不提交州或联邦法律要求的报告或记录,故意妨碍或阻挠提交,或诱使他人这样做。报告或记录只包括以证书持有人身份签署的报告或记录。

6.1.16 在患者-医师关系中施加影响,目的是让患者发生性行为。

6.1.17 在耳穴戒毒疗法实践中作出欺骗性、不真实或欺诈性的陈述,或在耳穴戒毒疗法实践中使用不符合东方医学界普遍治疗标准的诡计或计划。

6.1.18 通过使用欺诈、恐吓、不当影响,或通过过度接触或无理的行为,亲自或通过代理人来招揽患者。招揽系指直接或含蓄地要求接收方立即回应的任何讯息。

6.1.19 在未事先得患者充分知情和书面同意的情况下,实施了根据学界通行的耳穴戒毒疗法标准构成人体实验的任何程序或处方。

6.1.20 从事或提议从事《西弗吉尼亚州针灸实践法》许可范围之外的耳穴戒毒疗法实践,或接受并履行证书持有人知道或有理由知道其无法履行的专业职责。

6.1.21 违反或未能遵守委员会的合法命令,或违反根据委员会启动的任何程序作出的任何法院的命令;或

6.1.22 与根据《西弗吉尼亚州法典》第30章获得执照的任何类别的卫生保健从业者签订任何监督和/或合作协议,但不符合与之相关的实践标准。

6.2 当委员会发现任何申请人没有资格获得证书或发现任何证书持有人应根据《西弗吉尼亚州针灸实践法》或委员会的规则受到纪律处分时,委员会可采取以下任意一项或多项处分:

6.2.1 拒绝向申请人颁发证书。

6.2.2 公开申斥。

6.2.3 吊销或限制任何证书的期限,不得超过五年。

6.2.4 要求任何证书持有人参加委员会规定的教育计划。

6.2.5 撤销任何证书。

6.2.6 要求证书持有人接受医生或其他专业人员的护理、咨询或治疗。

6.2.7 要求证书持有人在另一执业者的指导或监督下实践;或

6.2.8 除上述处分外,委员会可作出不利于证书持有人或申请人的判决,但不执行判决和罚款;委员会亦可作出判决和罚款,但暂停执行罚款,并将耳穴戒毒治疗师列入察看期,如果不遵守委员会制定的任何条款,可撤销该察看期。委员会可根据《西弗吉尼亚州针灸实践法》《西弗吉尼亚州法典》第30－36－1条及其后各条酌情恢复并重新颁发证书。作为条件,委员会可以实施本规则或《西弗吉尼亚州针灸实践法》中规定的任何纪律处分或补救措施。

第32－14－7条　纪律和申诉程序

7.1 本条规定了与第32章立法规则第7节针灸师纪律和申诉程序所述耳穴戒毒证书持有人同样的申诉程序。一旦做出了最后的代理命令或决定,委员会应将本决定或命令通知本规则第5.1.2款所列的专业委员会。

第32－14－8条　有争议案件的听证程序

8.1 本规则规定了对耳穴戒毒证书持有人的有争议案件的听证程序,与第32章(程序规则)第8节(有争议案件的听证程序)中的规定相同。

第十五节　申请豁免特定人员的执照首年年费

第32－15－1条　总则

1.1 范围:本规则规定了免除低收入个人和军事人员及其配偶的执照年年费的程序。

1.2 权限:《西弗吉尼亚州法典》第30－1－23条,第30－36－7条。

1.3 申请日期:2020年4月20日。

1.4 生效日期:2020年4月30日。

1.5 失效条款:本规则自2030年4月30日到期时终止,不再具有效力。

第32－15－2条　定义

2.1 委员会系指西弗吉尼亚州针灸委员会。

2.2 Bo Acu－LIW 系指针灸委员会的豁免表格,用以申请免除低收入个人的初始执照费,如《西弗吉尼亚州法典》第30－1－23条所述。

2.3 Bo Acu－MFW 系指针灸委员会的豁免表格,用以申请免除兵役成员及其配偶的初始执照费,如《西弗吉尼亚州法典》第30－1－23条所述。

2.4 "初始"系指首次在西弗吉尼亚州获得针灸执业执照。

2.5 "当地劳动力市场"根据《西弗吉尼亚州法典》第21－1C－2条,系指西弗吉尼亚州内各县,以及存在任何地界距离西弗吉尼亚州边界五十英里范围内的西弗吉尼亚州以外的任何县。

2.6 "低收入个人"系指《西弗吉尼亚州法典》第21－1C－2条所界定的当地劳动力市

场中的个人,其调整后家庭总收入低于联邦贫困线的130%。这一术语还包括在州或联邦公共援助方案中注册的任何人,包括但不限于对贫困家庭的临时援助方案、医疗补助或补充营养援助方案。

2.7 "军人家属"系指美国武装部队、国民警卫队的现役军人、《美国法典》第38篇第101章所述预备役部队或这些部队的退伍军人及其配偶。这一术语还包括未再婚的已故军人的未亡配偶。

第 32‑15‑3 条　申请豁免初始执照费

3.1 委员会可向符合《西弗吉尼亚州法典》第30‑36‑3条及其后各条要求以及委员会颁布的规则的申请人颁发执照,如果申请人符合本规则所界定的"低收入个人"或一个或多个"军人家属"资格,委员会应豁免初始执照费。

3.2 本规则所界定的低收入个人,可向专业针灸师申请低收入免除初始执照费,提交由委员会提供的低收入免除初始执照费表格,以及委员会规定的所有必要核查文件。委员会应在收到完整申请后三十日内审查申请并作出决定。

3.3 按照本条规则所界定,军人家属可向委员会申请豁免专业针灸师的初始执照费,并提交由委员会提供的兵役核查表和委员会规定的所有必要的核查文件,并提交完整的申请。委员会应在收到完整申请后三十日内审查申请并作出决定。

第 32‑15‑4 条　豁免初始执照费所需文件

4.1 申请豁免低收入或兵役人员及其配偶初始执照费的个人,应向联委会提交初始执照费豁免 BoAcu‑LIW 或 BoAcu‑MFW 表格和本条规定的适当文件。

4.2 为确定低收入者有资格获得初始执照费豁免,申请人应向委员会提交证据,证明申请人调整后家庭总收入低于联邦贫困水平的130%,并提交资格证明文件:

4.2.1 贫困家庭临时援助方案。

4.2.2 医疗补助。

4.2.3 补充营养援助方案;或

4.2.4 联邦报税表。

4.3 为确定军人家属是否有资格获得初始执照费豁免,申请人应向委员会提交合格兵役证明和合格配偶或未亡配偶的资格证明,如下:

4.3.1 军人 DD‑214 表格。

4.3.2 军人 NGB‑22 表格。

4.3.3 军人 DD‑1300 表格;或

4.3.4 其现行军事命令的副本;或

4.3.5 经委员会确定适当的其他正式军事文件,证明该服役人员过去或现在合格服役;和

4.3.6 与合格军人的结婚证副本(如适用)、未亡配偶申请军人家属豁免的军人死亡证明副本,以及核实未亡配偶未再婚的公证宣誓书副本(如适用)。

4.4 光荣退伍的申请人应向委员会提交一份完整的申请和一份 DD‑214 表格或一份 NGB‑22 表格,表明申请人已光荣退伍。

第十六节　决定颁发初始执照时考虑刑事定罪记录

第 32－16－1 条　总则

1.1　范围：本规则规定了在决定颁发初始执照时考虑先前刑事定罪的程序。

1.2　权限：《西弗吉尼亚州法典》第 30－1－24 条,《西弗吉尼亚法典》第 30－36－7 条。

1.3　申请日期：2020 年 4 月 20 日。

1.4　生效日期：2020 年 4 月 30 日。

1.5　失效条款：本规则自 2030 年 4 月 30 日到期时终止,不再具有效力。

第 32－16－2 条　定义

2.1　"委员会"系指根据《西弗吉尼亚州法典》第 30－36－3 条设立的针灸委员会。

2.2　"初始执照"系指首次在西弗吉尼亚州获得的针灸执照。

2.3　"颁发执照"系指委员会正式授权从事针灸实践。

2.4　"未撤销的",在提及刑事定罪时,系指定罪未被驳回、撤销、赦免或取消。

第 32－16－3 条　与针灸实践的理性联系

3.1　委员会不得因先前的刑事定罪而取消申请人的初始执照资格,除非该定罪是与针灸实践具备理性联系的犯罪。在确定刑事定罪是否与针灸实践具备理性联系时,委员会应至少考虑：

3.1.1　其被判罪行的性质和严重性。

3.1.2　自犯罪发生以来的时间。

3.1.3　该罪行与履行执业针灸师职责所需的能力和健康状况的关系。

3.1.4　其进行康复或治疗的任何证据。

第 32－16－4 条　拒绝颁发执照后申请

4.1　尽管《西弗吉尼亚州法典》有其他相反的规定,如果申请人因先前的刑事定罪而被拒绝颁发执照,并满足以下条件,委员会应允许申请人申请初始执照：

4.1.1　自定罪之日起或从监禁释放之日起满五年,以较晚者为准。

4.1.2　在取消执照资格后的时间内未被判处任何其他罪行。

4.1.3　定罪并非暴力或性犯罪：但是如果犯有暴力或性犯罪,则取消执照资格的时间较长,这将由委员会根据个案决定。

第 32－16－5 条　申请执照资格确认

5.1　有犯罪记录的个人如先前未申请执照,可随时向委员会提出申请,以确认其犯罪记录是否会导致其丧失获得执照的资格。

5.2　该申请应使用委员会规定的申请表提交,其中应包括有关个人犯罪记录的充分细节,以便委员会能够确定进行定罪的司法管辖区、定罪日期和定罪的具体性质。

5.3　申请人可提交申请执照资格的康复证明,推荐信,和任何其他申请人认为相关的资料,以表明其健康状况和从事针灸实践的能力。

5.4　委员会应在收到申请人的申请后六十日内提供执照资格确认。

佐 治 亚 州

佐治亚州针灸法[①]

第 43‑34‑60 条　简称

本节应称为"佐治亚州针灸法"。

第 43‑34‑61 条　立法研究

大会认定并宣布,佐治亚州的针灸实践会影响公共健康、安全和福利,因此必须对其进行适当的管理和控制。

第 43‑34‑62 条　定义

本节使用的术语:

(1)"针灸"系指一种从传统和现代东方保健理念发展而来,采用东方医学技术、治疗方法和辅助疗法,旨在促进、维持和恢复健康并预防疾病的疗法。

(2)"耳穴戒毒疗法"系指仅以治疗化学依赖为目的,将一次性针灸针刺入国家针灸戒毒协会方案所规定的五个耳穴。

(3)"委员会"系指佐治亚州综合医学委员会。

(4)"针灸疗法"系指根据东方医学原理,在人体特定部位刺入一次性针灸针的治疗方式。干针是一种针灸实践技术。辅助疗法的范围可能包括手法治疗、器械治疗、草药治疗、温针治疗、电针治疗以及电磁治疗、膳食指南和功法的建议,但只有此类治疗、建议和运动是基于传统东方医学的理念,并与针灸疗法直接相关。

第 43‑34‑63 条　综合州立医学考试委员会的权力

委员会与咨询委员会协商后,有权并有责任:

(1)确定申请人申请执照和执照续期的资格及适宜性。

(2)通过和修改与本州法律相一致的规定,以开展事务、履行职责和执行本节内容。

(3)依照本文规定,审批、颁发、拒绝、撤销、吊销及续期针灸申请人和执业针灸师的执照,并就有关行为举行听证会。

[①]　根据《佐治亚州注释版法典》第 43 卷第 34 章第 3 节"针灸"译出。

（4）就关于违反本节及据本节通过的规定而提起的控诉，举行听证会，并起诉及禁止此类违反行为。

（5）确定申请费、考试费和执照费。

（6）要求并获得州教育机构或其他州机构的协助，并准备有关消费者利益的信息，以说明委员会的监管职能及向委员会提出和解决消费者控诉的程序。委员会应将信息提供给公众和适当的机构。

（7）制定继续教育的要求。

第43-34-64条 执照的要求

（a）每位针灸执照申请人均应满足以下要求：

（1）年满二十一岁。

（2）提交委员会要求的完整申请。

（3）缴纳委员会要求的任何费用。

（4）获得由国家能力保证组织批准并经委员会规定的国家认证机构颁发的针灸证书。

（5）顺利完成获委员会批准及国家认可的洁针技术课程。

（6）已购买不少于十万美元或三十万美元的职业责任保险。

（7）通过由国家能力保证组织认可的机构提供并经委员会批准的针灸考试。

（8）顺利取得针灸学位或完成正规的针灸学习和培训课程。申请人须向委员会提交符合要求的文件，以表明该教育或学习和培训的课程：

（A）在针灸和东方医学认证委员会认证的学校或在获委员会批准的机构完成；或

（B）与获委员会批准的经认证的针灸学校所提供的针灸教育具有基本同等效力。

（b）保留。

（c）任何根据本节获得针灸执照者，如其研究生临床经验不足一年，在可自行执业之前，必须在至少有四年临床执业经验的持证针灸师的监督下执业一年。此类针灸导师可以获得在佐治亚州或任何其他州或国家的执照，其执照要求基本同等于佐治亚州执业执照的要求，并且可能与佐治亚州的执照要求基本同等的其他州或国家累积从事四年的执业临床实践。

（d）每位申请授权成为耳穴戒毒技师从事耳穴戒毒治疗的人员均应满足以下要求：

（1）年满二十一岁。

（2）提交委员会要求的完整申请。

（3）缴纳委员会要求的任何费用。

（4）顺利完成获委员会批准且国家认可的治疗化学依赖的耳穴戒毒疗法培训计划；及

（5）顺利完成获委员会批准且国家认可的洁净针技术课程。

（e）耳穴戒毒疗法的实践可以在委员会规定的城市、县、州、联邦或私人化学依赖项目中进行，或由委员会授权从事针灸治疗，同时根据本章第2节获授权行医的人直接监督。

第43-34-65条 接受或拒绝执照申请的通知

在评估申请人提交的申请和其他证据后，委员会须通知申请人其提交的申请和证据是符合要求被接受或是不符合要求被驳回。如申请被驳回，通知书应当载明驳回理由。

第 43 - 34 - 66 条　交出执照;执照出示;地址更改

(a) 委员会颁发的任何证明执照的文件均为委员会财产,必须根据要求交出。

(b) 每位持有委员会依本节颁发的执照并积极从事针灸或作为耳穴戒毒技师积极从事耳穴戒毒治疗的,均应以适当和公开的方式出示证明其持有执照的文件。

(c) 每位持有委员会颁发的执照者,均应将地址变更通知委员会。

第 43 - 34 - 67 条　执照续期;非执业状态

(a) 对于依据本节颁发的执照,如持证人在申请续期时未违反本节规定,并且申请符合委员会现行的继续教育要求,则应每两年续期一次。

(b) 依据本节获得执照者有责任在执照到期前续期执照。

(c) 根据委员会制定的程序和条件,持证人可以要求将其执照列为非执业状态。持证人可以在满足委员会规定的条件后随时申请将执照恢复为执业状态。

第 43 - 34 - 68 条　知情同意书

(a) 任何接受针灸疗法者均须同意此程序,并且一般应告知其以下内容:

(1) 针灸疗法基于东方艺术,与传统的西方医学完全不同。

(2) 针灸师不能行医,不对患者的疾病或状况进行医学诊断,如该患者想获得医学诊断,则应去看医生。

(3) 针灸治疗的性质和目的。

(b) 委员会应制订一份标准的《知情同意书》,供依据本节取得执照者使用。该《知情同意书》须包括(a)款所规定的信息,以及委员会认为的任何其他适当的信息和补充信息。《知情同意书》中所载的信息应使用易于阅读和便于公众理解的语言。

第 43 - 34 - 69 条　禁止行为;制裁

委员会(尽管并非为专业许可委员会)在与咨询委员会协商后,可根据第 43 - 34 - 8 条(b)款的授权,对第 43 - 34 - 8 条(a)款规定的任何行为或涉及与转诊患者的任何人分摊或同意分摊针灸服务费用的行为实施任何制裁。

第 43 - 34 - 70 条　针灸咨询委员会

委员会应委任针灸咨询委员会。该咨询委员会应包括依照本节取得针灸执照的针灸专业人士、依照本章第 2 节获得医师执照的针灸师,以及委员会酌情决定的其他成员。咨询委员会成员不得因在委员会的服务而获得任何报酬。咨询委员会须承担委员会厘定的咨询职责及责任。针灸咨询委员会成员须根据本节取得执照。

第 43 - 34 - 71 条　禁止行为和声明;免责条款;处罚

(a) 除据本节获得执照或根据本法典第(b)款获得豁免,否则任何人都不得:

(1) 从事针灸或耳穴戒毒疗法;或

(2) 表示自己是据本节获得执照的针灸师或耳穴戒毒技师。

(b) 上述第(a)款中的禁令不适用于:

(1) 根据第 34 章第 2 节获得执照者。

(2) 针灸实践是针灸教育课程组成部分,参加针灸教育计划的学生受具有至少五年临床经验的持证针灸师的直接监督;或

（3）持有执照的针灸从业者在与本文相同或比本文更为严格的其他司法管辖区实施针灸行为，若是在经规定的针灸教育课程中定期进行授课或在经规定的针灸专业组织的教育研讨会的情况下，则其操作由依本文获得执照的针灸执业者或根据本章第 2 条获得执业资格的执业针灸师直接监督。

（c）任何违反上述第（a）款的人一经定罪，即属轻罪。

第 43－34－72 条　头衔的使用

（a）"执业针灸师"和"针灸师"的名称只能由根据本节获得执照者使用。

（b）"耳穴戒毒技师"的名称只能由据本节获得耳穴戒毒执照的人使用。拥有 A.D.T. 执照本身并不意味其有权证明自己是一名针灸师。耳穴戒毒技师被严格限制使用五个耳穴，用以治疗药物滥用、化学依赖或两者兼而有之的戒毒。

（c）据本节获得执照的人不得向公众宣传或声称自己根据本章第 2 节获授权而行医。

佐治亚州针灸行政法①

第 360－6－01 条　针灸；目的

本规则的目的是实施《佐治亚州针灸法案》（"法案"），授权综合州立医学考试委员会（"委员会"）通过规则和条例，实施针灸和耳穴戒毒治疗行政许可所需的一切行为。该规则确立发放针灸和耳穴戒毒治疗执照的标准，并通过纪律处分实施此类标准。此类规则还旨在向所有医师、其他相关的卫生保健专业人员以及所有希望获得执照的人告知该法案的相关要求。

第 360－6－02 条　定义

根据该法案颁布的本规则所使用的术语定义如下：

（1）"ACAOM"系指"针灸及东方医学教育审核委员会（ACAOM）"，是国家认可的针灸和东方医学项目认证机构。

（2）"法案"系指《佐治亚州针灸法案》，O.C.G.A. 第 43－34－60 节等。

（3）"针灸"系指一种从传统和现代东方保健理念发展而来，采用东方医学技术、治疗方法和辅助疗法，旨在促进、维持和恢复健康并预防疾病的疗法。

（4）"咨询委员会"系指佐治亚州综合医学委员会的针灸咨询委员会。

第 360－6－03 条　针灸执照要求

（1）每名获发针灸师执照的申请人必须符合以下规定：

（a）宣誓书：申请人是美国公民、美国合法永久居民或符合《联邦移民和国籍法》规定的合格外籍人士或非移民的宣誓书。如申请人不是美国公民，则必须提交文件，以确定其合格的外籍人士身份。该委员会参与了系统的外籍人士权利核查或救助（DHS－USCIS SAVE）项目，目的是核实非公民的公民身份和移民身份信息。如申请人是符合《联邦移民

---

① 根据《佐治亚州行政法典》第 360 卷第 360－6 章"针灸"译出。

和国籍法》规定的合格外籍人士或非移民,则必须提供由国土安全部或其他联邦移民机构签发的外籍人士号码。

（b）须至少年满二十一岁,并具有良好品德。

（c）提交委员会要求的完整申请。在支付所有费用和委员会收到所有要求的文件之前,不得视上述申请已完成。

（d）必须提交三份可接受的推荐信:一份是美国持证医师（医学博士或骨科医学博士）的推荐信,该医师在申请人执业的司法管辖区内且熟悉申请人执业状况,两份是熟悉申请人执业状况的针灸师的推荐信。

（e）已顺利取得针灸学位或完成正式的针灸学习及培训课程。申请人须向委员会提交符合要求的文件,以表明该教育或学习和培训的课程:

1. 在针灸和东方医学认证委员会认证的学校或在获委员会批准的机构完成;或

2. 与获委员会批准的经认证的针灸学校所提供的针灸教育具有基本同等效力。

（f）已通过由美国国家能力保证组织认可并获委员会批准的机构所提供的针灸考试。

（g）向国家针灸与东方医学认证委员会提交针灸认证证明。

（h）顺利完成获委员会批准的洁针技术课程。

（i）已提交证明,证实已购买至少十万美元或三十万美元的职业责任保险。

1. 如持证人变更责任承保人、取消责任保险或被责任承保人撤销,则持证人必须自变更或者撤销之日起三十日内通知委员会。

2. 根据该法案,未能持续购买责任保险可能会导致针灸执照被吊销。

（j）申请人须在委员会接获申请之日起 12 个月内,提交申请程序所需的所有文件。

（2）每名持有委员会颁发执照的人,如对地址及任何其他资料（包括但不限于专业法律责任范围的变更）进行更改,均应通知委员会,以便根据本规则或该法案获得执照。

（3）"执业针灸师"及"针灸师"的头衔,只可由获授权依据该法案及本规则行针的人使用。

第 360－6－04 条　名牌及针灸执照展示

（1）本州医院、诊所、疗养院提供服务的针灸师,于辅助生活社区或个人护理院时,应将针灸师的具体执照告知所有当前和未来患者,并应在接触患者时,佩戴标有持证人姓名和"针灸师"字样的清晰易读的身份标签。

（2）在所有与医疗机构相关的人员姓名广告中,获得佐治亚州针灸师执照的人员应表明自己是针灸师。

（3）任何依据该法案及本规则获发针灸执照者,如正在积极从事针灸或耳穴戒毒疗法,则须以公开和适当的方式展示委员会颁发的执照。

（4）委员会颁发的任何执照或文件,均属委员会财产,应在要求时交还。

第 360－6－05 条　受监督的针灸实践

（1）任何根据本节获得针灸执照者,如其研究生临床经验不足一年,在可自行执业之前,必须在持证针灸师的监督下执业一年。针灸导师（"导师"）目前应在佐治亚州取得执照,并在佐治亚州有四年执业的针灸临床经验,或者在其他州或国家有四年针灸师执业经验,只要该州或国家的针灸师执业标准基本等同于或超过佐治亚州的执照标准。

（2）针灸医师对研究生临床实习的监督，须符合以下规定和指南。

（a）定义：

1."医师"系指在研究生临床实习期间，受导师监督和监控的人员。

2."导师"系指符合本规则和适用法规定的针灸师，负责在监督研究生临床实习期间对医师进行监督。

3."受监督的研究生临床实习"系指在获批针灸师的直接监督下，经佐治亚州综合医学委员会（"委员会"）与针灸咨询委员会（"咨询委员会"）协商后按照 O.C.G.A.第 43－34－64（c）节和本规则进行的针灸实践。

（b）导师：委员会在对咨询委员会进行咨询后，须规定一名导师监督医师。导师必须为佐治亚州注册针灸师，并在该州执业。导师应具有不少于四年的针灸师执业经验。在佐治亚州或其他州或国家，有四年执业的临床经验，或总计四年执业的临床实践，只要这些州或国家的针灸师执照标准基本等同于或超过佐治亚州的执照标准。

（c）监督：从事监督后临床实践的导师和医师应当遵守下列准则：

1.监督计划：

（i）医师在监督下执业前，导师须向委员会呈交意向书及一份监督的书面大纲计划，委员会应与咨询委员会协商，对其进行审查和批准。

（ii）导师在医师为患者看病和治疗时，必须在场并时刻在场。医师应与导师在同一办公室内执业。

（iii）导师不得一次与两名以上的执业医生签订监督计划。

2.监控：导师不得少于一周或每两周监控一次医师在监督下对患者的治疗。监测应包括病例审查、安全程序监督、洁针技术和对医师职业水准的评估。

3.记录：

（i）患者治疗记录：导师须就医师在监督下的患者治疗备存书面记录，并须在咨询委员会的意见下，将患者治疗记录的摘要连同季度报告呈交委员会复核。记录应包括与患者治疗有关的任何信息，这些信息应包括在医师的导师所进行的监控中。

（ii）执业记录：

I.为监督之目的，执业被定义为在一年或十二个月的临床期间内，对至少一百名不同的患者进行至少五百次针灸服务。药物滥用或戒毒治疗不是为指导研究生临床针灸实践而进行的针灸治疗。

II.应随时在治疗地点保存所有相关和辅助文件的详尽和完整记录，以供委员会审查和检查。记录应包括但不限于：预约时间表、病历、治疗记录、收据和有关发票和支付针灸治疗费用的数据。

4.报告：

（i）季度报告：季度报告应由导师向委员会提交，报告应包括医师的表现、进展和对基本技能的理解。报告还应包括医师每月看的患者的数量及其提供的针灸治疗的数量。季度报告应在临时执照颁发日期后 3、6、9 和 12 个月提交委员会。

（ii）最终监督报告：在察看期结束时，须就医师的进展向委员会提交最终报告，并就医师是否适合单独执业,向委员会提出建议。该报告应由咨询委员会审查,并由咨询委员会就委员会的行为提出建议。

(d) 有关监督执业的条文亦可用作经委员会授权的人员对针灸服务的限制准则。

(e) 未遵守有关受监督的研究生临床执业的准则,可能导致委员会对持证人施加制裁、限制或纪律处分。

第360-6-06条　耳穴戒毒技师执照要求

(1) 每名申请以耳穴戒毒技师身份进行耳穴戒毒治疗的申请人,均须符合以下规定。如申请人不符合本规则所述的所有执照规定,委员会可酌情根据咨询委员会的建议,向申请人颁发执照。

(a) 至少二十一岁,并具有良好品德。

(b) 按照委员会的要求提交已完成的申请。

(c) 按委员会的要求缴纳申请费用。

(d) 已顺利完成获委员会批准的治疗化学依赖的耳穴戒毒治疗培训计划。

(e) 已顺利完成获委员会批准及国家认可的洁针技术课程。

(f) 提交雇主职业责任保险对申请人的保险范围的核实证明。

(g) 申请人须在委员会收到该项申请的日期起一年内完成所有执照规定。

(2) 耳穴戒毒疗法的做法只可在委员会规定的城市、县、州、联邦或私人化学依赖计划内进行,该方案须得到委员会规定,并由持证针灸师或委员会授权在佐治亚州行医者直接监督。

(3) "耳穴戒毒技师(ADT)"进行耳穴戒毒治疗,该头衔只可由依据该法案及本规则取得执照的人使用。持ADT执照并不允许任何人使用"针灸师"或"持证针灸师"的头衔。

(4) 每名持有委员会颁发执照的人,如对地址及任何其他资料(包括但不限于工作情况)进行更改,均应通知委员会。

(5) 耳穴戒毒技师执照只限于并只对在颁发执照时指定的雇主有效。ADT持证人应由其雇主为其购买职业责任保险。

(a) 如ADT持证人更改雇主,持证人须向委员会提交一份"更改雇主的要求"表格,并须得到委员会准许更改雇主。

(b) 如ADT持证人终止受雇于指定雇主,则该ADT执照自动失效,直至提出新的申请为止。

(6) 每位持有由委员会颁发的ADT执照者,在治疗时,必须时刻佩戴注明其姓名及职称的身份徽章。

第360-6-07条　耳穴戒毒技师执照展示

(1) 任何依据该法案及本规则获得执照进行耳穴戒毒治疗者,如正在积极进行耳穴戒毒治疗,须以公开而适当的方式展示委员会颁发的执照。

(2) 委员会颁发的任何执照或文件,均属委员会财产,应在要求时交还。

第360-6-08条　禁止针灸和耳穴戒毒治疗无证执业;豁免

(1) 任何人不得:

(a) 在无证的情况下,于佐治亚州实施针灸或耳穴戒毒治疗;或

（b）在未根据该法案获得执照的情况下，表明其是针灸师或耳穴戒毒技师。

（2）以下人士可不受委员会限制在佐治亚州接受针灸或耳穴戒毒治疗：

（a）将针灸作为学习计划的组成部分的学生，并在有至少五年临床经验的持证针灸师的直接临床监督下，参加获委员会批准的针灸教育计划的学生；或

（b）在委员会批准的针灸教育计划或委员会批准的针灸专业组织的教育研讨会的常规教学过程中进行针灸且在任何其他司法管辖区持有针灸执照或证书者；但在后一种情况下，执业须由依据该法案获发执照者或根据佐治亚州法律获发执业执照的针灸师直接监督。

第 360 - 6 - 09 条　医师

希望在佐治亚州从事针灸实践的医师，须顺利完成获委员会批准的三百学时课程，并在将此类疗法纳入其医疗实践前至少三十日以书面形式通知董事会其进行针灸治疗的意图。经委员会授权进行针灸治疗的医师享有与接受针灸和耳穴戒毒治疗的医师同等的权利和特权。

第 360 - 6 - 10 条　针灸咨询委员会的组成和职责

（1）委员会的意图及政策是在针灸咨询委员会（"咨询委员会"）组成中反映佐治亚州公民的文化多样性。咨询委员会的组成如下：

（a）至少四名被委任人，其中一名可能是业外人士或执业针灸师本人，三名执业针灸师及针灸专业代表的个人，以及委员会酌情决定的其他人士。

1. 在委员会委任时，这些人士须取得针灸执业执照。

2. 所有受聘于咨询委员会的人，均须向委员会行政主管或其指定的人提交一份简历及三封推荐信（其中一封可由熟悉被委任人针灸实践的医师提供）。

3. 为了保持咨询委员会的连续性，两名被委任人任期两年，两名被委任人任期一年，此为部分任期。在任命时，委员会行政主管将以书面方式通知每名被委任人其各自任期的开始和结束日期。各成员可重新向全体委员会申请再次申请连任，但连续任期不得超过两届。

4. 如咨询委员会成员在某一任期内被更换，则该替换成员将担任该任期剩余部分，担任部分任期的咨询委员会成员，在部分任期结束后，有资格连任两年。

5. 佐治亚州不对受委任人的时间和开支进行补偿。

（b）一名从事或教授针灸的执业医师：

1. 任期两年，并可由委员会多数票再委任两年，但连续任期不得超过两届。

2. 其工作时间和费用不由佐治亚州进行补偿。

（2）咨询委员会须就与任命咨询委员会成员有关的事宜，以及法案范围内的所有事项，向委员会提供意见。委员会与咨询委员会协商后，应：

（a）确定执照申请人和执照续期申请人的资格和适宜性。

（b）通过和修订符合佐治亚州法律的规则，而此类规则是履行其职责和管理该法案所需的。

（c）审查、批准、颁发、拒绝、撤销、吊销及续期申请人和持证人的执照，并就依照该法案履行的所有职责举行听证会。

（3）咨询委员会成员如非委员会成员，则必须在有需要时可出席会议，不得错过咨询委

员会连续举行的三次会议,或在一个日历年内缺席四次会议,且委员会行政主管或委员会主席不得无故缺席。

(a)咨询委员会可建议委员会因违反出席规则将一名成员免职。咨询委员会可向委员会建议将违反出席规则的成员免职。这项建议应由咨询委员会以多数票通过。

(b)委员会在收到撤职建议后,可以多数票罢免咨询委员会的一名成员。

(4)委员会可根据咨询委员会的建议,在委员会的网页上刊登广告或以任何其他适当方法填补咨询委员会的空缺。所有申请人必须在委员会所规定的任何截止日期前提交申请,并须向委员会行政主管或其指定的人提交一份简历及三封推荐信(其中一封可以来自熟悉申请人针灸实践的医师)。

第360-6-11条　执照续期

(1)根据本法案颁发的所有执照应每两年续期一次。执照将在申请人生日的最后一日到期。

(2)如在有效期届满前不能续期执照,将受到委员会要求的延期续签的处罚。

(3)有效期届满后三个月内仍未续期的执照,因未续期而被行政撤销,并向公众公布,并公布在委员会的网站上。

(4)尽管本规则第(3)款另有规定,任何第 O.C.G.A.第 15-12-1 节所界定的服务成员,如在州外的执业时,其执照已届满,则须获准凭该已届满的执照执业,该服务成员六个月内在不得因已届满的执照被控告违反有关该执业的规定,直至其解除执业或调任至本州境内的另一地点为止。该服务成员有权在其从解除执业或调任之日起六个月内,免费将期满的执照续期到本州境内的一个地点。服务成员必须向委员会提交一份由服务成员指挥官签署的正式军事命令或书面核实的副本,以免除任何费用。

(5)持证人须提供符合要求的证据,证明已符合委员会所规定的继续教育规定,包括至少一学时的传染病课程。

(6)持证人必须在续期表格上证明其已阅读、理解和熟悉疾病控制及预防中心(CDC)的指导,以防止人类免疫缺陷病毒、乙型病毒性肝炎及丙型病毒性肝炎及其他传染病的传播。

(7)持证人须接受审计,以决定是否符合委员会所颁布的规则所规定的继续教育规定。

(8)如未能满足继续教育的要求,则不续期和撤销根据该法案颁发的执照。

(9)所有续期申请人必须提供一份宣誓书和一份安全、可验证且符合 O.C.G.A.50-36-1(f)规定的文件。如申请人曾提供过安全的、可验证的美国公民身份证明和宣誓书,则续期时不需要其他美国公民身份证明。如申请续期的申请人不是美国公民,则其必须提交文件,以确定其合格的外籍人士身份。该委员会已参与 DHS-USCIS SAVE(系统的外籍人士权利核查或储蓄)项目,目的是验证非美国公民和移民身份信息。如申请续期的人为符合《联邦移民和国籍法》规定的外籍人士或非移民,则其必须提供由国土安全部或其他联邦机构签发的外籍人士号码。

第360-6-12条　处置生物危害物质和洁针库存记录和使用针灸针库存记录

(1)针灸实践及耳穴戒毒,对公众健康、安全及福利均有影响,是合适的监管对象。

(2)针灸和耳穴戒毒是采用锋利器具对人体皮肤进行长期侵入性治疗,应采取一切必要的预防措施,防止人类免疫缺陷病毒(引起获得性免疫缺陷综合征的病毒)、乙型病毒性肝炎和丙型肝炎及其他传染病的传播。根据该法案获得执照的人员和从事针灸的豁免人员应采取一切措施,以符合疾病控制及预防中心(CDC)的最新建议,该建议为防止长期侵入性治疗过程中,将人类免疫缺陷病毒、乙型病毒性肝炎和丙型病毒性肝炎及其他传染性疾病传播给患者,该建议载于《1991年发病率和死亡率周报》40(第RR-8号)第1~9页。所有目前获得委员会批准的人都有责任熟悉此类建议,委员会认为此类建议是可接受的和现行医疗实践的最低标准。如不符合这些最低标准,委员会可判定这是不专业的行为,并会受到委员会的检讨和纪律处分。

(3)一次性针灸针被视为生物危害废物,必须按照所有适用的联邦和州法律、法规予以处置。为了进一步确保佐治亚公民的公共卫生和安全,根据该法案获得执照的人和不从事针灸的个人必须保存反映以下详细信息的准确医疗记录和办公室记录:

(a)购买一次性针灸针的发票。

(b)所有一次性针灸针的处置文件及处置方法。

(4)与购买一次性针灸针及处置一次性针灸针有关的记录,必须保存不少于五年,并须在委员会获授权代表以书面要求或委员会代理人就委员会的申诉、指控和/或调查提出要求时,交还委员会。

(5)所有依据本法案获得执照的持证人,必须提交经委员会设计和规定的经公证的文件,承认其已阅读、理解和熟悉疾病控制及预防中心(CDC)的指导,以防止人类免疫缺陷病毒、乙型病毒性肝炎及丙型病毒性肝炎及其他传染病的传播。本文件必须在申请时和每一个续期周期内向委员会提交。

第360-6-13条 临时执照

针灸师和耳穴戒毒技师执照的临时执照可由委员会颁发。

第360-6-14条 整脊疗法医师必须满足针灸师的执照要求

如O.C.G.A.43-9-16所述,如该法案第1.1节修订,欲施行针灸的整脊疗法医师必须符合该法案和委员会颁布的针灸规则的许可要求。整脊疗法医师的申请人必须在佐治亚州获得整脊疗法医师执业执照,持有效整脊疗法医师执照,并在佐治亚州整脊疗法医师考试委员会中信誉良好。根据佐治亚州大会的意图,本规则不得解释为禁止根据第3条获发在佐治亚州进行针灸的执照的整脊疗法医师从事针灸实践。佐治亚州综合医学委员会,以及任何其他考试委员会,对获准在本州从事针灸的整脊疗法医师拥有唯一、专属和原始管辖权,以便为针灸师执照制定标准,并通过纪律处分强制执行此类针灸标准。

第360-6-15条 无证执业

(1)根据本法案取得执照的人,除非获得委员会准许在佐治亚州执业,否则不得以执业医生身份在佐治亚州执业。

(2)任何人不得向公众宣传或自称为"执业针灸师"或"耳穴戒毒技师",除非本人已根据本法案取得执照或在其他方面获法律豁免。

第360-6-16条 治疗知情同意书

(1)任何接受针灸治疗的人,必须在该等程序之前以书面方式表示同意,并须知晓以下

一般条款:

（a）针灸师未持有在佐治亚州执业的执照。

（b）针灸师不得在佐治亚州行医。

（c）针灸师未对患者的疾病或身体状况做出医学诊断。

（d）如患者欲取得医疗诊断,则患者须访问执业医师,并向执业医师寻求医疗意见。

（e）正在进行的针灸治疗的性质及目的。

（2）任何人在进行耳穴戒毒手术前,必须以书面方式表示同意,并须获告知以下一般条款:

（a）耳穴戒毒技师未持有在佐治亚州执业的执照。

（b）耳穴戒毒技师不得在佐治亚州行医。

（c）耳穴戒毒技师未持有在佐治亚州执业针灸的执照。

（d）耳穴戒毒技师未就患者的疾病或身体状况做出医疗诊断。

（e）如患者欲取得医疗诊断,则患者须访问执业医师,并向执业医师寻求医疗意见。

（f）正在做出的耳穴戒毒治疗程序的性质及目的。

（g）耳穴戒毒技师严格限制使用五个以内的耳穴,以治疗因物质滥用或化学依赖,或两者兼而有之的戒毒。

（h）持证从事针灸时间或耳穴戒毒者,必须为每名接受治疗的人使用获批的、标准化的"知情同意书"表格。表格须由医生及患者在提供服务前签署及注明日期。

第 360-6-17 条　制裁的实施;禁止使用转诊费

委员会与咨询委员会协商后,可:

（1）发现 O.C.G.A.43-1-19(a)款中规定的任何行为后,可根据 O.C.G.A.43-1-19(d)款授权进行任何处罚;或

（2）调查表明这种行为涉及与任何介绍患者的人分摊或同意分摊针灸服务的费用。

第 360-6-18 条　非执业状态

（1）任何人如欲维持其针灸师执照,但不打算从事针灸实践,可向委员会递交申请及费用,以申请非执业状态。

（a）持有非执业状态执照的人不得在本州作为针灸师执业。

（b）为重新获得针灸师执照,必须将已填写完成的申请及恢复费用递交委员会。申请人必须能够向委员会证明,其具有针灸方面的知识、技能和熟练度,而且其在精神和身体上都能以合理的技巧安全执业。

（2）任何人如欲维持其耳穴戒毒技师执照,但不打算施行耳穴戒毒治疗,可向委员会提交申请及费用,以申请非执业状态。

（a）持有非执业状态执照的个人不得在本州作为耳穴戒毒技师执业。

（b）为重新获得耳穴戒毒技师执业执照,必须将已填写完成的申请及恢复费用递交委员会。申请人必须能够向委员会证明,其具有在耳穴戒毒治疗方面的知识、技能及熟练度,而且其在精神及身体上都能以合理的技巧安全执业。

（3）由委员会酌情决定恢复执照。

ARKANSAS

ARKANSAS CODE ANNOTATED

Subchapter 1.   General Provisions

§ 17 – 102 – 101.   Short title

This chapter shall be known as the "Arkansas Acupuncture Practices Act".

§ 17 – 102 – 102.   Definitions

As used in this chapter:

(1) "Acupuncture" means the insertion, manipulation, and removal of needles from the body and the use of other modalities and procedures at specific locations on the body for the prevention, cure, or correction of a malady, illness, injury, pain, or other condition or disorder by controlling and regulating the flow and balance of energy and functioning of the patient to restore and maintain health, but acupuncture shall not be considered surgery;

(2) "Acupuncturist" means a person licensed under this chapter to practice acupuncture and related techniques in this state and includes the terms "licensed acupuncturist", "certified acupuncturist", "acupuncture practitioner", and "Oriental acupuncture practitioner";

(3) "Board" means the Arkansas State Board of Acupuncture and Related Techniques;

(4) "Chiropractic physician" means a person licensed under the Arkansas Chiropractic Practices Act, § 17 – 81 – 101 et seq.;

(5) "Moxibustion" means the use of heat on, or above, or on acupuncture needles, at specific locations on the body for the prevention, cure, or correction of a malady, illness, injury, pain, or other condition or disorder; and

(6) (A) "Related techniques" means the distinct system of basic health care that uses all allied diagnostic and treatment techniques of acupuncture, Oriental, traditional, and modern, for the prevention or correction of a malady, illness, injury, pain, or other condition or disorder by controlling and regulating the flow and balance of energy and functioning of the patient to restore

and maintain health.

(B) As used in this subdivision (6), "related techniques" includes, but is not limited to, acupuncture, moxibustion or other heating modalities, cupping, magnets, cold laser, electroacupuncture including electrodermal assessment, application of cold packs, ion pumping cord, lifestyle counseling, including general eating guidelines, tui na, massage incidental to acupuncture, breathing and exercising techniques, and the recommendation of Chinese herbal medicine lawfully and commercially available in the United States. Provided, "related techniques", including, but not limited to, tui na, shall not involve manipulation, mobilization, or adjustment to the spine or extraspinal articulations.

§ 17 – 102 – 103. Disposition of funds

(a) (1) All fees authorized by this chapter are the property of the Arkansas State Board of Acupuncture and Related Techniques and shall be provided to the Treasurer of the Arkansas State Board of Acupuncture and Related Techniques to be disposed of as provided in this chapter.

(2) Any surplus in the treasury of the board at the end of the fiscal year shall remain in the treasury and may be expended in succeeding years for the purposes herein set out.

(b) All funds received by the board shall be deposited into a financial institution designated by the board and expended in the furtherance of the purposes of this chapter and the board's duties thereunder, which include, but are not limited to:

(1) The publication and distribution of the Arkansas Acupuncture Practices Act, § 17 – 102 – 101 et seq.;

(2) The publication and yearly distribution of a directory of all licensed acupuncturists;

(3) Investigations of violations of this chapter;

(4) Institution of actions to compel compliance with the provisions of this chapter; and

(5) Defense of actions brought against it as a result of its actions under the provisions of this chapter.

§ 17 – 102 – 104. False advertising

(a) A person defined in § 17 – 102 – 102(4) shall not solicit for patronage or advertise for patronage by any means whatever that are misleading, fraudulent, deceptive, or dishonest.

(b) It constitutes false advertising under this section for an acupuncturist as defined in § 17 – 102 – 102(2) to refer to himself or herself other than as a licensed acupuncturist, certified acupuncturist, acupuncture practitioner, or Oriental acupuncture practitioner.

(c) A person licensed or certified under this chapter shall not identify himself or herself as a doctor or physician.

(d) A violation of this section is grounds for disciplinary action under § 17 – 102 – 309(a)(4).

§ 17 – 102 – 105. Public health and sanitation

(a) Acupuncturists shall use only presterilized, disposable needles in their administration of acupuncture treatments. The use of staples in the practice of acupuncture is unlawful.

(b) Sanitation practices shall include:

(1) Hands shall be washed with soap and water or other disinfectant before handling needles and between treatment of different patients; and

(2) Skin in the area of penetration shall be thoroughly swabbed with alcohol or other germicidal solution before inserting needles.

(c) No person shall be allowed to practice acupuncture and related techniques without first having passed a nationally recognized clean-needle-technique course.

§ 17 - 102 - 106.   Prosecution of violations

It shall be the duty of the several prosecuting attorneys of the State of Arkansas to prosecute to final judgment every criminal violation of this chapter committed within their jurisdictions when requested and authorized by the Arkansas State Board of Acupuncture and Related Techniques.

§ 17 - 102 - 107.   Redesignated as § 17 - 102 - 205

§ 17 - 102 - 108.   Redesignated as § 17 - 102 - 206

§ 17 - 102 - 109.   Redesignated as § 17 - 102 - 103

§ 17 - 102 - 110.   Redesignated as § 17 - 102 - 106

Subchapter 2.   Board of Acupuncture and Related Techniques

§ 17 - 102 - 201.   Creation of board — Members — Appointment

(a) (1) There is created the Arkansas State Board of Acupuncture and Related Techniques. The board shall consist of five (5) persons appointed by the Governor as full members and one (1) person appointed by the Governor as an ex officio member.

(2) Three (3) full members of the board shall be qualified acupuncturists.

(3) (A) Two (2) full members shall be appointed to represent the public and shall not have practiced acupuncture and related techniques in this or any other jurisdiction nor be retired from or have any financial interest in the occupation regulated.

(B) The public members shall be subject to confirmation by the Senate.

(C) The public members shall be full voting members but shall not participate in the grading of examinations.

(4) (A) The ex officio member shall be a physician licensed pursuant to the Arkansas Medical Practices Act, § 17 - 95 - 201 et seq., § 17 - 95 - 301 et seq., and § 17 - 95 - 401 et seq., and shall be entitled to be notified of all board meetings and to participate in the deliberations of the board.

(B) However, the ex officio member shall have no vote, shall not serve as an officer of the board, and shall not be counted to establish a quorum or a majority necessary to conduct business.

(5) (A) On a biennial basis beginning in October 2010, the board shall file a written

report with the House Committee on Public Heath,[1] Welfare, and Labor and the Senate Committee on Public Health, Welfare, and Labor.

(B) The report shall contain a certified copy of the minutes of all board meetings as required by § 17 – 102 – 205 for the calendar years 2009 through October 2010 and thereafter covering the period of time since the last report.

(C) The report shall contain a comprehensive assessment of the board's functionality, including without limitation staff and office site adequacy and any other information as may be requested by the House Committee on Public Health, Welfare, and Labor and the Senate Committee on Public Health, Welfare, and Labor sufficient for the House Committee on Public Health, Welfare, and Labor and the Senate Committee on Public Health, Welfare, and Labor to make a recommendation to the Governor regarding whether the board should be continued or whether the board should be disbanded and abolished in accordance with a proclamation issued by the Governor.

(b) (1) The initial full members of the board shall be appointed by the Governor for staggered terms as follows:

(A) One (1) member's term shall expire after one (1) year;

(B) One (1) member's term shall expire after two (2) years; and

(C) One (1) member's term shall expire after three (3) years.

(2) Of the two (2) additional members appointed pursuant to Acts 1999, No. 536, one (1) shall be appointed for a two-year term and the other for a three-year term.

(3) The initial ex officio board member shall be appointed to a term of three (3) years.

(4) Successors shall be appointed for three-year terms.

(5) Vacancies shall be filled by appointment by the Governor for the unexpired term.

(6) Board members shall serve until their successors have been appointed and qualified.

(c) The Governor may remove any full member from the board for any reason that would justify the suspension or revocation of his or her license to practice acupuncture and related techniques.

(d) A person who is or has been in the preceding two (2) years on the faculty of a school which is subject to review by the board may not serve on the board.

§ 17 – 102 – 202.   Board members — Qualifications

(a) Each member of the Arkansas State Board of Acupuncture and Related Techniques shall be a citizen of the United States, a resident of this state, and, before entering upon the duties of the office, shall take the oath prescribed by the Arkansas Constitution for state officers and shall file it with the Secretary of State who shall thereupon issue to each person so appointed a certificate of appointment.

(b) Each full professional member also shall be a graduate of a reputable school or institute of acupuncture or Oriental medicine and be certified by the National Certification Commission for Acupuncture and Oriental Medicine.

§ 17 – 102 – 203.　Board members — Liability

No member of the Arkansas State Board of Acupuncture and Related Techniques during the term of his or her office or thereafter shall be liable for damages as a result of any official act in the performance of his or her duty as such a member. Any action therefor shall upon motion be dismissed with prejudice at the cost of the plaintiff.

§ 17 – 102 – 204.　Board organization — Meetings

（a）The Arkansas State Board of Acupuncture and Related Techniques shall within sixty （60）days of August 1, 1997, and every May thereafter hold a meeting and elect from its membership a president, a secretary, and a treasurer for terms set by the board.

（b）（1）It shall be the duty of the board to meet regularly one （1）time in every six （6）months.

（2）Special meetings of the board may be called at any time at the pleasure of the President of the Arkansas State Board of Acupuncture and Related Techniques or by the Secretary of the Arkansas State Board of Acupuncture and Related Techniques on the request of any two （2）full members of the board.

（3）Three （3）full members shall constitute a quorum at any meeting of the board.

（c）The board shall determine by its own rules the time and manner of giving notice to members of meetings and other matters.

（d）Any action of the board shall require an affirmative vote of a majority of the full membership of the board, excluding the ex officio member.

§ 17 – 102 – 205.　Board minutes — Records

（a）The Secretary of the Arkansas State Board of Acupuncture and Related Techniques shall keep a record of the minutes of its meetings and a record of all persons making application for license and the action of the Arkansas State Board of Acupuncture and Related Techniques thereon.

（b）The secretary shall also keep a record of the names, addresses, and license numbers of all acupuncturists licensed by the board, together with a record of license renewals, suspensions, and revocations.

§ 17 – 102 – 206.　Board duties and powers

（a）（1）The Arkansas State Board of Acupuncture and Related Techniques is empowered to incur whatever expenses it may deem necessary or expedient in performing its functions.

（2）All of the disbursements provided for in this section shall be out of the fees and fines collected by the Arkansas State Board of Acupuncture and Related Techniques.

（b）The Arkansas State Board of Acupuncture and Related Techniques is authorized to：

（1）Make suitable bylaws for carrying out the duties of the Arkansas State Board of Acupuncture and Related Techniques under the provisions of this chapter；

(2) Sue and be sued;

(3) Have an official seal that shall bear the words "Arkansas State Board of Acupuncture and Related Techniques";

(4) (A) Provide a secretary's certificate.

(B) The certificate of the Secretary of the Arkansas State Board of Acupuncture and Related Techniques under seal shall be accepted in the courts of the state as the best evidence as to the minutes of the Arkansas State Board of Acupuncture and Related Techniques and shall likewise be accepted in the courts of the state as the best evidence as to the licensure or nonlicensure of any person under the requirements of this chapter;

(5) (A) Adopt, publish, and, from time to time, revise rules consistent with the law as may be necessary to enable the Arkansas State Board of Acupuncture and Related Techniques to carry into effect the provisions of this chapter.

(B) Within thirty (30) days after the effective date of this act, the Arkansas State Board of Acupuncture and Related Techniques shall promulgate new rules to replace the following existing rules: Title I, Title II, Title III, Title IV, Title V, and Title VI.

(C) All proposed rules after the effective date of this act shall be approved in writing by the Arkansas State Medical Board under the Arkansas Administrative Procedure Act, § 25 – 15 – 201 et seq., but before submission to the Administrative Rules Subcommittee of the Legislative Council;

(6) Keep a record of all proceedings, receipts, and disbursements of the Arkansas State Board of Acupuncture and Related Techniques;

(7) Adopt standards for applicants wishing to take the licensing examination and conduct examinations or contract with persons or entities to conduct examinations of applicants;

(8) (A) Grant, deny, renew, suspend, or revoke licenses to practice acupuncture and related techniques for any cause stated in this chapter.

(B) Except as otherwise provided by this chapter, the Arkansas State Board of Acupuncture and Related Techniques shall have exclusive jurisdiction to determine who shall be permitted to practice acupuncture and related techniques in the State of Arkansas; and

(9) Conduct disciplinary proceedings under this chapter.

(c) (1) In the performance of the duties of the Arkansas State Board of Acupuncture and Related Techniques, the Arkansas State Board of Acupuncture and Related Techniques may administer oaths and take testimony on any matters within the Arkansas State Board of Acupuncture and Related Techniques' jurisdiction and issue subpoenas and thereby compel the attendance of persons before the Arkansas State Board of Acupuncture and Related Techniques for the purpose of examining any facts or conditions properly pending before the Arkansas State Board of Acupuncture and Related Techniques for action of the Arkansas State Board of Acupuncture and Related Techniques.

(2) All subpoenas issued by the Arkansas State Board of Acupuncture and Related Techniques shall be served in the manner prescribed by law for the service of subpoenas issuing from the courts, and all persons so served shall obey the subpoenas or be subject to the penalties provided by law for the disobedience of subpoenas issuing from the courts.

§ 17 - 102 - 207.   Redesignated as § 17 - 102 - 307

§ 17 - 102 - 208.   Redesignated as § 17 - 102 - 308

§ 17 - 102 - 209.   Redesignated as § 17 - 102 - 309

§ 17 - 102 - 210.   Redesignated as § 17 - 102 - 310

§ 17 - 102 - 211.   Redesignated as § 17 - 102 - 311

Subchapter 3.   Licensing

§ 17 - 102 - 301.   License required

In order to safeguard life and health, any person practicing acupuncture and related techniques in the state for compensation or gratuitously shall be required to submit evidence that he or she is qualified to practice and licensed as provided in this chapter.

§ 17 - 102 - 302.   Repealed by Acts of 2013, Act 1147, § 3, eff. Aug. 16, 2013

§ 17 - 102 - 303.   Unlawful practice — Penalty — Injunction

(a) Except as otherwise provided in this chapter, it shall be unlawful for any person not licensed under the provisions of this chapter:

(1) To practice or offer to practice acupuncture and related techniques; or

(2) To use any sign, card, or device to indicate that the person is an acupuncturist.

(b) Except as otherwise provided in this chapter, any person who shall attempt to practice acupuncture and related techniques as defined in this chapter without having first been licensed or otherwise permitted under the provisions of this chapter to do so, shall be deemed guilty of a misdemeanor. Upon conviction, he or she shall be punished by a fine of not less than one thousand dollars ($1,000) nor more than five thousand dollars ($5,000) or by imprisonment in the county jail for a period of not less than one (1) month nor more than eleven (11) months, or by both fine and imprisonment. Each day shall constitute a separate offense.

(c) The courts of this state having general equity jurisdiction are vested with jurisdiction and power to enjoin the unlawful practice of acupuncture and related techniques in a proceeding by the Arkansas State Board of Acupuncture and Related Techniques or any member thereof or by any citizen of this state in the county in which the alleged unlawful practice occurred or in which the defendant resides or in Pulaski County. The issuance of an injunction shall not relieve a person from criminal prosecution for violation of the provisions of this chapter, but the remedy of injunction shall be in addition to liability to criminal prosecution.

§ 17 - 102 - 304.   Applications — Fees — Qualifications

(a) (1) No person shall be licensed to practice acupuncture and related techniques unless he or she has passed an examination and has been found to have the necessary qualifications as prescribed in the rules adopted by the Arkansas State Board of Acupuncture and Related Techniques.

(2) (A) Applications for a license to practice acupuncture and related techniques in the State of Arkansas pursuant to this chapter shall be made to the Secretary of the Arkansas State Board of Acupuncture and Related Techniques in writing on forms furnished by the board.

(B) The application shall be signed by the applicant in his or her own handwriting and acknowledged before an officer authorized to administer oaths.

(3) Before any applicant shall be eligible for an examination, the applicant shall furnish satisfactory proof to the board that he or she:

(A) Has successfully completed not fewer than sixty (60) semester credit hours of college education, to include a minimum of thirty (30) semester credit hours in the field of science; and

(B) Has completed a program in acupuncture and related techniques and has received a certificate or diploma from an institute approved by the board as described in this section. The training received in the program shall be for a period of no fewer than four (4) academic years and shall include a minimum of eight hundred (800) hours of supervised clinical practice.

(b) Before approval of an institute of acupuncture and related techniques, the board shall determine that the institute meets standards of professional education. These standards shall provide that the institute:

(1) Require, as a prerequisite to graduation, a program of study of at least four (4) academic years;

(2) Meet the minimum requirements of a board-approved national accrediting body;

(3) Require participation in a carefully supervised clinical or internship program; and

(4) Confer a certificate, diploma, or degree in acupuncture and related techniques only after personal attendance in classes and clinics.

(c) To qualify to take the examination, an applicant additionally must:

(1) Be at least twenty-one (21) years of age;

(2) Be a citizen of the United States or a legal resident;

(3) Not have had a license to practice acupuncture and related techniques in any other state suspended or revoked nor have been placed on probation for any cause;

(4) Not have been convicted of a felony listed under § 17 − 3 − 102; and

(5) Not be a habitual user of intoxicants, drugs, or hallucinatory preparations.

(d) The board may charge the following fees:

(1) Initial application for licensing, a fee not to exceed two hundred fifty dollars ($250);

(2) Written and practical examination not including the cost of the nationally recognized examination, a fee not to exceed three hundred fifty dollars ($350);

(3) Biennial licensing renewal, a fee not to exceed four hundred dollars ($400);

（4）Late renewal more than thirty （30） days, but not later than one （1） year, after expiration of a license, which late fee is in addition to any other fees, a fee not to exceed one hundred dollars （$100）;

（5）Reciprocal licensing, a fee not to exceed seven hundred fifty dollars （$750）;

（6）Annual continuing education provider registration, a fee not to exceed two hundred dollars （$200）; and

（7）Any and all fees to cover reasonable and necessary administrative expenses.

（e）（1）（A）If the applicant is approved, the applicant shall be admitted for examination.

（B）Should the applicant pass the examination, no part of the fee shall be returned, and the applicant shall be issued a license to practice acupuncture and related techniques in accordance with this chapter.

（C）Should an applicant be approved but fail to appear for the examination, no part of his or her fee shall be returned, but the applicant shall be eligible for examination at a later date.

（D）Should the approved applicant fail the examination, no part of his or her fee shall be returned, and the applicant shall be eligible for reexamination at a later date, at the discretion of the board, upon paying an examination fee of fifty dollars （$50.00）per failed subject up to one hundred fifty dollars （$150）.

（2）If the applicant is not approved, the application and one-half （½）of the examination fee shall be returned to the applicant with the reasons for the disapproval clearly stated.

§ 17‐102‐305.　Examinations

（a）Examinations shall be given in English and in writing and shall include the following subjects:

（1）Anatomy and physiology;

（2）Pathology;

（3）Diagnosis;

（4）Hygiene, sanitation, and sterilization techniques;

（5）Acupuncture and related principles, practices, and techniques; and

（6）Chinese herbal medicine.

（b）The Arkansas State Board of Acupuncture and Related Techniques shall hold an examination at least one （1） time each calendar year, and all applicants shall be notified in writing of the date and time of all examinations. The board may utilize a nationally recognized examination if it deems the national exam is sufficient to qualify a practitioner for licensure in this state.

（c）The board shall issue a license to every applicant whose application has been filed with and approved by the board and who has paid the required fees and who either:

（1）Has passed the board's examination with a score on each subject of not less than seventy percent （70%）; or

(2) Has achieved a passing score on a board-approved nationally recognized examination.

§ 17 – 102 – 306.   Display of license

A person licensed under this chapter shall post his or her license in a conspicuous location in his or her place of practice.

§ 17 – 102 – 307.   License renewal

Each licensee shall be required to pay biennial license renewal fees and meet continuing education requirements as specified in this chapter. A licensee who fails to renew his or her license within one (1) year after its expiration may not renew it, and it may not be restored, reissued, or reinstated thereafter, but that person may apply for and obtain a new license if he or she meets the following requirements:

(1) Meets all current standards of the Arkansas State Board of Acupuncture and Related Techniques; and

(2) Takes and passes the examination and pays all fees associated therewith as if seeking a license for the first time.

§ 17 – 102 – 308.   Continuing education

(a) The Arkansas State Board of Acupuncture and Related Techniques shall not renew the license of any person engaged in the practice of acupuncture and related techniques unless the licensee presents to the board evidence of attendance at a board-approved educational session or sessions of not fewer than twenty-four (24) hours of continuing education within the previous biennial period.

(b) Licensees residing out of state shall comply with the continuing education requirements.

(c) The presentation of a fraudulent or forged evidence of attendance at an educational session shall be a cause for suspension or revocation of the holder's license.

§ 17 – 102 – 309.   Disciplinary actions — Grounds — Action by the board

(a) The following acts by an applicant for a license or by a licensed acupuncturist shall constitute grounds for which the disciplinary actions specified in subsection (b) of this section may be taken by the Arkansas State Board of Acupuncture and Related Techniques:

(1) Attempting to obtain, obtaining, or renewing a license to practice acupuncture and related techniques by bribery, fraud, or deceit;

(2) Having pled guilty or nolo contendere to, or having been found guilty of, a crime in any jurisdiction which directly relates to the practice of acupuncture and related techniques or to the ability to practice same;

(3) Advertising, practicing, or attempting to practice under a name other than one's own;

(4) Making deceptive, untrue, or fraudulent representations in the practice of acupuncture and related techniques;

(5) Becoming mentally incompetent or unfit or incompetent by reason of negligence, habits, or other causes;

(6) Becoming habitually intemperate or addicted to the use of habit-forming drugs, illegal drugs, or alcohol;

(7) Acting unprofessionally in the practice of acupuncture and related techniques;

(8) Committing fraud or deceit in filing insurance forms, documents, or information pertaining to the health or welfare of a patient; or

(9) Willfully or repeatedly violating any of the provisions of this chapter or any rule or order of the board.

(b) When the board finds any person guilty of any of the acts set forth in subsection (a) of this section, it has the sole authority to:

(1) Refuse to issue a license to the offender;

(2) Revoke or suspend the offender's license;

(3) Restrict the practice of the offender;

(4) Impose an administrative fine not to exceed five thousand dollars ($5,000) for each count or separate offense;

(5) Reprimand the offender; or

(6) Place the offender on probation for a period of time and subject to such conditions as the board may specify.

(c) The board shall not reinstate the license of an acupuncturist or cause a license to be issued to a person it has deemed to be unqualified until such time as the board is satisfied that he or she has complied with all the terms and conditions set forth in the final order and that he or she is capable of safely engaging in the practice of acupuncture and related techniques.

(d) Disciplinary proceedings taken under this section shall be as provided in the Arkansas Administrative Procedure Act, § 25 - 15 - 201 et seq.

§ 17 - 102 - 310.　Exempted activities

Nothing herein shall be construed to prohibit or to require a license hereunder with respect to the practice of medicine and surgery, chiropractic, osteopathy, dentistry, podiatry, optometry, Christian Science, physical therapy, cosmetology, massage therapy, or any branch of the healing arts as defined by the laws of this state as now or hereafter enacted, it not being intended by this chapter to limit, restrict, enlarge, or alter the privileges and practices of any of these professions or branches of the healing arts.

§ 17 - 102 - 311.　Exemptions

(a) This chapter does not limit, interfere with, or prevent any other class of licensed healthcare professionals from practicing acupuncture and related techniques when permitted by its state licensing board.

(b) However, a chiropractic physician may practice acupuncture as part of chiropractic practice after completing an educational program in acupuncture from a college accredited by the Council on Chiropractic Education.

(c) A massage therapist may practice cupping therapy as part of massage therapy after completing an educational program in cupping therapy.

§ 17 – 102 – 312.   Legend drugs

An acupuncturist as defined in § 17 – 102 – 102(2) shall not prescribe, dispense, or administer a legend drug as defined under § 20 – 64 – 503.

§ 17 – 102 – 313.   Injections

An acupuncturist as defined in § 17 – 102 – 102(2) shall not administer an injection of a substance.

ARKANSAS ADMINISTRATIVE CODE

007.37.1 – I.   TITLE I

A. DEFINITIONS: For the purpose of these rules the following definitions apply in addition to those in the Act.

1. "Act" is the Arkansas Acupuncture Practices Act, as found in Ark. Code Ann. § 17 – 102 – 101 et seq.

2. "Acupuncture" means the insertion, manipulation, and removal of acupuncture needles from the body, and the use of other modalities and procedures at specific locations on the body, for the prevention, cure, or correction of a malady, illness, injury, pain, or other condition or disorder by controlling and regulating the flow and balance of energy and functioning of the patient to restore and maintain health. Acupuncture shall not be considered surgery.

3. "Acupuncturist" means a person licensed under the Act to practice acupuncture and related techniques in the State of Arkansas, and includes the term licensed acupuncturist, and the abbreviation "L.Ac."

4. "Applicant" is a person who has submitted to the Board an application for licensure.

5. "Board" is the Arkansas State Board of Acupuncture and Related Techniques.

6. "Clinical Experience" is the practice of acupuncture and related techniques as defined in the Act, after graduation from an educational program in acupuncture and related techniques as required herein. A year of clinical experience shall be consistent with the National Commission for the Certification of Acupuncture and Oriental Medicine's (NCCAOM) requirements.

7. "Institution" is a school that teaches an educational program in acupuncture and related techniques, certified by the Accreditation Commission for Acupuncture and Oriental Medicine (ACAOM) and that has been approved by the Board, pursuant to Ark. Code Ann. § 17 – 102 – 304(b).

8. "Licensee" is an individual licensed pursuant to the Act and defined as an acupuncturist under Title I. A.3. of these Rules. Those persons exempted under § 17 – 102 – 311 shall not be

considered as licensed under the Act and shall not use the descriptive term "licensed" referring to an acupuncture practice in Arkansas.

9. "Moxibustion" means the use of heat on, or above, or on acupuncture needles, at specific locations on the body for the prevention, cure, or correction of a malady, illness, injury, pain, or other condition or disorder.

10. "Office" is the physical facility used for the practice of acupuncture and related techniques.

11. "Related Techniques" are the techniques used in the Chinese and Asian traditional healing arts in addition to acupuncture as set out in Title I, Section B, Scope of Practice herein, including Chinese herbs.

12. "Rules" are the rules promulgated pursuant to the Act, governing acupuncturists, applicants, educational programs, educational institutions, and all matters covered by the Act.

13. "Supervised Clinical Practice" is the observation and application of acupuncture and related techniques in actual treatment situations under appropriate supervision, as defined by NCCAOM.

14. "Supervision" is the coordination, direction and continued evaluation at first hand of the person in training or engaged in obtaining clinical practice and shall be provided by a qualified instructor or tutor as set forth in a board-approved institute of acupuncture and related techniques.

B. SCOPE OF PRACTICE: The practice of acupuncture and related techniques in Arkansas is a distinct system of primary health care with the goal of prevention, cure, or correction of any illness, injury pain or other disorder or condition by controlling and regulating the flow and balance of energy and functioning of the person to restore and maintain health. Acupuncture and related techniques include all of the allied traditional and modern diagnostic, treatment, and therapeutic methods of the Chinese/Asian healing arts. The scope of practice of acupuncturists shall include but is not limited to:

1. Evaluation and management services.

2. Examination and diagnostic testing.

3. The ordering of radiological, laboratory or other diagnostic tests.

4. The stimulation of points or areas of the body using needles, moxabustion and other heating modalities, cold, light, lasers, sound, vibration, magnetism, electricity, cupping, bleeding, suction, pressure, ion pumping cords, or other devices or means.

5. Physical medicine modalities and techniques, including, tui na, gua sha, shiatsu, anmo, and other massage incidental to acupuncture and related techniques.

6. Therapeutic exercises, breathing techniques, meditation, and the use of biofeedback and other devices that utilize color, light, sound, electromagnetic energy and other means therapeutically.

7. Dietary and nutritional counseling and the administration of food, beverages and dietary

supplements therapeutically.

8. The recommendation of any Chinese herbal medicine, Western herbal medicine, or substances such as vitamins, minerals, enzymes, amino acids, nutritional supplements, and glandulars, lawfully and commercially available in the United States.

9. Counseling regarding physical, emotional and spiritual lifestyle balance.

C. Provided, however, the practice of acupuncture in Arkansas shall not involve:

a. Manipulation, mobilization or adjustment to the spine or extra-spinal articulations;

b. The prescribing, dispensing, injection or administering of any substance or legend drug as defined under A.C.A. 20 – 64 – 503;

007.37.1 – II.   TITLE II

A.1   BOARD COMPOSITION AND DUTIES: In addition to its duties described in the Act, the Board shall:

1. Meet in special meetings at any time. Notice of special meetings shall be provided to Board members, the media which have requested notification, and all other interested parties who have requested notification of such meeting at least twenty-four (24) hours in advance of such special meetings.

2. Meet in regular meetings upon such a schedule as shall be set by the Board. Notice of regular meetings shall be provided to Board members, the media, and all interested parties who have requested notification of such meeting at least three (3) days in advance of such regular meetings.

3. Keep a file of all approved educational programs.

4. Keep a file of all licensees and provisional licensees.

5. Issue certificates of approval of educational programs and educational institutions.

6. Delegate its ministerial duties if it so chooses, as provided by the Act.

7. Notify the Governor when any board member has missed three consecutive regular meetings without attending any intermediate special meeting.

8. Elect a President, Secretary, and Treasurer at the first Board meeting held each May.

9. Perform such other duties and shall exercise such other powers as may be conferred upon it by statute, or as may be reasonably implied from such statutory powers and duties and as may be reasonably necessary in the performance of its responsibilities under the Act, pursuant to Ark. Code Ann. § 17 – 102 – 108.

A.2   PUBLIC RECORDS: All records kept by the Board shall be available for public inspection pursuant to the Arkansas Freedom of Information Act and the Arkansas Administrative Procedures Act.

B. MEETINGS OF THE BOARD

(a) Regular Meetings. The Board shall meet at least once in every six (6) months, and may meet more often.

(b) Special Meetings. The Board may meet in special meetings called at any time at the pleasure of the President or by the Secretary upon the request of any two (2) full members of the Board.

(c) Quorum. A quorum of the Board shall consist of three (3) full members of the Board in attendance at any meeting. For purposes of determining a quorum, the ex officio member shall not be considered a full member.

(d) Voting. Any and every official action taken by the Board shall require an affirmative vote of a majority of the full membership of the Board that is three (3) out of the five (5) full members. No vote on any official action shall include a vote by the ex officio member.

C. ADOPTION OF RULES

The Board may adopt such rules as are necessary to conduct its business and administer its duties as found in the Act. All rules shall be adopted pursuant to the provisions of the Arkansas Administrative Procedures Act. Prior to any proposed rule being submitted to the Administrative Rules and Regulations Committee of the Arkansas Legislative Council, said rule shall be approved in writing by the Arkansas State Medical Board.

In addition to rules proposed by the Board, interested parties may petition the Board for a change in or addition to the rules pursuant to the Arkansas Administrative Procedure Act. The Board shall consider such written request at its next regular meeting.

007.37.1 - Ⅲ.   TITLE Ⅲ

A.1   GENERAL

All agency action regarding licensure shall be governed by the Arkansas Acupuncture Practice Act, A.C.A. 17 - 102 - 101 and, when applicable, A.C.A. §§ 25 - 15 - 201 et seq.

A.2   REQUIREMENT TO KEEP CURRENT ADDRESSES ON FILE

All persons holding a license issued by Arkansas State Board of Acupuncture and Related Techniques are required to provide the board with information so that the board can remain in contact and provide notice of complaints and/or hearings. The licensee is required to provide written notice to the board of any change in business and/or residence address within 10 working days of the change. Service of notices of hearing sent by mail will be addressed to the latest address on file with the board.

A.3   APPLICATION FOR ORIGINAL LICENSURE

(a) The Board shall not cause a license to be issued to any person it has deemed to be unqualified pursuant to the provisions of the Act and these rules.

(b) All applicants are required to be at least 21 years of age, be a citizen of the United States and/or a legal resident, not have had a license to practice acupuncture and related techniques in any other state suspended or revoked nor have been placed on probation for any cause, not have been convicted of a felony listed in Ark. Code Ann. § 17 - 3 - 102, and not be a habitual user of intoxicants, drugs or hallucinatory preparations.

(c) Every Applicant must provide a statement signed by the Applicant and the signature verified by a Notary Public as to whether he or she:

(1) Has had had a license to practice acupuncture and related techniques in any other state suspended or revoked or been placed on probation for any cause; and

(2) Has been convicted of a felony listed in Ark. Code Ann. § 17 – 3 – 102.

A.4   Every person seeking an original Arkansas license to practice acupuncture and related techniques shall file an application on the current form provided by the Board. All applications must be complete and in English.

(a) EXHIBITS REQUIRED: Every application shall be accompanied by:

1. The fee for application for licensure specified in Title Ⅲ, C.

2. A notarized form signed by the Applicant authorizing the release to the Board of additional information regarding the Applicant and his or her qualifications for licensure, including but not limited to educational background, criminal background check, transcripts, credentials, and accreditation information on educational institutions.

(b) VERIFICATION: Verification of the Applicant's education shall include:

1. A certified copy of the Applicant's certificate or diploma from an accredited educational institution evidencing completion of the required program of study in acupuncture and related techniques.

2. An official copy of the Applicant's transcript that shall be sent directly to the Board by the approved educational institution from which the Applicant received the certificate or diploma, and that shall verify the Applicant's satisfactory completion of the required academic and clinical education and that shall designate the completed subjects and the hours of study completed in each subject; and

(c) SUFFICIENCY OF DOCUMENT: The Board shall determine the sufficiency of the documentation to support the application for licensure. The Board may, in its sole discretion, request further documentation, proof of qualifications and/or require a personal interview with any Applicant to establish his or her qualifications.

B. AUTHORIZED FORMS

The Board shall authorize such forms as are necessary from time to time for the application for licenses, and the renewal of licenses. The authorized forms may be reproduced without permission from the Board but shall not be altered or changed in any way by any prospective Licensee. Authorized forms shall be available from the Board to any member of the public or any prospective Licensee. Requests for forms may be made in writing or by telephone call to the Board at its offices, or to the Board Secretary.

C.1   REQUIREMENTS FOR LICENSING

(a) EDUCATIONAL REQUIREMENTS: Every Applicant shall provide satisfactory proof that he or she has completed and graduated from an approved four year academic educational program in acupuncture and related techniques and has received a certificate or diploma for completion of the approved educational program from an institute approved under C.1.(a)1. The program must include an education in Chinese herbal medicine, as required by ACAOM.

(1) APPROVED EDUCATIONAL INSTITUTION AND PROGRAM. For the Board to determine that an institution meets the standards of professional education, the institution must require a program of study of at least four (4) academic years which must meet Accreditation Commission for Acupuncture and Oriental Medicine's (ACAOM) level of education and standards or other criteria as found reasonable by the Board, require participation by students in a supervised clinical or internship program which includes a minimum of eight hundred (800) hours of supervised clinical practice, and confer a certificate, diploma, or degree only after personal attendance in classes and clinics. An applicant from a foreign institution shall provide documentation to show that the institution and program meets the same or higher standards.

(2) PREREQUISITES: Has successfully completed not fewer than sixty (60) semester credit hours of college education, to include a minimum of thirty (30) semester credit hours in a relevant field of science, including but not limited to biology, chemistry, anatomy, physiology, and psychology.

(b) EXAMINATION REQUIREMENT.

An applicant shall be required to pass a Board-approved nationally recognized examination on Oriental Medicine or on both acupuncture and Chinese herbal medicine.

C.2   FEES: The Board shall charge fees for the following, in compliance with A.C.A. Section 17 - 102 - 304(d)(1)-(7):

(a) Initial/reciprocal application for licensing, set at $250.00;

(b) Biennial licensing renewal or original and reciprocal licensees, set at $400.00;

(c) Late renewal (in addition to the application fee), set at $100.00;

(d) Continuing education provider one-time registration fee, set at $200.00;

(e) Administrative support fee (annual), set at $100.00;

D. RECIPROCAL LICENSING:

(a) Required Qualifications. An applicant applying for reciprocal licensure shall hold a substantially similar license in another United States' jurisdiction.

(1) A license from another state is substantially similar to an Arkansas license if applicant has, or the other state's licensure qualifications require an applicant to have, passed an examination(s) given by NCCAOM in either:

i. Oriental Medicine; or

ii. Both acupuncture and Chinese herbal medicine.

(2) The applicant shall hold his or her occupational licensure in good standing;

(3) The applicant shall not have had a license revoked for:

i. An act of bad faith; or

ii. A violation of law, rule, or ethics;

(4) The applicant shall not hold a suspended or probationary license in a United States' jurisdiction.

(b) Required documentation. An applicant shall submit a fully-executed application, the required fee, and the documentation described below.

(1) As evidence that the applicant's license from another jurisdiction is substantially similar to Arkansas's, the applicant shall submit the following information:

i. Evidence of current and active licensure in that state. The Board may verify this information online or by telephone; and

ii. Evidence that the applicant has passed an examination(s) given by NCCAOM in either Oriental Medicine or both acupuncture and Chinese herbal medicine. The Board may verify this information online or by telephone.

(2) To demonstrate that the applicant has not had a license revoked for bad faith or a violation of law, rule, or ethics, as required by subsection III.D.(a)(3), and that the applicant does not hold a license on suspended or probationary status, as required by subsection III.D.(a)(4), the applicant shall provide the Board with:

i. The names of all states in which the applicant is currently licensed or has been previously licensed;

ii. Letters of good standing or other information from each state in which the applicant is currently or has ever been licensed showing that the applicant has not had his license revoked for the reasons listed in subsection III.D.(a)(3) and does not hold a license on suspended or probationary status as described in subsection III.D.(a)(4). The Board may verify this information online or by telephone.

(c) Temporary License

(1) The Board shall issue a temporary license immediately upon receipt of the application, the required fee, and the documentation required under subsection III.D.(b)(1).i. and ii. to show that the applicant has a license in good standing from another jurisdiction that is substantially similar to an Arkansas license.

(2) An applicant shall submit a completed the application with all required remaining documentation in order to receive a license.

(3) The temporary license shall be effective for at least 90 days or until the Board makes a decision on the application, whichever occurs first.

E. ACUPUNCTURE DETOX SPECIALISTS.

(a) Detox specialists shall register with the Board by providing either:

(1) A certified copy of documentation of the completion of the National Acupuncture Detoxification Association (NADA) certification course; or

(2) Evidence of active certification (or registration or licensure) as an acupuncture detox

specialist in another state.

(b) An acupuncture detox specialist shall be permitted to practice only under the supervision of an acupuncturist who is licensed by the Arkansas State Board of Acupuncture and Related Techniques.

(c) An acupuncture detox specialist shall be permitted to use only the five (5) point ear protocol of NADA for substance abuse and shall not treat or offer treatment in any other capacity.

F. Acupuncture Applicants from States that Do Not Licensee[1] Acupuncturists

(a) An applicant from a state that does not license acupuncturists shall be sufficiently competent in the field of acupuncture and related techniques.

(b) Required documentation.

(1) An applicant shall submit a fully-executed application and the required fee; and

(2) As evidence that the applicant is sufficiently competent in the field of acupuncture and related techniques, the applicant shall provide evidence that the applicant has passed an examination(s) given by NCCAOM in either Oriental Medicine or both acupuncture and Chinese herbal medicine. The Board may verify this information online or by telephone.

G. Military Licensure

(a) (1) "Automatic licensure" means the granting of occupational licensure without an individual's having met occupational licensure requirements provided under Title 17 of the Arkansas Code or by these Rules.

(2) As used in this subsection, "returning military veteran" means a former member of the United States Armed Forces who was discharged from active duty under circumstances other than dishonorable.

(b) The Board shall grant automatic licensure to an individual who holds a substantially equivalent license in another U.S. jurisdiction and is:

(1) An active duty military service member stationed in the State of Arkansas;

(2) A returning military veteran applying for licensure within one (1) year of his or discharge from active duty; or

(3) The spouse of a person under subsection III.G.(b)(1) or (2).

(c) The Board shall grant such automatic licensure upon receipt of all of the below:

(1) Payment of the initial licensure fee;

(2) Evidence that the individual holds a substantially equivalent license in another state; and

(3) Evidence that the applicant is a qualified applicant under subsection III.G.(b)(1), (2), or (3).

H. Pre-Licensure Criminal Background Check

(a) Pursuant to Act 990 of 2019, an individual may petition for a pre-licensure determination of whether the individual's criminal record will disqualify the individual from licensure.

(b) The individual must obtain the pre-licensure criminal background check petition form from the Board.

(c) The Board's staff will respond with a decision in writing to a completed petition within a reasonable time.

(d) The Board staff's response will state the reasons for the decision.

(e) All decisions of the Board's staff in response to the petition will be determined by the information provided by the individual.

(f) A decision of the Board's staff in response to a pre-licensure criminal background check petition is not subject to appeal.

(g) The Board will retain a copy of the petition and response and it will be reviewed during the formal application process.

I. Waiver Request

(a) If an individual has been convicted of an offense listed in A.C.A. §17 – 3 – 102(a), except those permanently disqualifying offenses found in subsection A.C.A. §17 – 3 – 102(e), the Board may waive disqualification of a potential applicant or revocation of a license based on the conviction if a request for a waiver is made by:

(1) An affected applicant for a license; or

(2) An individual holding a license subject to revocation.

(b) The Board may grant a waiver upon consideration of the following, without limitation:

(1) The age at which the offense was committed;

(2) The circumstances surrounding the offense;

(3) The length of time since the offense was committed;

(4) Subsequent work history since the offense was committed;

(5) Employment references since the offense was committed;

(6) Character references since the offense was committed;

(7) Relevance of the offense to the occupational license; and

(8) Other evidence demonstrating that licensure of the applicant does not pose a threat to the health or safety of the public.

(c) A request for a waiver, if made by an applicant, must be in writing and accompany the completed application and fees.

(d) The Board will respond with a decision in writing and will state the reasons for the decision.

(e) An appeal of a determination under this section will be subject to the Administrative Procedures Act §25 – 15 – 201 et seq.

007.37.1 – IV.   TITLE IV

A.1   LICENSE RENEWAL: Every Applicant for license renewal must provide a statement as to whether he or she, since applying for licensure or since last applying for license renewal, which ever occurred most recently:

(a) Has been subject to any disciplinary action in any jurisdiction related to the practice of acupuncture and related techniques, or related to any other health care professions for which the Applicant for license renewal is licensed, certified, registered or legally recognized to practice; and

(b) Has been convicted of a felony listed under Ark. Code Ann. § 17 – 3 – 102 in any jurisdiction.

Any Applicant for license renewal who has been subject to any action or proceeding comprehended by Title III.A.1 may be subject to disciplinary action, including denial, suspension or revocation of licensure.

A.2 LICENSING PERIOD: The licensing period shall run from January 1 to the second consecutive December 31. A newly licensed acupuncturist shall be issued a license that shall be required to be renewed on the second December 31 following the initial date of licensure. If license is not renewed by this date, license shall expire and licensee shall not practice until such time that renewal requirements have been met. The Board shall send renewal notifications to licensees no later than December 1.

A.3 LICENSE RENEWAL: Except as provided otherwise in the Act, or in these Rules, or pursuant to other State law, each licensed acupuncturist shall be granted renewal of his or her license for two years upon receipt by the Board of his or her renewal application that shall include any continuing education documentation required by Ark. Code Ann. 17 – 102 – 308 and Title IV.B. of these Rules and the fee for the biennial license renewal specified in Title III.C.2.

A.4 LATE LICENSE RENEWAL:

(a) Each licensee shall be required to pay biennial license renewal fees and meet continuing education requirements as specified in the Act and in these Rules. During a grace period of 30 days after the expiration of the license (December 31), no late fee will be required. However, if a license is expired for thirty (30) days to one (1) year, the late renewal fee shall be assessed and the licensee shall meet all of requirements of renewal. Practice of acupuncture and related techniques is not allowed during any period of expiration.

(b) An individual who meets the conditions established in A.C.A. § 17 – 1 – 107 and can demonstrate that the individual passed the applicable examination(s) with scores sufficient for licensure at the time the individual's initial license was issued shall, in order to be re-licensed furnish evidence of completion of the number of hours of acceptable continuing professional education (CPE) computed by multiplying twelve (12) times the number of years the licensee has held an inactive or invalid license, not to exceed 60 hours.

A.5 EXPIRED LICENSE: A licensee shall not practice acupuncture and related techniques following the expiration of the license, until such time that the expired license is renewed pursuant to Title IV.A.3 and Title IV.A.4.

B.1   CONTINUING EDUCATION: The Board shall not renew the license of any licensee unless the licensee presents to the Board evidence of attendance at a board-approved educational session or sessions of not less than twenty-four (24) hours of continuing education within the previous biennial period, which shall include a CPR course for healthcare professionals, to be considered as two (2) hours of the required twenty-four (24) hours of continuing education.

Approved continuing education courses may not be retaken for credit in consecutive biennial periods. Proof of teaching courses related to acupuncture or related techniques may be applied to a maximum of four (4) hours of continuing education, subject to approval by the board.

B.2   The Board may accept hours from Board approved courses or NCCAOM approved courses as valid continuing education hours, provided that documentation contains: provider contact information, course information (including any relevant NCCAOM reference), and official seal or signature.

(a) If the course has not been approved by NCCAOM or the Board for continuing education, the licensee shall submit information to the Board about the course, including the person or organization sponsoring or presenting the course, an outline of the subject matter covered by the course and the length of the course in hours.

(b) It is the Board's intention to respond to all submissions of continuing education courses for approval in a timely manner. If the submission is not specifically denied in writing by the Board within 60 days after the postmark of the applicant's submission, the submission shall be approved.

(c) Applications for approval of providers of continuing education shall be on an individual course basis. Provider applicants shall be responsible for obtaining and submitting the proper information and fees to the Board.

(d) If the Board denies approval for any course or courses upon application for license renewal, the applicant shall have an additional 90 days to obtain the required hours during which time the applicant can continue to practice. Failure to acquire the proper hours within said 90 days shall result in non-renewal of the license.

007.37.1 – V.   TITLE V

A. HEARING PROCEDURES ON DENIED APPLICATIONS

(a) If a preliminary determination is made by the board that an application for license should be denied the board will inform the applicant of the grounds or basis of the proposed denial in writing. Any Applicant who is denied the issuance of a license by the Board may appeal such decision and request a hearing before the full Board on the application. The Applicant shall file the appeal in writing with the Board within thirty (30) days of receipt of the notice of denial.

(b) Within thirty (30) days of the filing of the appeal on the denial of a license, the Board shall hold a hearing on the application. The Applicant shall be notified in writing of the date, time, and location of the hearing at least twenty (20) days in advance of the hearing on the appeal.

(c) The Board and the Applicant shall disclose no later than ten (10) days before the hearing on the merits the names, addresses and telephone numbers of all persons who they intend to call as witnesses at the hearing, and shall provide a list of exhibits which will be offered for introduction into evidence.

(d) The Applicant shall not engage in communications with any member of the Board on any matter related to the application or the appeal prior to the date set for the hearing, nor shall the Board members engage in communications in violation of the Arkansas Administrative Procedures Act or the Arkansas Freedom of Information Act.

(e) At the hearing, the Applicant shall be provided the opportunity to present evidence, by testimony or by documents, cross examine all witnesses, and call witnesses for the Board to consider with respect to the grant or denial of the license sought by the Applicant.

(f) Hearings before the Board are governed by the Arkansas Administrative Procedures Act, and the Board shall not be bound by the Arkansas Rules of Evidence or the Arkansas Rules of Civil Procedure in its proceedings. However, the Rules may serve as a guide to the presiding officer for the conduct of the hearing. The President of the Board shall rule on all motions as well as all evidentiary and procedural matters that arise during the hearing. The Board may appoint an impartial hearing officer to preside at or assist the Board.

(g) The Board shall not cause a license to be issued to a person it has deemed to be unqualified until and unless the Board has been satisfied that the Applicant has complied with all the terms, conditions, and requirements set forth in the Act and these rules, and that the Applicant is capable of safely and ethically engaging in the practice of acupuncture and related techniques.

(h) When an Applicant has been denied a license, he or she may not reapply for a license until one of the following has taken place:

(1) one full year has passed since the date the license was denied; or

(2) there has been a significant change in circumstances or facts with respect to the applicant's credentials and/or qualifications.

B.1　COMPLAINT AND DISCIPLINARY PROCEDURES

(a) A complaint may be initiated by any person by a telephone call, a written complaint, or a walk-in complaint presented to any Board Member or the Board's representative. The Board shall prepare a complaint form. This form shall be available at the office of the Board or from the Secretary of the Board. A written complaint form shall be submitted to the Board to initiate the review process. If a complaint is made by telephone, a complaint form shall be mailed to the complainant.

(b) The Secretary of the Board shall maintain a written log of all complaints received which records the date of the complaint, the name, address and telephone number of the Complainant, the name of the subject of the complaint (Respondent), the method by which the complaint was made (e. g., telephone, letter, sworn written complaint, etc.), and other pertinent data as the Board may direct.

(c) Acupuncturists shall have every patient sign a form that contains the following information: "All licensed acupuncturists are governed by Arkansas statutes A.C.A. § 17 – 102 – 101 et seq, and the Rules of the Arkansas State Board of Acupuncture and Related Techniques (ASBART). Patients may contact ASBART for information or complaints."

B.2   PROCEDURES FOR RECEIPT OF A COMPLAINT

(a) Upon receipt of a written, signed complaint, or upon the Board's own action as initiated by a vote of the majority of the members of the Board acting at a duly convened meeting of the Board, and as then reduced to a written complaint, if the Board has reasonable cause to believe that the Act or the Rules promulgated pursuant thereto have been or are being violated, the Board Secretary shall:

1. Log in the date of receipt of any complaint initiated by the Board or any other party.

2. Determine whether the Respondent is licensed by the Board to practice acupuncture and related techniques in the State of Arkansas, or is an Applicant for licensure.

3. Assign a complaint number and create an individual file. Complaint numbering shall begin with the last two digits of the year in which the complaint is filed and shall then continue sequentially (e.g. 11 – 001).

4. Within seven (7) working days of the date of receipt of the complaint, send written acknowledgment of receipt of the complaint to the Complainant.

(b) Furnish the Respondent with a copy of the complaint and all documents filed in relation to the complaint by certified mail within seven (7) working days of the receipt of the complaint by the Board. The Respondent shall also be informed in writing at this time that the Board has initiated an investigation into the complaint, and that the Respondent may furnish the Board documents relevant to the complaint.

(c) Both parties shall refrain from contacting any member of the Board while the complaint is under investigation, and until the matter has been resolved.

B.3   REVIEW OF THE COMPLAINT

(a) The Board will review all written, signed complaints filed against a Licensee or Applicant.

(b) The Respondent shall be provided at least twenty (20) calendar days in which to file a written response to the complaint, and shall be advised that he or she is required to provide all documents and exhibits in support of his or her position.

(c) If the Board determines that further information is needed, it may issue subpoenas, or employ an investigator, or experts, or other persons whose services are determined to be necessary, in order to assist in the processing and investigation of the complaint.

(d) Upon completion of the investigation, the Board will prepare a written summary of its initial findings. The summary shall not identify any of the parties by name, but by case number only until the issue has been set for a hearing. The Board shall provide a copy of its findings to the Complainant and Respondent prior to the matter being set for a hearing.

(e) If the Board determines that it does not have jurisdiction, or if it does have jurisdiction but finds that no violation exists, both the Complainant and Respondent will be notified in writing. The letter will explain why the case cannot be accepted for investigation and/or action (e.g. due to the statute of limitations, or the nature of the complaint being a fee dispute, or there being no violation of the Act or the Rules), or it may note that the complaint can be referred to another agency. A letter from the Board will be sent within thirty (30) days of the date of the Board's decision to both the Complainant and Respondent. The letter will state the Board's action and the reasons for its decision. The letter will be signed by the President.

B.4   HEARING BY THE BOARD

(a) Unless the Board dismisses the complaint pursuant to Title V. B.3(e), above, the complaint shall be set for a hearing before the full Board. The matter shall be referred to only by the assigned case number, and shall be brought pursuant to the provisions of the Arkansas Administrative Procedure Act.

(b) The Respondent shall be notified of the hearing at least thirty (30) days in advance of the date set for the hearing. The Complainant shall also receive a copy of the notice of hearing. The notice of hearing shall set forth the charges and allegations against Respondent in sufficient detail so as to provide full disclosure and notice of all violations of the Act and rules.

(c) The Respondent may file a response to the notice of hearing, but is not required to do so. Any written response to the charges must be filed with the Board ten (10) days in advance of the date set for the hearing on the complaint.

(d) The Respondent may waive a hearing on the notice and complaint. Such waiver of the right to a hearing must be in writing, signed by the Respondent, and filed with the Board.

(e) At any time the Board may enter into a settlement agreement with the Licensee as a means of resolving a complaint. Any proposed settlement agreement must be approved by the Board upon a majority vote of those qualified to vote, and must be approved further by the Licensee or Applicant, upon a knowing and intentional waiver by the Licensee or Applicant of his or her right to a hearing.

(f) The Board is empowered to issue subpoenas pursuant to the Ark. Code Ann. § 17 – 102 – 206(c) and Ark. Code Ann. § 17 – 80 – 102.

(g) The Board may appoint an impartial hearing officer to preside at or assist the Board in any hearing.

B.5   DISCIPLINARY PROCEEDINGS

(a) The parties shall disclose to each other no later than ten (10) days before the hearing on the merits the names, addresses and telephone numbers of all persons who they intend to call as witnesses at the hearing, and shall provide a list of exhibits which each intends to offer for introduction into evidence. If the opposing party is not in possession of a copy of any of the listed exhibits, the party which intends to offer the exhibits shall provide copies of all such exhibits at the time the written exhibit list is provided.

(b) The Respondent shall not engage in communications with any member of the Board on any matter after a notice of hearing has been issued by the Board, nor shall the Board members engage in ex-parte communications in violation of the Arkansas Administrative Procedures Act or the Arkansas Freedom of Information Act.

(c) At the hearing, each party shall be provided the opportunity to present evidence, by testimony or by documents, cross examine witnesses and call witnesses.

(d) Hearings before the Board are governed by the Arkansas Administrative Procedures Act and shall not be bound by the Arkansas Rules of Evidence or the Arkansas Rules of Civil Procedure in its proceedings. However, the Rules may serve as a guide to the presiding officer for the conduct of the hearing. The President of the Board or its duly appointed hearing officer shall rule on all motions as well as all evidentiary and procedural matters that arise during the hearing.

(e) When a Licensee is found guilty of any of the acts set forth in the Act or a violation of any Order of the Board, or of a violation of these rules, the Board may impose the following sanctions:

1. Refuse to issue a license to the Applicant;

2. Revoke or suspend the license of the Licensee;

3. Restrict the practice of the Licensee;

4. Impose an administrative fine not to exceed five thousand dollars ($5,000.00) for each count or separate offense of which the Licensee is found guilty;

5. Reprimand the Licensee; or

6. Place the Licensee on probation for such period of time as the Board deems is appropriate and impose such conditions as the Board may specify for the conduct of the Licensee's practice.

In the event that the Board revokes or suspends the license of an acupuncturist, the license shall not be reinstated until such time as the Board is satisfied that the Licensee has complied with all the terms and conditions set forth in the final disciplinary order of the Board, and that the Licensee is capable of safely and ethically engaging in the practice of acupuncture and related techniques. Upon written request by the Licensee for reinstatement, the Board shall review the case to determine whether a license should be reissued.

007.37.1 – VI. TITLE VI

A. PROHIBITED ACTS AND CONDUCT OF LICENSED PROFESSIONALS: Any Applicant for license renewal who provides the Board with false information or makes a false statement to the Board with regard to any action or proceeding comprehended by the Act or these rules may be subject to disciplinary action, including denial, suspension or revocation of licensure. Prior to the entry of a final order to suspend or revoke a license, or to impose other sanctions upon a licensee, the Board will serve the licensee a complaint and notice hearing in writing. The licensee shall be afforded the opportunity for a hearing and the Board has the burden of proving the alleged facts and violations of law stated in the complaint.

The following acts or omissions may be considered as grounds for disciplinary action by the Board, following notice and hearing, or for the denial of application for licensure:

(1) PROFESSIONAL INCOMPETENCE: Failure to possess or apply the knowledge, or to use the skill and care ordinarily used by reasonably well-qualified acupuncturists practicing under similar circumstances, giving due consideration to the locality involved.

(2) FAILURE TO FOLLOW PROPER INSTRUMENT STERILIZATION PROCEDURE: Failure to use sterile instruments or failure to follow proper instrument sterilization procedures including the use of biological monitors and the keeping of accurate records of sterilization cycles and equipment service maintenance as described in the manufacturer's instruction manual, and the current edition of "Clean Needle Technique For Acupuncturists — A Manual" published by the National Commission For The Certification Of Acupuncturists. This provision shall not apply to needles, which may not be re-used or sterilized for a subsequent use on more than one patient under any circumstances.

(3) FAILURE TO FOLLOW CLEAN NEEDLE TECHNIQUE: Failure to follow clean needle technique as defined in the current edition of "Clean Needle Technique For Acupuncturist — A Manual" published by the National Commission For The Certification Of Acupuncturists.

(4) FALSE REPORTING: Willfully making or filing false reports or records in his or her practice as an acupuncturist, or filing false statements for collection of fees for services that were not rendered.

(5) OUT OF STATE DISCIPLINARY ACTION: Committing any act or omission which has resulted in disciplinary action against the acupuncturist or applicant by the acupuncture licensing or disciplinary authority or court in another state, territory, or country.

(6) PROCURING LICENSE BY BRIBERY, FRAUD, OR DECEIT: Committing fraud or deceit in procuring or attempting to procure or renew a license or a provisional license to practice in the profession of acupuncture and related techniques by making false statements, or providing false information the application for licensure. An acupuncturist or an applicant shall be guilty of bribery if he or she attempts to pay money or provide anything of value to a member of the licensing Board in return for having a license issued.

(7) MISREPRESENTATION: Advertising, practicing, or attempting to practice under a name other than one's own.

(8) FALSE ADVERTISING: Soliciting or advertising for patronage by any means which

is misleading, fraudulent, deceptive, or dishonest. It also constitutes false advertising for an acupuncturist to identify himself or herself as a doctor or physician.

(9) EDUCATIONAL FRAUD: Practicing fraud, deceit, gross negligence, or misconduct in the operation of an educational program in acupuncture and related techniques.

(10) FAILURE TO KEEP RECORDS: Failure to keep written records reflecting the course of treatment of the patient. Records shall be kept for a period of no less than five (5) years, and shall be subject to review by the Board.

(11) FAILURE TO PROVIDE RECORDS TO PATIENT: Failure to make available to a patient or client, upon request, copies of documents in the possession or under the control of the Licensee that have been prepared for and paid for by the patient or client.

(12) BREACH OF CONFIDENTIALITY: Revealing personally identifiable facts, data or information obtained in a professional capacity, without the prior consent of the patient or client, except as authorized or required by law.

(13) DELEGATING RESPONSIBILITIES TO UNQUALIFIED PERSONS:

a. Delegating professional responsibilities to a person when the acupuncturist delegating such responsibilities knows or has reason to know that the person is not qualified by education, by experience or by licensure or certification to perform the responsibilities; or

b. Failure to exercise appropriate supervision over Provisional Licensees or students who are authorized to practice only under the supervision of the acupuncturist.

(14) EXERCISING INFLUENCE WITHIN A PATIENT – DOCTOR RELATIONSHIP FOR PURPOSES OF ENGAGING A PATIENT IN SEXUAL ACTIVITY: Exercising influence within a patient-doctor relationship for the purpose of engaging in sexual activity with a patient.

(15) LACK OF FITNESS TO PRACTICE: Continuing to practice and provide treatment for patients when the Licensee:

a. Has become mentally incompetent or unfit, or has become incompetent by reason of negligence, habits, or other related causes; or

b. Has become habitually intemperate or addicted to the use of habit-forming drugs, illegal drugs, and/or alcohol.

(16) INSURANCE FRAUD: Knowingly committing fraud or deceit in the filing of insurance forms, documents, or information pertaining to the health or welfare of a patient, or knowingly allows an employee to file insurance forms, documents, or information pertaining to health or welfare benefits which are false.

(17) WILLFUL VIOLATIONS: Willfully or repeatedly violating any of the provisions of the Act or any of the provisions of these rules, or any lawful order of the Board.

(18) POSTING OF LICENSE: An acupuncturist who has been licensed by this Board shall post his or her license in a conspicuous location at his or her office or place of practice; failure to post the license may be considered unprofessional conduct.

(19) PUBLIC HEALTH AND SANITATION:

a. Failure to use only pre-sterilized, disposable needles in the administration of acupuncture;

b. Using staples in the practice of acupuncture;

c. Failing to wash hands with soap and water or other disinfectants before handling needles and between treatments of different patients;

d. Re-using the same needles on more than one patient in the administration of acupuncture.

(20) CRIMES LISTED UNDER A. C. A. § 17 - 3 - 102: Having pled guilty or nolo contendere to, or having been found guilty of, a crime listed in A.C.A. § 17 - 3 - 102.

(21) INCOMPETENCE AND UNPROFESSIONAL CONDUCT: The foregoing specifications of unprofessional conduct shall not be exclusive of the types of acts and omissions that may be found by the Board to constitute incompetence or unprofessional conduct.

B. EMERGENCY ACTION

(1) If the Board finds that the public health, safety, or welfare imperatively requires emergency action and incorporates that finding in its order, the Board can summarily suspend, limit, or restrict a license. The notice requirement in Title V. B.4 does not apply and must not be construed to prevent a hearing at the earliest time practicable.

(2) Emergency Order:

An emergency adjudicative order must contain findings that the public health, safety, and welfare imperatively require emergency action to be taken by the Board. The written order must include notification of the date on which Board proceedings are scheduled for completion.

Written Notice:

The written emergency adjudicative order will be immediately delivered to persons who are required to comply with the order. One or more of the following procedures will be used:

a. Personal delivery;

b. Certified mail, return receipt requested, to the last address on file with the Board;

c. First class mail to the last address on file with the Board

d. Fax. Fax may be used as the sole method of delivery if the person required to comply with the order has filed a written request that Board orders be sent by fax and has provided a fax number for that purpose

e. Oral Notice. Unless the written emergency order is served by personal delivery on the same day that the order issues, the Board shall make reasonable immediate efforts to contact by telephone the persons who are required to comply with the order.

f. Electronic mail (email) to the last known email address, with a request for an immediate acknowledgement of receipt by the persons.

(3) Unless otherwise provided by law, within 10 days after emergency action taken pursuant to paragraph B. (1) of this rule, the Board must initiate a formal suspension or revocation proceeding.

C. VOLUNTARY SURRENDER OF LICENSE

The licensee, in lieu of formal disciplinary proceedings, may offer to surrender his or her license, subject to the Board's determination to accept the proffered surrender, rather than conducting a formal disciplinary proceeding.

D. REINSTATEMENT AFTER SUSPENSION

(1) An order suspending a license may provide that a person desiring reinstatement may file with the Board a verified petition requesting reinstatement.

(2) The petition for reinstatement must set out the following:

a. That the individual has fully and promptly complied with the requirements of Title V.B.5(e) of these rules pertaining to the duty of a sanctioned professional;

b. That the individual has refrained from practicing in this profession during the period of suspension;

c. That the individual's license fee is current or has been tendered to the Board; and

d. That the individual has fully complied with the requirements imposed as conditions for reinstatement.

(3) Any knowing misstatement of fact may constitute grounds for denial or revocation of reinstatement.

(4) Failure to comply with the provisions of these Rules precludes consideration for reinstatement.

(5) No individual will be reinstated unless the Arkansas State Board of Acupuncture and Related Techniques approves reinstatement by majority vote.

E. RE – LICENSURE FOR REVOKED OR SURRENDERED LICENSE

(1) No individual who has had his or her license revoked or who has surrendered his or her license will be licensed, except on petition made to the Board. The petition for re-licensure is not allowed until at least two years after the revocation or surrender of license took effect.

(2) The applicant bears the burden of proof that he or she is rehabilitated following the revocation or surrender of his or her license, that he or she can engage in the conduct authorized by the license without undue risk to the public health, safety, and welfare, and that he or she is otherwise qualified for the license pursuant to § 17 – 102 – 101 et seq.

(3) The Board may impose any appropriate conditions or limitations on a license to protect the public health, safety, and welfare.

(4) The Board may require that the person seeking re-licensure take the licensing examination.

NORTH CAROLINA

NORTH CAROLINA GENERAL STATUTES ANNOTATED

§ 90 – 450. Purpose

It is the purpose of this Article to promote the health, safety, and welfare of the people of North Carolina by establishing an orderly system of acupuncture licensing and to provide a valid, effective means of establishing licensing requirements.

§ 90 – 451. Definitions

The following definitions apply in this Article:

(1) Acupuncture. — A form of health care developed from traditional and modern Chinese medical concepts that employ acupuncture diagnosis and treatment, and adjunctive therapies and diagnostic techniques, for the promotion, maintenance, and restoration of health and the prevention of disease.

(2) Board. — The Acupuncture Licensing Board.

(3) Practice of acupuncture or practice acupuncture. — The insertion of acupuncture needles and the application of moxibustion to specific areas of the human body based upon acupuncture diagnosis as a primary mode of therapy. Adjunctive therapies within the scope of acupuncture may include massage, mechanical, thermal, electrical, and electromagnetic treatment and the recommendation of herbs, dietary guidelines, and therapeutic exercise.

§ 90 – 452. Practice of acupuncture without license prohibited

(a) Unlawful Acts. — It is unlawful to engage in the practice of acupuncture without a license issued pursuant to this Article. It is unlawful to advertise or otherwise represent oneself as qualified or authorized to engage in the practice of acupuncture without having the license required by this Article. A violation of this subsection is a Class 1 misdemeanor.

(b) Exemptions. — This section shall not apply to any of the following persons:

(1) A physician licensed under Article 1 of this Chapter.

（2）A student practicing acupuncture under the direct supervision of a licensed acupuncturist as part of a course of study approved by the Board.

（3）A chiropractor licensed under Article 8 of this Chapter.

§ 90 – 453. Acupuncture Licensing Board

（a）Membership. — The Acupuncture Licensing Board shall consist of nine members, three appointed by the Governor and six by the General Assembly. The six members appointed by the General Assembly shall be licensed to practice acupuncture in this State and shall not be licensed physicians under Article 1 of this Chapter. The persons initially appointed to those positions by the General Assembly need not be licensed at the time of selection but shall have met the qualifications under G. S. 90 – 455 (a) (4) and (5). Of the Governor's three appointments, one shall be a layperson who is not employed in a health care profession; one shall be a physician licensed under Article 1 of this Chapter who has successfully completed 200 hours of Category I American Medical Association credit in medical acupuncture training as recommended by the American Academy of Medical Acupuncture; and one shall be licensed to practice acupuncture in this State. Of the members to be appointed by the General Assembly, three shall be appointed upon the recommendation of the Speaker of the House of Representatives, and three shall be appointed upon the recommendation of the President Pro Tempore of the Senate. The members appointed by the General Assembly must be appointed in accordance with G.S. 120 – 121.

Members serve at the pleasure of the appointing authority. Vacancies shall be filled by the original appointing authority and the term shall be for the balance of the unexpired term. A vacancy by a member appointed by the General Assembly must be filled in accordance with G.S. 120 – 122.

（b）Terms. — The members appointed initially by the Governor shall each serve a term ending on June 30, 1994. Of the General Assembly's initial appointments upon the recommendation of the Speaker of the House of Representatives, one shall serve a term ending June 30, 1995, and the other shall serve a term ending June 30, 1996. Of the General Assembly's initial appointments upon the recommendation of the President Pro Tempore of the Senate, one shall serve a term ending June 30, 1995, and the other shall serve a term ending June 30, 1996. After the initial appointments, all members shall be appointed for terms of three years beginning on July 1. No person may serve more than two consecutive full terms as a member of the Board.

（c）Meetings. — The Board shall meet at least once each year within 45 days after the appointment of the new members. At the Board's first meeting each year after the new members have been appointed, the members shall elect a chair of the Board and a secretary for the year. No person shall chair the Board for more than five consecutive years. The Board shall meet at other times as needed to perform its duties. A majority of the Board shall constitute a quorum for the transaction of business.

（d）Compensation. — Members of the Board are entitled to compensation and to reimbursement for travel and subsistence as provided in G.S. 93B - 5.

§ 90 - 454. Powers and duties of Board

The Board may:

(1) Deny, issue, suspend, and revoke licenses in accordance with rules adopted by the Board, and may collect fees, investigate violations of this Article, and otherwise administer the provisions of this Article.

(2) Sponsor or authorize other entities to offer continuing education programs, and approve continuing education requirements for license renewal.

(3) Establish requirements for, collect fees from, and approve schools of acupuncture in this State. The requirements shall be at least as stringent as the core curricula standards of the Council of Colleges of Acupuncture and Oriental Medicine.

(4) Sue to enjoin violations of G.S. 90 - 452. The court may issue an injunction even though no person has yet been injured as a result of the unauthorized practice.

(5) Adopt and use a seal to authenticate official documents of the Board.

(6) Employ and fix the compensation of personnel and professional advisors, including legal counsel, as may be needed to carry out its functions, and purchase, lease, rent, sell, or otherwise dispose of personal and real property for the operations of the Board.

(7) Expend funds as necessary to carry out the provisions of this Article from revenues and interest generated by fees collected under this Article.

(8) Adopt rules to implement this Article in accordance with Chapter 150B of the General Statutes.

(9) Establish practice parameters to become effective July 1, 1995. The practice parameters shall be applicable to general and specialty areas of practice. The Board shall review the parameters on a regular basis and shall require licensees to identify parameters being utilized, the plan of care, and treatment modalities utilized in accordance with the plan of care.

§ 90 - 455. Qualifications for license; renewal; inactive, suspended, expired, or lapsed license

(a) Initial License. — To receive a license to practice acupuncture, a person shall meet all of the following requirements:

(1) Submit a completed application as required by the Board.

(2) Submit any fees required by the Board.

(3) Submit proof of successful completion of a licensing examination administered or approved by the Board.

(4) Provide documentary evidence of having met one of the following standards of education, training, or demonstrated experience:

a. Successful completion of a three-year postgraduate acupuncture college or training program approved by the Board.

b. Continuous licensure to practice acupuncture by an agency of another state or another state whose qualifications for licensure meet or exceed those of this State for at least 10 years before application for licensure in this State during which time no disciplinary actions were taken or are pending against the applicant and submitting proof to the Board that the applicant has fulfilled at least an average of 20 continuing education units in acupuncture or health care-related studies for each of the 10 years preceding application for licensure.

(5) Submit proof of successful completion of the Clean Needle Technique Course offered by the Council of Colleges of Acupuncture and Oriental Medicine.

(6) Be of good moral character.

(7) Is not currently or has not engaged in any practice or conduct that would constitute grounds for disciplinary action pursuant to G.S. 90 – 456.

(8) Submit a form signed by the applicant attesting to the intention of the applicant to adhere fully to the ethical standards adopted by the Board.

(b) Renewal of License. — The license to practice acupuncture shall be renewed every two years. Upon submitting all required declarations, documents, and fees required by the Board for renewal, the applicant's license shall remain in good standing for a period of up to 120 days during which time the Board shall meet to review and act upon the application for renewal. To renew a license, an applicant shall:

(1) Submit a completed application as required by the Board.

(2) Submit any fees required by the Board.

(3) Upon request by the Board, submit proof of completion of 40 hours of Board-approved continuing education units within each renewal period.

(c) Inactive License. — A licensed acupuncturist who is not actively engaged in the practice of acupuncture in this State and who does not wish to renew the license may direct the Board to place the license on inactive status. A license may remain on inactive status for a period not to exceed eight years from the date the license was placed on inactive status. Upon an applicant's proof of completion of 40 hours of Board-approved continuing education units, payment of all fees, a determination by the Board that the applicant is not engaged in any prohibited activities that would constitute the basis for discipline as set forth in G.S. 90 – 456, and has not engaged in any of those prohibited activities during the period of time the license has been on inactive status, the Board may activate the license of the applicant.

(d) Suspended License. — A suspended license is subject to the renewal requirements of this section and may be renewed as provided in this section. This renewal does not entitle the licensed person to engage in the licensed activity or in any other conduct or activity in violation of the order or judgment by which the license was suspended, until the license is reinstated. If a license revoked on disciplinary grounds is reinstated and requires renewal, the licensed person shall pay the renewal fee and any applicable late fee.

(e) Expired License. — A license that has expired as a result of failure to renew pursuant to subsection (b) of this section may be renewed no later than two years after its expiration. The date of renewal shall be the date the Board acts to approve the renewal. To apply for renewal of an expired license, the applicant shall:

(1) File an application for renewal on a form provided by the Board.

(2) Submit proof of completion of all continuing education requirements.

(3) Pay all accrued renewal fees, along with an expired license fee.

(f) Lapsed License. — A license that has lapsed as a result of not being renewed within two years after the license expired or not reactivated within eight years after the license lapsed is deemed inactive. A lapsed license may not be renewed, reactivated, or reinstated. A person with a lapsed license may apply to obtain a new license pursuant to subsection (a) of this section.

§ 90 – 456. Prohibited activities

The Board may deny, suspend, or revoke a license, require remedial education, or issue a letter of reprimand, if a licensed acupuncturist or applicant:

(1) Engages in false or fraudulent conduct which demonstrates an unfitness to practice acupuncture, including any of the following activities:

a. Misrepresentation in connection with an application for a license or an investigation by the Board.

b. Attempting to collect fees for services which were not performed.

c. False advertising, including guaranteeing that a cure will result from an acupuncture treatment.

d. Dividing, or agreeing to divide, a fee for acupuncture services with anyone for referring a patient.

(2) Fails to exercise proper control over one's practice by any of the following activities:

a. Aiding an unlicensed person in practicing acupuncture.

b. Delegating professional responsibilities to a person the acupuncturist knows or should know is not qualified to perform.

c. Failing to exercise proper control over unlicensed personnel working with the acupuncturist in the practice.

(3) Fails to maintain records in a proper manner by any of the following:

a. Failing to keep written records describing the course of treatment for each patient.

b. Refusing to provide to a patient upon request records that have been prepared for or paid for by the patient.

c. Revealing personally identifiable information about a patient, without consent, unless otherwise allowed by law.

(4) Fails to exercise proper care for a patient, including either of the following:

a. Abandoning or neglecting a patient without making reasonable arrangements for the continuation of care.

b. Exercising, or attempting to exercise, undue influence within the acupuncturist/patient relationship by making sexual advances or requests for sexual activity or making submission to such conduct a condition of treatment.

(5) Displays habitual substance abuse or mental impairment so as to interfere with the ability to provide effective treatment.

(6) Is convicted of or pleads guilty or no contest to any crime which demonstrates an unfitness to practice acupuncture.

(7) Negligently fails to practice acupuncture with the level of skill recognized within the profession as acceptable under such circumstances.

(8) Willfully violates any provision of this Article or rule of the Board.

(9) Has had a license denied, suspended, or revoked in another jurisdiction for any reason which would be grounds for this action in this State.

§ 90 – 457. Fees

The Board may establish fees, not to exceed the following amounts:

(1) Application and an examination, one hundred dollars ($100.00).

(2) Issuance of a license, five hundred dollars ($500.00).

(3) Renewal of a license, three hundred dollars ($300.00).

(4) Renewal of a license, an additional late fee of two hundred dollars ($200.00).

(5) Duplicate license fee, twenty-five dollars ($25.00).

(6) Duplicate wall certificate fee, fifty dollars ($50.00).

(7) Labels for licensed acupuncturists, one hundred fifty dollars ($150.00).

(8) Returned check fee, forty dollars ($40.00).

(9) Licensure verification, forty dollars ($40.00).

(10) Name change, twenty-five dollars ($25.00).

(11) Continuing education program approval fee, fifty dollars ($50.00).

(12) Continuing education provider approval fee, two hundred dollars ($200.00).

(13) Initial school application fee, one thousand dollars ($1,000).

(14) Renewal school approval fee, seven hundred fifty dollars ($750.00).

(15) Inactive license renewal fee, fifty dollars ($50.00), payment due for each two-year extension.

§ 90 – 457.1. Continuing education

(a) Applicants for license renewal shall complete all required continuing education units during the two calendar years immediately preceding the license renewal date.

(b) The Board shall set the minimum hours for study of specific subjects within the scope of practice of acupuncture. The Board shall set the maximum hours for subjects that have content relating to any health service and are relevant to the practice of acupuncture. In addition to formally organized courses, the Board may approve courses, such as personal training in nonaccredited programs and teaching diagnosis and treatment, as long as these courses have received prior approval by the Board.

(c) For purposes of this Article, one continuing education unit is defined as one contact hour or 50 minutes.

(d) The Board may choose to audit the records of any licensee who has reported and sworn compliance with the continuing education requirement. The audit of any licensee shall not take place more than every two years.

(e) Failure to comply with the continuing education requirements shall prohibit license renewal and result in the license reverting to expired status at the end of the renewal period.

(f) A licensee may apply to the Board for an extension of time to complete the portion of continuing education requirements that the licensee is unable to meet due to such unforeseeable events as military duty, family emergency, or prolonged illness. The Board may, at its discretion, grant an extension for a maximum of one licensing period. The Board shall receive the request no later than 30 days before the license renewal date. The applicant shall attest that the request is a complete and accurate statement, and the request shall contain the following:

(1) An explanation of the licensee's failure to complete the continuing education requirements.

(2) A list of continuing education courses and hours that the licensee has completed.

(3) The licensee's plan for satisfying the continuing education requirements.

§ 90 – 458. Use of titles and display of license

The titles "Licensed Acupuncturist" or "Acupuncturist" shall be used only by persons licensed under this Article. Possession of a license under this Article does not by itself entitle a person to identify oneself as a doctor or physician. Each person licensed to practice acupuncture shall post the license in a conspicuous location at the person's place of practice.

§ 90 – 459. Third-party reimbursements

Nothing in this Article shall be construed to require direct third-party reimbursement to persons licensed under this Article.

§§ 90 – 460 to 90 – 469. Reserved

§§ 90 – 460 to 90 – 469. Reserved

NORTH CAROLINA ADMINISTRATIVE CODE

Section .0100. Licensure

.0101 APPLICATION AND PRACTICE REQUIREMENTS FOR LICENSURE

In addition to and for the purposes of meeting the requirements of G. S. 90 – 455, an applicant for licensure to practice acupuncture shall satisfy requirements one through six and eight listed below or requirements one through five and requirements seven and eight listed below:

(1) Submit a completed application;

(2) Submit fees as required by Rule .0103 of this Section;

(3) Ensure that an official copy of a diploma, transcript, license or certificate, examination score, or other document required for application is forwarded directly to the Board by the issuing entity or its successor organization or designated state agency. Documents shall have an official or government seal or written verification authenticating the document;

(4) If the applicant sat for the National Certification Commission for Acupuncture and Oriental Medicine (NCCAOM) examination on or before June 30, 2004, the applicant shall submit proof that he or she passed the acupuncture written exam and the point location exam as established and determined by NCCAOM or its successor organization. If the applicant sat for the licensing examination after June 30, 2004, the applicant shall submit proof that he or she passed, as determined by NCCAOM, the following four NCCAOM modules: Foundations of Oriental Medicine, Acupuncture, Biomedicine and Point Location;

(5) Submit proof that he or she passed the Clean Needle Technique course as offered and determined by the Council of Colleges of Acupuncture and Oriental Medicine (CCAOM) or its successor organization;

(6) Submit proof of satisfying the education requirements listed below:

(a) US Trained Applicants. All U.S. trained applicants shall graduate from a three-year postgraduate acupuncture college, accredited by or in candidacy status by the Accreditation Commission for Acupuncture and Oriental Medicine (ACAOM) or its successor organization.

(b) Foreign Trained Applicants. All foreign trained applicants shall graduate from a postgraduate acupuncture college that meets the curricular requirements of ACAOM. The college shall also be approved by either:

(i) A foreign government's Ministry of Education;

(ii) A foreign government's Ministry of Health;

(iii) A governmental agency that is comparable to a division or department of the US Government charged with educational accreditation; or

(iv) A private foreign accreditation agency that has an accreditation process and standards substantially equivalent to that of ACAOM, and that is recognized for that purpose by the substantially equivalent governmental entity in that foreign country. The educational institutions shall meet the curricular requirements of ACAOM.

(c) The documents substantiating that the U.S. trained applicant has met the specified requirements shall be submitted as follows:

(i) The educational program or governmental agency from which the applicant received the certificate or diploma shall send an official copy of the applicant's transcript directly to the Board in a sealed envelope.

(ii) By its submission of this transcript, the program or agency shall verify the applicant's satisfactory completion of the required ACAOM academic and clinical education and designate the completed courses and the hours of study completed in each subject.

(d) The documents substantiating that the Foreign trained applicant has met the specified requirements shall be submitted as follows:

(i) The educational program or governmental agency from which the applicant received the certificate or diploma shall send an official copy of the applicant's transcript directly to the Board in a sealed envelope;

(ii) By submission of this transcript, the program or agency shall verify the applicant's satisfactory completion of his or her clinical education and designate the completed courses and hours of study earned in each subject;

(iii) The applicant, at his or her own expense, shall submit an accurate English translation that interprets all documents submitted in a foreign language. Each translated document shall bear the affidavit of the translator certifying that he or she is competent in both the language of the document and the English language and that the translation is a true and complete translation of the foreign language original. Each translated document shall also bear the affidavit of the applicant, certifying that the translation is a true and complete translation of the original. Each affidavit shall be signed before a notary public; and

(iv) All foreign trained applicants, at his or her expense, shall submit their transcripts for evaluation by a foreign credential evaluation service to determine if the applicant's course work is equivalent to that required of an applicant from a three-year postgraduate acupuncture college accredited by the Accreditation Commission for Acupuncture and Oriental Medicine (ACAOM). This includes a subject-by-subject analysis that meets the curricular requirements of ACAOM in effect at the time of certification by the National Certification Commission for Acupuncture and Oriental Medicine (NCCAOM) in the acupuncture written and point location examinations. The applicant may use a current member of the National Association of Credential Evaluation Services (NACES) or the American Association of Collegiate Registrars and Admissions Offices (AACRAO);

(7) Practice Requirements:

(a) The applicant shall fulfill the requirements set forth in G.S. 90 - 455.

(b) Disciplinary action, as used in Article 30 of Chapter 90 of the General Statutes, means censure, suspension, or revocation but does not include a letter of caution, warning or admonition; and

(8) Submit a license history stating the disciplinary record of the applicant to reflect any censure, suspension or revocation. The record shall be sent directly to the Board by each state board in which the applicant has been licensed to practice acupuncture.

.0102 REQUIREMENTS/WAIVER/QUALIFICATIONS/LICENSURE DETAILED IN G.S. 90 – 455

An applicant for licensing seeking a waiver of the requirements of Rule .0101 of this Section shall:

(1) Submit a completed application before December 31, 1994, and

(2) Submit non-refundable fees as required by Rule .0103 of this Section, and

(3) Provide proof of North Carolina residency as of January 1, 1993, and

(4) Fulfill one of the following:

(a) Submit a certified copy, certified by the issuing institution, of a transcript including evidence of graduation from an acupuncture college approved by the Board (an approved acupuncture college is one that is a minimum of two academic years of training and is certified or approved by the state or country in which it operates), or

(b) Submit evidence of successful completion of the Clean Needle Technique (CNT) course and achieve a score of not less than 15 points as outlined in the Sub-items (4)(b)(i) and (ii) of this Rule to satisfy requirements for a Board approved training program.

(i) Submit proof of a score of not less than 70% on the National Commission for the Certification of Acupuncturists examination: 15 points; or

(ii) Training: Accrue 15 points (a minimum of 5 points in both categories in Sub-items) (4)(b)(ii)(A) and (B) of this Rule.

(A) Education:

(I) Structured — For each 100 hours of documented completion of a formal training program approved by the Board: 1 point. A formal training program is an acupuncture college certified or approved by the state or country in which it operates.

(II) Apprenticeship — For each 150 hours of supervised apprenticeship training with an acupuncturist [and which is verified by such acupuncturist(s)]: 1 point.

(B) Experience: An applicant must accrue a minimum of five points in any combination of Sub-items (4)(ii)(B)(I) and (II) of this Rule. Acupuncture must comprise at least 90% of the applicant's practice. Treatments for cessation of smoking and weight loss shall not be adequate to satisfy the experience requirements if such therapies comprise more than 40% of the applicant's practice.

(I) Treatment of not fewer than 100 different patients for not less than 2000 patient hours within the last three years prior to application for licensure: 5 points.

(II) Treatment of not fewer than 100 patients for not less than 4000 patient hours within the last three years prior to application for licensure: 10 points.

(5) Submit all correspondence, including application, in writing, typed or printed only, to the North Carolina Acupuncture Licensing Board, P.O. Box 25171, Asheville, North Carolina 28803.

.0103　FEES

The following fees shall apply：

（1）	Application（non-refundable）	$100.00
（2）	Initial biennial licensing	$500.00
（3）	Renewal of biennial licensing	$300.00
（4）	Late license renewal（additional）	$200.00
（5）	Inactive license renewal，biennial extension	$50.00
（6）	Duplicate license	$25.00
（7）	Duplicate wall certificate	$50.00
（8）	Mailing Labels	$150.00
（9）	Returned check	$40.00
（10）	Verification of North Carolina licensure to another state	$25.00
（11）	Name change	$5.00
（12）	Continuing education per single program approval	$50.00
（13）	Continuing education provider approval	$50.00
（14）	Initial school application	$1,000.00
（15）	Biennial renewal school approval application	$500.00

.0104　DEFINITIONS

In addition to the definitions contained in G. S. 90 - 451, the following shall apply throughout this Chapter：

（1）"Licensed Acupuncturist" or "Acupuncturist" is the title conveyed by the North Carolina Acupuncture Licensing Board pursuant to Article 30 of Chapter 90 of the North Carolina General Statutes. Licensed Acupuncturists or Acupuncturists may only refer to him or herself as a doctor in the state of North Carolina, if he or she has earned an educational degree of "doctor" or "doctorate" in accordance with G.S. 90 - 458.

（2）"Acupuncture adjunctive therapies" include the adjunctive therapies listed in G.S. 90 - 451（3）. It also includes stimulation to acupuncture points and channels by any of the following：cupping, thermal methods, magnets, and gwa-sha scraping techniques.

（3）"Acupuncture diagnostic techniques" include the use of observation, listening, smelling, inquiring, palpation, pulse diagnosis, tongue diagnosis, hara diagnosis, physiognomy, five element correspondence, ryodoraku, akabani, and electro-acupuncture.

(4) "Acupuncture needles" mean the same as in 21 CFR 880.5580, which is hereby incorporated by reference, including subsequent amendments and editions, and can be found at https://www.gpo.gov/fdsys/pkg/CFR-2016-title21-vol8/pdf/CFR-2016-title21-vol8-sec880-5580. pdf at no cost. "Acupuncture needles" include solid filiform needles, intradermal, plum blossom, press tacks, and prismatic needles.

(5) "Dietary guidelines" include nutritional counseling and the recommendation of food and supplemental substances.

(6) "Electrical stimulation" includes the treatment or diagnosis of energetic imbalances using TENS, Piezo electrical stimulation, acuscope therapy, auricular therapy devices, percutaneous and transcutaneous electrical nerve stimulation and Class IIIa, 5 milliwatt laser devices. All laser products shall meet the performance standards for light-emitting products as set forth in 21 CFR 1040.10 and 1040.11, including subsequent amendments and editions, which can be found at https://www.gpo.gov/fdsys/pkg/CFR-2012-title21-vol8/pdf/CFR-2012-title21-vol8-part1040.pdf at no cost.

(7) "Herbal medicine" includes tinctures, patent remedies, decoction, powders, diluted herbal remedies, freeze dried herbs, salves, poultices, medicated oils, and liniments.

(8) "Massage and manual techniques" include acupressure, shiatsu, Tui-Na, qi healing, and medical qi gong.

(9) "Therapeutic exercise" includes qi gong, Taoist self-cultivation exercises, dao yin, tai qi chuan, bagua, and meditative exercises.

(10) "Thermal methods" include moxibustion, hot and cold packs and infrared lamps. The use of infrared heat lamps shall be done in accordance with 21 CFR 890.5500, including subsequent amendments and editions, which can be found at https://www.gpo.gov/fdsys/pkg/CFR-2017-title21-vol8/pdf/CFR-2017-title21-vol8-sec890-5500.pdf at no cost.

.0105 QUALIFICATIONS FOR LICENSURE THROUGH LICENSE RECIPROCITY

An applicant for licensure to practice acupuncture in North Carolina shall:

(1) Submit a completed application;

(2) Submit fees as required by Rule .0103 of this Section;

(3) Have submitted directly to the North Carolina Acupuncture Licensing Board, an official letter from the licensing board of another jurisdiction with whom the North Carolina Acupuncture Licensing Board has a reciprocal licensing agreement, verifying that the applicant is currently licensed and in good standing in such jurisdiction.

.0106 CHANGE OF NAME OR ADDRESS

Every person licensed under the provisions of this Article shall give written notice to the Board of any change in his or her name or address within 60 calendar days after the change takes place.

.0107 BOARD MAILING ADDRESS

All correspondence shall be mailed to the following address:

North Carolina Acupuncture Licensing Board

P.O. Box 10686

Raleigh, North Carolina 27605

Section .0200. Renewal of Licensure

.0201 RENEWAL OF LICENSURE

The procedure and requirements for renewal of license are as follows:

(1) Biennial Renewal. A licensee shall renew his or her license by the second July 1 following initial licensure and thereafter renew his or her license by July 1 every two years.

(2) Continuing Education. Licensees seeking renewal of their license shall verify on a renewal form prepared by the Board that the licensee has completed the required continuing education units in accordance with Rule .0301 of this Chapter. The renewal form shall include the following information:

(a) licensee's: identity and contact information;

(b) requested action from the Board;

(c) statements pertaining to renewal and fitness for licensure; and

(d) information pertaining to courses taken including the number of units completed and each of the courses completed.

(3) Fees. The licensee shall pay the renewal fee prescribed in Rule .0103 of this Chapter.

(4) Suspended license. The holder of a suspended license shall meet the renewal requirements pursuant to G.S. 90 - 455(b) and this Rule for the duration of the suspension or the license shall expire pursuant to G.S. 90 - 457.1(e).

(5) Expired license. Failure to receive notification that a license has expired does not relieve the holder of an expired license of the responsibility of meeting the continuing education requirements that would have been required if the license had continued to be in effect. These continuing education units shall not apply to the renewal requirements for the subsequent renewal period. In order to renew an expired license pursuant to G.S. 90 - 455(e), the applicant shall file the renewal form prepared by the Board, submit proof of completion of continuing education, and pay the late license renewal (additional) fee resulting from the expired license as well as the renewal of biennial licensing fee. Expired licenses not renewed within two years after the license expired or not reactivated within eight years after the license is placed on inactive status, pursuant to G.S. 90 - 455(c), shall be deemed lapsed, pursuant to G.S. 90 - 455(f).

.0202 PROCESS TO OBTAIN INACTIVE LICENSE; ACTIVATE LICENSE

(a) The procedure and requirements for inactive status are as follows:

(1) Written request for inactive license. A licensed acupuncturist not engaged in the practice

of acupuncture may request that his or her license be placed in inactive status by submitting the request in writing to the Board.

(2) Following a period of eight years, the Board shall treat an inactive license as lapsed.

(b) The procedure and requirements to activate a license are as follows:

(1) Submit an application to activate a license on a form provided by the Board.

(2) The applicant meeting the requirements to activate his or her license as set out in G.S. 90-455(c) shall submit a signed statement to the Board establishing that he or she has not been involved in any prohibited activities set forth in G.S. 90-456 during the period of inactive status.

(3) To make this determination, the Board may hold a hearing in accordance with the requirements followed for revocation and suspension of a license as set out in 21 NCAC 1 .0710.

(4) The applicant shall satisfy the Board that he or she completed 40 hours of continuing education units within the preceding two-year period as set out in G.S. 90-455.

(c) Fees: An applicant shall submit payment of an inactive license fee extension every two years upon notice by the Board.

(d) The Board shall activate a license upon a finding that the applicant has paid the sum total fee, completed the continuing education requirements, and not engaged in any prohibited activities that would constitute the basis for discipline as set forth in G.S. 90-456.

Section .0300. Continuing Education

.0301 STANDARDS FOR CONTINUING EDUCATION

(a) Unless otherwise indicated, one CEU, as used in this Rule, shall be equal to one contact hour or 50 minutes of instruction.

(b) All licensees shall complete 40 Continuing Education Units (CEU) every two years as follows:

(1) 25 CEUs shall be obtained from courses that have content relating to the scope of the practice of acupuncture. Fifteen of these 25 hours shall contain course content related to the insertion of acupuncture needles and the application of moxibustion to the human body. The remaining 10 hours of CEUs may be obtained from course content related to adjunctive therapies including massage, mechanical, thermal, electrical, and electromagnetic treatment and the recommendation of herbs, dietary guidelines, and therapeutic exercise; and

(2) the remaining 15 CEUs may be comprised of any combination of the following:

(A) 15 CEUs related to any of the content contained in Subparagraph (b)(1) of this Rule;

(B) up to 10 CEUs for acupuncture or Chinese medicine research studies in hospitals or institutions as set forth in Paragraph (e) of this Rule;

(C) up to 10 CEUs for teaching of Chinese medicine in a formally organized course as set forth in Paragraph (c)(2) of this Rule;

(D) up to 10 CEUs for published work in peer-reviewed journals as set forth in Paragraph (g) of this Rule; or

(E) two CEUs for obtaining or maintaining CPR certification.

(c) All courses completed for purposes of CEUs shall meet the following requirements:

(1) be approved by one or more of the following organizations or their successor organizations:

(A) Acupuncture schools in candidacy status or accredited by the Accreditation Commission for Acupuncture and Oriental Medicine.(ACAOM);

(B) National Certification Commission for Acupuncture and Oriental Medicine;

(C) The Society for Acupuncture Research;

(D) National Acupuncture Detoxification Association;

(E) American Academy of Medical Acupuncture (AAMA); or

(F) North Carolina Acupuncture Licensing Board (NCALB); and

(2) be formally organized. A formally organized course shall meet the following requirements:

(A) the sponsor shall maintain a record of attendance for four years. Records shall be made available to the Board upon request;

(B) the instructor shall hold credentials to practice in the field that is the subject of the course or the instructor shall be competent to teach the designated course and be permitted to perform acupuncture needling techniques for the purposes of demonstration, as determined by the Board based upon the instructor's educations, training, and experience;

(C) the course shall have stated objectives and a syllabus or a description of the content of the course with a class outline;

(D) the course shall be evaluated by each participant on an evaluation form provided by the instructor; and

(E) upon completion of each course, the provider shall issue a certificate of completion to each participant to include the following information:

(i) the title of the course;

(ii) the name of the participant;

(iii) the name of the instructors;

(iv) the name of the provider;

(v) the date and location of the course;

(vi) the number of CEUs completed.

(d) Licensees may obtain up to 28 hours of CEUs by completing online courses approved by an organization set forth in Subparagraph (c)(1) of this Rule.

(e) 10 CEUs may be obtained in each renewal period by licensees who are involved in acupuncture or Chinese medicine research studies in accredited hospitals or educational institutions. A research project may only be submitted once for the purpose of obtaining CEU credit. In order to obtain Research approved CEUs the following must be submitted to the Board for review and approval:

(1) The Institutional Review Board (IRB) approval;

(2) A summary of the study; and

(3) The names and credentials of researchers involved.

(f) A maximum of 10 CEUs may be obtained in each renewal period by teaching acupuncture education in an educational institution accredited by the Accreditation Commission for Acupuncture and Oriental Medicine (ACAOM) or a CEU course approved by the NCALB. One hour of CEU credit shall be awarded for every three hours of teaching up to 30 hours. All CEUs for teaching shall be approved in advance by the Board prior to the date of the class. For approval the licensee shall submit the following information:

(1) the title of the course;

(2) a summary of course content or class syllabus;

(3) the location of the course;

(4) the dates of the course;

(5) the total number of classroom hours taught;

(6) a copy of course evaluation to be provided students; and

(7) the course fees and refund policy.

(g) 10 CEUs may be obtained by authoring an article in a peer-reviewed journal of acupuncture or Chinese medicine. Examples of journals that shall be considered by the Board include:

(1) The Journal of Traditional Chinese Medicine;

(2) The American Journal of Chinese Medicine; and

(3) The World Journal of Traditional Chinese Medicine.

(h) CEUs from any given course may be used to satisfy the requirements of only one renewal period.

(i) Each licensee shall retain for four years records of all continuing education programs attended, indicating:

(1) the title of the course or program;

(2) the name of the participant;

(3) the name of all instructors;

(4) the name of the provider;

(5) the date and location of the course; and

(6) the number of CEUs completed.

(j) Pursuant to G.S. 90 – 457.1(b), the Board may audit the records of any licensee to ensure compliance with the continuing education requirements of this Rule. No licensee shall be subject to audit more than once every two years.

(k) All applications for pre-approval for CEU courses must be submitted 60 days prior to the date of the course.

(1) A licensee may apply to the Board for an extension of time to complete continuing education requirements in accordance with G.S. 90 – 457.1(f).

Section .0400. Practice Parameters and Procedures

.0401 PRACTICE PARAMETERS

The following are the practice parameters for acupuncturists in North Carolina:

(1) A licensed acupuncturist shall practice within the scope of training offered by a college accredited, or in candidacy status, by the National Accreditation Commission for Schools and Colleges of Acupuncture and Oriental Medicine.

(2) A licensed acupuncturist must practice within the confines of his training. Parameters for diagnosis and treatment of patients include, Five Elements, Eight Principles, Yin Yang Theory, Channel Theory, Zang Fu Organ Theory, Six Stages and Four Aspects of Disease Progressions.

.0402 ACUPUNCTURE PROCEDURES

The following procedures shall be followed within the practice of acupuncture:

(1) Practice Setting:

(a) Treatments shall be given in surroundings that provide privacy and confidentiality.

(b) Community acupuncture practices that perform acupuncture treatment in a group setting shall obtain and retain a signed consent waiving the right to a private treatment setting from every patient prior to his or her first treatment.

(c) Every acupuncture office shall be maintained in a clean and sanitary condition at all times, and shall have an accessible bathroom facility.

(d) All applicable OSHA Standards, as amended or replaced, shall be met including those pertaining to blood borne pathogens, which can be found at https://www.gpo.gov/fdsys/pkg/CFR-2017-title29-vol6/pdf/CFR-2017-title29-vol6-sec1910-1030.pdf at no cost.

(e) All acupuncture practice and recordkeeping shall be compliant with all State and federal laws and regulations pertaining to the confidentiality of medical records including security and privacy regulations enacted under HIPAA, as amended or replaced, including 45 C.F.R Part 160, which can be found at https://www.gpo.gov/fdsys/pkg/CFR-2017-title45-vol1/pdf/CFR-2017-title45-vol1-part160.pdf at no cost, and subparts A and E of Part 164, which can be found at https://www.gpo.gov/fdsys/pkg/CFR-2017-title45-vol1/pdf/CFR-2017-title45-vol1-part164-subpartA.pdf and https://www.gpo.gov/fdsys/pkg/CFR-2017-title45-vol1/pdf/CFR-2017-title45-vol1-part164-subpartE.pdf respectively and at no cost.

(2) Prior to treatment, a licensee shall obtain a written or oral medical history that includes the following information:

(a) Current and past conditions, illnesses, treatments, hospitalizations, and current medications, and allergies to medications;

(b) A social history that shall include the use of tobacco, alcohol, caffeine, and recreational drugs;

(c) The names of health practitioners;

(d) The presenting complaints, along with remedies and treatments tried and in progress;

(e) Whether the patient is pregnant and whether the patient has any biomedical devices, such as artificial joints or cardiac pacemaker.

(3) Fees. Information concerning treatment fees shall be made available to the patient prior to treatment.

(4) Guarantees. No express or implied guarantee about the success of treatment shall be given to the patient. Reasonable indication of the length of treatment and usual outcome shall be given to the patient.

(5) Diagnosis:

(a) Licensees shall diagnose each patient employing methods used by the traditions represented in Asian medicine as reflected in Rule .0104 (2) of this Chapter and within the context of Accreditation Commission for Acupuncture and Oriental Medicine (ACAOM) educational programs.

(b) All acupuncture diagnostic techniques utilized shall be recorded at each visit.

(6) Treatment. The specifics of all treatment shall be recorded at each visit. Treatments shall be in accordance with Asian and biomedical knowledge obtained in acupuncture training programs.

(7) Medical Records. Dated notes of each patient visit and communication shall be kept seven years. Authorization for release of medical records shall be obtained prior to sharing of any patient information. Medical records shall be released to patient upon receipt of the authorization. G.S. 90 – 411 sets forth the amounts healthcare providers can charge for copies of patient medical records. In charging patients for their records, licensees shall follow G.S. 90 – 411 as written, or as subsequently amended.

(8) Failure to Progress:

(a) If a patient fails to respond to treatments, the licensee shall initiate a discussion with the patient about other forms of treatment available or make a referral to another health care professional.

(b) In the case of persistent or unexplained pain, or the unexplained worsening of any condition while receiving treatment, the licensee shall initiate a referral or seek a consultation with other health care providers. In choosing a referral source, the licensee shall give priority to practitioners who have previously seen or treated the patient.

(c) Licensees shall honor and consider all requests by a patient for information about other forms of treatment available or for referral to another health care practitioner.

Section .0500. Schools and Colleges of Acupuncture

.0501 QUALIFICATIONS FOR ESTABLISHING A SCHOOL FOR ACUPUNCTURE IN NORTH CAROLINA

(a) For the purposes of this Rule "Acupuncture program" means training in acupuncture offered by an academic institution on a continuing basis.

(b) In addition to and for the purposes of meeting the requirements of G.S. 90 - 454(3), in order to be approved as a school of acupuncture an institution must meet the following standards:

(1) submit a completed application;

(2) submit fees as required by Rule .0103 of this Chapter;

(3) offer an Acupuncture program that extends over a minimum of three academic years, six semesters, nine quarters or 27 months, which consists of a minimum of 1800 clock hours with a minimum of 900 hours of didactic and theoretical training and 650 hours of supervised clinic. A minimum of 400 hours of the 650 hours of clinical training must be actual treatments;

(4) achieve candidacy status with the National Accreditation Commission for Schools and Colleges of Acupuncture and Oriental Medicine within one year of beginning classes and maintain accreditation throughout years of operation;

(5) provide a transcript of grades, as part of the student's record, that includes the following: name, address, date of birth, course titles, grades received, number of clock hours per course;

(6) grant a diploma only after the student has successfully completed the educational program in acupuncture, personally attended all required classes and completed the program requirements.

Section .0700. Administrative Procedures

.0701 ADMINISTRATIVE REVIEW OF BOARD'S DECISION DENYING ISSUANCE OF A LICENSE

Whenever the North Carolina Acupuncture Licensing Board has determined that a person has failed to satisfy the Board of his qualifications and has failed to be issued a license, the Board shall immediately notify such person of its decision, and indicate in what respect the applicant has so failed to satisfy the Board. Such applicant shall be given a contested case hearing before the Board upon request of such applicant filed with or mailed by registered mail to the secretary of the Board at 1418 Aversboro Rd., Garner, North Carolina 27529 within 60 days after receipt of the Board's decision, stating the reasons for such request. The Board shall within 20 days of receipt of such request notify such applicant of the time and place of a public hearing, which shall be held within 60 days. The burden of satisfying the Board of his qualifications for licensure shall be upon the applicant. Following such hearing, the Board shall determine whether the applicant is entitled to be licensed.

.0702 FILING COMPLAINTS

(a) General. Any person who has reason to believe that a licensed acupuncturist has violated the laws governing acupuncture may file a complaint with the North Carolina Acupuncture Licensing Board. Complaints shall be filed with the secretary of the North Carolina Acupuncture Licensing Board at 1418 Aversboro Road, Garner, North Carolina 27529.

(b) Form of Complaint. Complaints may be formal or informal, but must be in writing:

(1) Informal Complaint. The Board shall consider any written communication, construed most favorably to the complainant, which appears to allege a violation of the laws governing acupuncture an informal complaint.

(2) Formal Complaint. A complainant shall execute a formal complaint in writing under oath upon a form provided by the secretary. The complaint shall specify the statute or rule allegedly violated and shall contain a short statement of the acts or omissions constituting the alleged violation including the dates of said acts or omissions.

(c) Secretary's Response to Complaints. The secretary shall review any complaint to determine whether a major or minor violation has been alleged. If the secretary determines that the alleged violation is minor, he shall attempt to resolve the complaint by informal communication with the complainant and the acupuncturist complained of. If the secretary determines that the alleged violation is major, he shall assist the complainant in filing a formal complaint, if one has not already been filed.

.0703 DETERMINATION OF PROBABLE CAUSE

(a) General. Formal complaints shall be investigated by the North Carolina Acupuncture Licensing Board. The Board shall hold a hearing to determine whether there is probable cause to believe a violation of the laws governing acupuncture has occurred.

(b) Notice of Hearing. The secretary shall provide notice of the probable cause hearing to the acupuncturist complained against by certified mail at least 15 days in advance of the hearing.

(c) Conduct of Probable Cause Hearing. The probable cause hearing shall be informal, and the secretary may establish at his discretion such procedures as are necessary to facilitate examination of the evidence. The Board may consider evidence at the probable cause hearing which would not be admissible if offered at the hearing in a contested case.

(d) Action by the Board. After examining the evidence presented at the probable cause hearing, the Board may dispose of each charge in the formal complaint as follows:

(1) If no probable cause exists to believe that a violation of G.S. 90 – 456 has occurred, the charge may be dismissed.

(2) If the respondent admits the charge, he may be directed to cease and desist from commission of those acts which violate the provisions of G.S. 90 – 456.

(3) If a charge is denied and probable cause is found, or if a charge, while admitted, is of such gravity as to make the imposition of punitive sanctions appropriate, the complaint shall be

presented to the Board for its decision on the merits in accordance with G.S. 150B, Article 3A.

.0704 INFORMAL PROCEEDINGS

(a) In addition to formal hearings pursuant to G.S. 90 – 456, the Board may conduct informal proceedings in order to settle on an informal basis matters of dispute. A person practicing acupuncture pursuant to a license or other authority granted by the Board may be invited to attend a meeting with the Board or a committee of the Board on an informal basis to discuss any matter the Board deems appropriate. No public record of such proceeding shall be made nor shall any individual be placed under oath to give testimony. Matters discussed by a person appearing informally before the Board may, however, be used against such person in a formal hearing if a formal hearing is subsequently initiated.

(b) As a result of such informal meeting, the Board may recommend that certain actions be taken by such person, may offer such person the opportunity to enter into a consent order which will be a matter of public record, may institute a contested case concerning such person, or may take other action as the Board may deem appropriate in each case.

(c) Attendance at such an informal meeting is not required and is at the sole discretion of the person so invited. A person invited to attend an informal meeting may have counsel present at such meeting.

.0705 INITIATION OF FORMAL HEARINGS

(a) The North Carolina Acupuncture Licensing Board may initiate a disciplinary action against a licensed acupuncturist or applicant pursuant to G.S. 90 – 456.

(b) Upon receipt of a written request and substantiating information from any person in a position to present information as a basis for the action, the North Carolina Acupuncture Licensing Board shall conduct an investigation sufficient to determine whether reasonable cause exists to initiate disciplinary action(s).

(c) An opportunity will be given the person for a hearing before the Board at the next meeting.

.0706 CONTINUANCES

Any person summoned to appear before the Board at a contested case hearing may seek to obtain a continuance of that hearing by filing with the Executive Secretary of the Board, as soon as the reason for continuance is known, a motion for continuance setting forth with specificity the reason the continuance is desired. Continuances shall be granted for reasons such as personal or family illness, death, or an act of God. Motions for continuances shall be ruled upon by the President and Executive Secretary of the Board or in the absence of the President, by the Secretary and Executive Secretary.

.0707 DISQUALIFICATION FOR PERSONAL BIAS

Any person summoned to appear before the Board at a contested case hearing may challenge on the basis of personal bias or other reason for disqualification the fitness and competency of any member of the Board to hear and weigh evidence concerning that person. Challenges shall be stated by way of motion accompanied by affidavit setting forth with specificity the grounds for such challenge and shall be filed with the Executive Secretary of the Board within 14 days of receipt of letter. Nothing contained in this Rule shall prevent a person appearing before the Board at a contested case hearing from making personal inquiry of members of the Board as to their knowledge of and personal bias concerning that person's case.

.0708 RESERVED FOR FUTURE CODIFICATION

.0709 PROCEDURE OF REVOCATION OF LICENSURE

(a) If the North Carolina Acupuncture Licensing Board determines that reasonable cause exists to initiate a disciplinary action pursuant to G.S. 90 – 456, the Board shall prepare written charges and determine what action(s) shall be taken.

(b) The Board shall provide the person with a copy of the written charges and notify the person that it shall take the determined action(s) unless the person, within 60 days of receipt of notice, initiates administrative proceedings under G.S. 150B, Article 3A. The notice will be sent certified mail, return receipt requested.

(c) If the person initiates administrative proceedings the North Carolina Acupuncture Licensing Board shall defer final action on the matter until the proceedings are completed. If the person does not initiate administrative proceedings within 60 days of receipt of notice, the North Carolina Acupuncture Licensing Board may implement the action(s) at its next meeting.

(d) The North Carolina Acupuncture Licensing Board may reinstate a suspended or revoked license or may grant a new license upon application and demonstration of satisfactory compliance with Board requirements.

.0710 HEARING BEFORE REVOCATION OR SUSPENSION OF A LICENSE

Before the Board shall revoke, restrict or suspend any license granted by it, the licensee shall be given a written notice indicating the general nature of the charges, accusation, or complaint made against him. This notice may be prepared by a committee of one or more members of the Board designated by the Board, and stating that such licensee will be given an opportunity to be heard concerning such charges or complaint at a time and place stated in such notice, or at a time and place to be thereafter designated by the Board. The Board shall hold a hearing not less than 30 days from the date of the service of such notice upon such licensee, at which such licensee may appear personally and through counsel, may cross examine witnesses and present evidence in his own behalf.

.0711 PROVISIONS FOR PETITION FOR A RULE CHANGE

Each person desiring to petition for the adoption, amendment or repeal of a rule shall submit the following information to the Board:

(1) draft of the proposed rule or amendment to a rule;

(2) reasons for the proposal;

(3) effect of the existing rule;

(4) data supporting the proposal;

(5) effect on existing practices in the area involved, including costs;

(6) names of those most likely to be affected, with addresses if known; and

(7) the name and address of the petitioner. The North Carolina Acupuncture Licensing Board shall render a decision regarding the denial of a petition or the initiation of rule-making proceedings.

FLORIDA

FLORIDA STATUTES ANNOTATED

457.01. Renumbered as 485.011 in Fla.St.1955

See, now, F.S.A. § 485.011

457.011. Repealed by Laws 1976, c. 76 – 168, § 3; Laws 1979, c. 79 – 165, § 1

457.02. Renumbered as 485.021 in Fla.St.1955

See, now, F.S.A. § 485.021

457.021. Repealed by Laws 1976, c. 76 – 168, § 3; Laws 1979, c. 79 – 165, § 1

457.03. Renumbered as 485.031 in Fla.St.1955

See, now, F.S.A. § 485.031

457.031. Repealed by Laws 1976, c. 76 – 168, § 3; Laws 1979, c. 79 – 165, § 1

457.04. Renumbered as 485.041 in Fla.St.1955

See, now, F.S.A. § 485.041

457.041. Repealed by Laws 1976, c. 76 – 168, § 3; Laws 1979, c. 79 – 165, § 1

457.05. Renumbered as 485.051 in Fla.St.1955

See, now, F.S.A. § 485.051

457.051. Repealed by Laws 1976, c. 76 – 168, § 3; Laws 1979, c. 79 – 165, § 1

457.06. Renumbered as 485.061 in Fla.St.1955

See, now, F.S.A. § 485.061

457.061. Repealed by Laws 1976, c. 76 – 168, § 3; Laws 1979, c. 79 – 165, § 1

457.07. Renumbered as 485.071 in Fla.St.1955

See, now, F.S.A. § 485.071

457.071. Repealed by Laws 1976, c. 76 – 168, § 3; Laws 1979, c. 79 – 165, § 1

457.08. Renumbered as 485.081 in Fla.St.1955

See, now, F.S.A. § 485.081

457.081. Repealed by Laws 1976, c. 76 - 168, § 3; Laws 1979, c. 79 - 165, § 1

457.09. Renumbered as 485.091 in Fla.St.1955

See, now, F.S.A. § 485.091

457.091. Repealed by Laws 1976, c. 76 - 168, § 3; Laws 1978, c. 78 - 95, § 9; Laws 1979, c. 79 - 165, § 1

457.10. Repealed by Laws 1976, c. 76 - 168, § 3; Laws 1979, c. 79 - 165, § 1

457.101. Legislative intent

The Legislature finds that the interests of the public health require the regulation of the practice of acupuncture in this state for the purpose of protecting the health, safety, and welfare of our citizens while making this healing art available to those who seek it.

457.102. Definitions

As used in this chapter:

(1) "Acupuncture" means a form of primary health care, based on traditional Chinese medical concepts and modern oriental medical techniques, that employs acupuncture diagnosis and treatment, as well as adjunctive therapies and diagnostic techniques, for the promotion, maintenance, and restoration of health and the prevention of disease. Acupuncture shall include, but not be limited to, the insertion of acupuncture needles and the application of moxibustion to specific areas of the human body and the use of electroacupuncture, Qi Gong, oriental massage, herbal therapy, dietary guidelines, and other adjunctive therapies, as defined by board rule.

(2) "Acupuncturist" means any person licensed as provided in this chapter to practice acupuncture as a primary health care provider.

(3) "Board" means the Board of Acupuncture.

(4) "License" means the document of authorization issued by the department for a person to engage in the practice of acupuncture.

(5) "Department" means the Department of Health.

(6) "Oriental medicine" means the use of acupuncture, electroacupuncture, Qi Gong, oriental massage, herbal therapy, dietary guidelines, and other adjunctive therapies.

(7) "Prescriptive rights" means the prescription, administration, and use of needles and devices, restricted devices, and prescription devices that are used in the practice of acupuncture and oriental medicine.

457.103. Board of Acupuncture; membership; appointment and terms

(1) The Board of Acupuncture is created within the department and shall consist of seven members, to be appointed by the Governor and confirmed by the Senate. Five members of the board must be licensed Florida acupuncturists. Two members must be laypersons who are not and who have never been acupuncturists or members of any closely related profession. Members shall be appointed for 4-year terms or for the remainder of the unexpired term of a vacancy.

(2) All provisions of chapter 456 relating to the board shall apply.

457.104. Rulemaking authority

The board has authority to adopt rules pursuant to ss. 120.536(1) and 120.54 to implement provisions of this chapter conferring duties upon it.

457.105. Licensure qualifications and fees

(1) It is unlawful for any person to practice acupuncture in this state unless such person has been licensed by the board, is in a board-approved course of study, or is otherwise exempted by this chapter.

(2) A person may become licensed to practice acupuncture if the person applies to the department and:

(a) Is 21 years of age or older, has good moral character, and has the ability to communicate in English, which is demonstrated by having passed the national written examination in English or, if such examination was passed in a foreign language, by also having passed a nationally recognized English proficiency examination;

(b) Has completed 60 college credits from an accredited postsecondary institution as a prerequisite to enrollment in an authorized 3-year course of study in acupuncture and oriental medicine, and has completed a 3-year course of study in acupuncture and oriental medicine, and effective July 31, 2001, a 4-year course of study in acupuncture and oriental medicine, which meets standards established by the board by rule, which standards include, but are not limited to, successful completion of academic courses in western anatomy, western physiology, western pathology, western biomedical terminology, first aid, and cardiopulmonary resuscitation (CPR). However, any person who enrolled in an authorized course of study in acupuncture before August 1, 1997, must have completed only a 2-year course of study which meets standards established by the board by rule, which standards must include, but are not limited to, successful completion of academic courses in western anatomy, western physiology, and western pathology;

(c) Has successfully completed a board-approved national certification process, is actively licensed in a state that has examination requirements that are substantially equivalent to or more stringent than those of this state, or passes an examination administered by the department, which examination tests the applicant's competency and knowledge of the practice of acupuncture and oriental medicine. At the request of any applicant, oriental nomenclature for the points shall be used in the examination. The examination shall include a practical examination of the knowledge and skills required to practice modern and traditional acupuncture and oriental medicine, covering diagnostic and treatment techniques and procedures; and

(d) Pays the required fees set by the board by rule not to exceed the following amounts:

1. Examination fee: $500 plus the actual per applicant cost to the department for purchase of the written and practical portions of the examination from a national organization approved by the board.

2. Application fee: $300.

3. Reexamination fee: $500 plus the actual per applicant cost to the department for purchase of the written and practical portions of the examination from a national organization approved by the board.

4. Initial biennial licensure fee: $400, if licensed in the first half of the biennium, and $200, if licensed in the second half of the biennium.

457.107. Renewal of licenses; continuing education

(1) The department shall renew a license upon receipt of the renewal application and the required fee set by the board by rule, not to exceed $500.

(2) The department shall adopt rules establishing a procedure for the biennial renewal of licenses.

(3) The board shall prescribe by rule continuing education requirements of up to 30 hours biennially as a condition for renewal of a license. All education programs that contribute to the advancement, extension, or enhancement of professional skills and knowledge related to the practice of acupuncture, whether conducted by a nonprofit or profitmaking entity, are eligible for approval. The continuing professional education requirements must be in acupuncture or oriental medicine subjects, including, but not limited to, anatomy, biological sciences, adjunctive therapies, sanitation and sterilization, emergency protocols, and diseases. The board may set a fee of up to $100 for each continuing education provider. The licensee shall retain in his or her records the certificates of completion of continuing professional education requirements. All national and state acupuncture and oriental medicine organizations and acupuncture and oriental medicine schools are approved to provide continuing professional education in accordance with this subsection.

457.108. Inactive status; expiration; reactivation of licenses

(1) A license that has become inactive may be reactivated under this section upon application to the department. The board shall prescribe by rule continuing education requirements as a condition of reactivating a license. The continuing education requirements for reactivating a license must not exceed 10 classroom hours for each year the license was inactive, in addition to completion of the number of hours required for renewal on the date the license became inactive.

(2) The board shall adopt rules relating to application procedures for inactive status, renewal of inactive licenses, and reactivation of licenses. The board shall prescribe by rule an application fee for inactive status, a renewal fee for inactive status, a delinquency fee, and a fee for the reactivation of a license. None of these fees may exceed the biennial renewal fee established by the board for an active license.

(3) The department shall not reactivate a license unless the inactive or delinquent licensee has paid any applicable biennial renewal or delinquency fee, or both, and a reactivation fee.

457.1085. Infection control

Prior to November 1, 1986, the board shall adopt rules relating to the prevention of infection, the safe disposal of any potentially infectious materials, and other requirements to protect the health, safety, and welfare of the public. Beginning October 1, 1997, all acupuncture needles that are to be used on a patient must be sterile and disposable, and each needle may be used only once.

457.109. Disciplinary actions; grounds; action by the board

(1) The following acts constitute grounds for denial of a license or disciplinary action, as specified in s. 456.072(2):

(a) Attempting to obtain, obtaining, or renewing a license to practice acupuncture by bribery, by fraudulent misrepresentations, or through an error of the department.

(b) Having a license to practice acupuncture revoked, suspended, or otherwise acted against, including the denial of licensure, by the licensing authority of another state, territory, or country.

(c) Being convicted or found guilty, regardless of adjudication, in any jurisdiction of a crime which directly relates to the practice of acupuncture or to the ability to practice acupuncture. Any plea of nolo contendere shall be considered a conviction for purposes of this chapter.

(d) False, deceptive, or misleading advertising or advertising which claims that acupuncture is useful in curing any disease.

(e) Advertising, practicing, or attempting to practice under a name other than one's own.

(f) Failing to report to the department any person who the licensee knows is in violation of this chapter or of the rules of the department. However, a person who the licensee knows is unable to practice acupuncture with reasonable skill and safety to patients by reason of illness or use of alcohol, drugs, narcotics, chemicals, or any other type of material, or as a result of a mental or physical condition, may be reported to a consultant operating an impaired practitioner program as described in s. 456.076 rather than to the department.

(g) Aiding, assisting, procuring, employing, or advising any unlicensed person to practice acupuncture contrary to this chapter or to a rule of the department.

(h) Failing to perform any statutory or legal obligation placed upon a licensed acupuncturist.

(i) Making or filing a report which the licensee knows to be false, intentionally or negligently failing to file a report or record required by state or federal law, willfully impeding or obstructing such filing or inducing another person to do so. Such reports or records shall include only those which are signed in the capacity as a licensed acupuncturist.

(j) Exercising influence within a patient-acupuncturist relationship for purposes of engaging a patient in sexual activity. A patient shall be presumed to be incapable of giving free, full, and informed consent to sexual activity with his or her acupuncturist.

(k) Making deceptive, untrue, or fraudulent representations in the practice of acupuncture or employing a trick or scheme in the practice of acupuncture when such scheme or trick fails to conform to the generally prevailing standards of treatment in the community.

(1) Soliciting patients, either personally or through an agent, through the use of fraud, intimidation, undue influence, or a form of overreaching or vexatious conduct. A solicitation is any communication which directly or implicitly requests an immediate oral response from the recipient.

(m) Failing to keep written medical records justifying the course of treatment of the patient.

(n) Exercising influence on the patient to exploit the patient for the financial gain of the licensee or of a third party.

(o) Being unable to practice acupuncture with reasonable skill and safety to patients by reason of illness or use of alcohol, drugs, narcotics, chemicals, or any other type of material or as a result of any mental or physical condition. In enforcing this paragraph, upon a finding of the State Surgeon General or the State Surgeon General's designee that probable cause exists to believe that the licensee is unable to serve as an acupuncturist due to the reasons stated in this paragraph, the department shall have the authority to issue an order to compel the licensee to submit to a mental or physical examination by a physician designated by the department. If the licensee refuses to comply with such order, the department's order directing such examination may be enforced by filing a petition for enforcement in the circuit court where the licensee resides or serves as an acupuncturist. The licensee against whom the petition is filed shall not be named or identified by initials in any public court record or document, and the proceedings shall be closed to the public. The department shall be entitled to the summary procedure provided in s. 51.011. An acupuncturist affected under this paragraph shall at reasonable intervals be afforded an opportunity to demonstrate that he or she can resume the competent practice of acupuncture with reasonable skill and safety to patients. In any proceeding under this paragraph, neither the record of proceedings nor the orders entered by the department shall be used against an acupuncturist in any other proceeding.

(p) Gross or repeated malpractice or the failure to practice acupuncture with that level of care, skill, and treatment which is recognized by a reasonably prudent similar acupuncturist as being acceptable under similar conditions and circumstances.

(q) Practicing or offering to practice beyond the scope permitted by law or accepting and performing professional responsibilities which the licensee knows or has reason to know that he or she is not competent to perform.

(r) Delegating professional responsibilities to a person when the licensee delegating such responsibilities knows or has reason to know that such person is not qualified by training, experience, or licensure to perform them.

(s) Violating a lawful order of the board previously entered in a disciplinary hearing or failing to comply with a lawfully issued subpoena of the department.

(t) Conspiring with another to commit an act, or committing an act, which would tend to coerce, intimidate, or preclude another licensee from lawfully advertising his or her services.

(u) Fraud or deceit or gross negligence, incompetence, or misconduct in the operation of a course of study.

(v) Failing to comply with state, county, or municipal regulations or reporting requirements relating to public health and the control of contagious and infectious diseases.

(w) Failing to comply with any rule of the board relating to health and safety, including, but not limited to, the sterilization of needles and equipment and the disposal of potentially infectious materials.

(x) Violating any provision of this chapter or chapter 456, or any rules adopted pursuant thereto.

(2) The board may enter an order denying licensure or imposing any of the penalties in s. 456.072(2) against any applicant for licensure or licensee who is found guilty of violating any provision of subsection (1) of this section or who is found guilty of violating any provision of s. 456.072(1).

(3) The department shall not reinstate the license of an acupuncturist, or cause a license to be issued to a person it has deemed to be unqualified, until such time as the board is satisfied that he or she has complied with all the terms and conditions set forth in the final order and is capable of safely engaging in the practice of acupuncture.

457.11. Repealed by Laws 1976, c. 76 – 168, § 3; Laws 1979, c. 79 – 165, § 1

457.111. Repealed by Laws 1986, c. 86 – 265, § 12, eff. Oct. 1, 1986

457.116. Prohibited acts; penalty

(1) A person may not:

(a) Practice acupuncture unless the person is licensed under ss. 457.101 – 457.118;

(b) Use, in connection with his or her name or place of business, any title or description of services which incorporates the words "acupuncture," "acupuncturist," "certified acupuncturist," "licensed acupuncturist," "oriental medical practitioner"; the letters "L. Ac.," "R. Ac.," "A.P.," or "D.O.M."; or any other words, letters, abbreviations, or insignia indicating or implying that he or she practices acupuncture unless he or she is a holder of a valid license issued pursuant to ss. 457.101 – 457.118;

(c) Present as his or her own the license of another;

(d) Knowingly give false or forged evidence to the board or a member thereof;

(e) Use or attempt to use a license that has been suspended, revoked, or placed on inactive or delinquent status;

(f) Employ any person who is not licensed pursuant to ss. 457.101 – 457.118 to engage in the practice of acupuncture; or

(g) Conceal information relating to any violation of ss. 457.101 – 457.118.

(2) A person who violates this section commits a misdemeanor of the second degree, punishable as provided in s. 775.082 or s. 775.083.

457.118. Effect of chapter on other health care practices

This chapter shall not be construed to expand or limit the scope of practice authorized for any health care professional licensed under chapter 458, chapter 459, chapter 460, chapter 461, chapter 466, chapter 474, or chapter 486, as such scope of practice is defined by statute or rule.

457.119. Repealed by Laws 1986, c. 86 – 265, § 12, eff. Oct. 1, 1986

457.12. Repealed by Laws 1976, c. 76 – 168, § 3; Laws 1979, c. 79 – 165, § 1

457.13. Repealed by Laws 1976, c. 76 – 168, § 3; Laws 1979, c. 79 – 165, § 1

457.14. Repealed by Laws 1976, c. 76 – 168, § 3; Laws 1979, c. 79 – 165, § 1

457.15. Repealed by Laws 1976, c. 76 – 168, § 3; Laws 1978, c. 78 – 323, § 4; Laws 1979, c. 79 – 165, § 1

457.16. Repealed by Laws 1976, c. 76 – 168, § 3; Laws 1979, c. 79 – 165, § 1

FLORIDA ADMINISTRATIVE CODE

Chapter 64B1 – 1. Organization

64B1 – 1.003. Other Business Involving the Board.

For the purposes of Board member compensation under subsection (4) of Section 456.011, F.S., "other business involving the Board" is defined to include:

(1) Board meetings;

(2) Meetings of committees of the Board;

(3) Meetings of a Board member with Department staff or contractors of the Department at the Department or Board's request. Any participation or meeting of members noticed or unnoticed will be on file in the Board office;

(4) Probable cause panel meetings;

(5) All participation in board-authorized meetings with professional associations of which the board is a member or invitee. This would include, but not be limited to, all meetings of national associations of which the board is a member as well as board-authorized participation in meetings of national or professional associations or organizations involved in educating, regulating, or reviewing the profession over which the board has statutory authority; and,

(6) Conference calls for which licensing or disciplinary action is agendaed and which exceed four hours in duration; or which are called on an emergency basis.

64B1 – 1.0035. Excused Absences.

Excused absences of board members are defined as absences caused by:

(1) Illness or injury of the board member;

(2) Illness, injury or death of a board member's immediate family;

(3) Jury duty;

(4) State or federal military service.

64B1 – 1.008.   Public Comment.

The Board of Acupuncture invites and encourages all members of the public to provide comment on matters or propositions before the Board or a committee of the Board. The opportunity to provide comment shall be subject to the following:

(1) Members of the public will be given an opportunity to provide comment on subject matters before the Board after an agenda item is introduced at a properly noticed board meeting.

(2) Members of the public shall be limited to five (5) minutes to provide comment. This time shall not include time spent by the presenter responding to questions posed by Board members, staff or board counsel. The chair of the Board may extend the time to provide comment if time permits.

(3) Members of the public shall notify board staff in writing of their interest to be heard on a proposition or matter before the Board. The notification shall identify the person or entity, indicate support, opposition, or neutrality, and identify who will speak on behalf of a group or faction of persons consisting of five (5) or more persons. Any person or entity appearing before the Board may use a pseudonym if he or she does not wish to be identified.

Chapter 64B1 – 2.   Fees

64B1 – 2.001.   Fees.

(1) The initial application fee is $200.

(2) The initial license fee is $200.

(3) The biennial renewal fee for an active license is $275.

(4) The biennial renewal fee for an inactive license is $150.

(5) The application fee for inactive status is $200.

(6) The application fee for retired license is $50.

(7) The retired status fee is $50.

(8) Change of status fee for any time other than renewal is $200.

(9) The fee for reactivation of a license is $275.

(10) The deliquency fee is $200.

(11) The initial continuing education provider registration fee is $100.

(12) The biennial continuing education provider registration fee is $100.

(13) The fee for a duplicate wall certificate or license is $25.

64B1 – 2.0015.   Repealed

64B1 – 2.004.   Repealed

64B1 – 2.005.   Repealed

64B1 – 2.006.   Repealed

64B1 – 2.009. Repealed

64B1 – 2.0095. Repealed

64B1 – 2.010. Repealed

64B1 – 2.011. Repealed

64B1 – 2.012. Repealed

64B1 – 2.014. Repealed

64B1 – 2.015. Fee for Certification of a Public Record.

The Board shall charge a fee of twenty-five dollars ($25.00) for the certification of a public record.

64B1 – 2.016. Repealed

64B1 – 2.018. Repealed

Chapter 64B1 – 3. Definition; Examination of Acupuncturists

64B1 – 3.001. Definitions.

(1) Acupuncture means a form of primary health care based on traditional Chinese medical concepts, that employs acupuncture diagnosis and treatment, as well as adjunctive therapies and diagnostic techniques, for the promotion, maintenance, and restoration of health and the prevention of disease. Acupuncture shall include but not be limited to the insertion of acupuncture needles and the application of moxibustion to specific areas of the human body.

(2) Acupuncture shall include, but not be limited to:

(a) Auricular, hand, nose, face, foot and/or scalp acupuncture therapy;

(b) Stimulation to acupuncture points and channels by use of any of the following:

1. Needles, moxibustion, cupping, thermal methods, magnets, gwa-sha scraping techniques, acupatches, and acuform,

2. Manual stimulation including acutotement (which is defined as stimulation by an instrument that does not pierce the skin), massage, acupressure, reflexology, shiatsu, and tui-na,

3. Electrical stimulation including electro-acupuncture, percutaneous and transcutaneous electrical nerve stimulation,

4. Laser biostimulation in accordance with relevant federal law including Food and Drug Administration rules and regulations, providing written notice of such intended use together with proof of compliance with federal requirements are received by the Board of Acupuncture not less than 14 days prior to first time use.

(3) Acupuncture diagnostic techniques shall include but not be limited to the use of observation, listening, smelling, inquiring, palpation, pulses, tongue, physiognomy, five element correspondence, ryodoraku, akabani, German electro acupuncture, Kirlian photography, and thermography.

(4) The needles used in acupuncture shall be solid filiform instruments which shall include but not be limited to: dermal needles, plum blossom needles, press needles, prismatic needles and disposable lancets. The use of staples in the practice of acupuncture shall be prohibited.

(5) Adjunctive therapies shall include but not be limited to:

(a) Nutritional counseling and the recommendation of nonprescription substances which meet the Food and Drug Administration labeling requirements, as dietary supplements to promote health;

(b) Recommendation of breathing techniques and therapeutic exercises;

(c) Lifestyle and stress counseling;

(d) The recommendation of all homeopathic preparations approved by the Food and Drug Administration and the United States Homeopathic Pharmacopeia Committee; and,

(e) Herbology.

64B1 – 3.003.   Repealed

64B1 – 3.004.   Acupuncture Examination.

The NCCAOM examination consisting of the Foundations of Oriental Medicine Module, the Acupuncture with Point Location Module, the Biomedicine Module and the Chinese Herbology Module is approved by the Board.

64B1 – 3.008.   Repealed

64B1 – 3.009.   Licensure by Endorsement Through National Certification.

Pursuant to Section 457.105(2)(c), F.S., the Board of Acupuncture will certify for licensure by endorsement those applicants who:

(1) Provide proof of an active certification in Oriental Medicine from the National Certification Commission for Acupuncture and Oriental Medicine (NCCAOM).

(2) Meet the requirements of Sections 457.105(2)(a) and (d), F.S.

(3) Meet the requirements of set forth in subsections 64B1 – 4.001(4), (5) and (6), F.A.C.

64B1 – 3.010.   Licensure by Endorsement Through Another State License.

Pursuant to Section 457.105(2)(c), F.S., the Board of Acupuncture will certify for licensure those applicants who:

(1) Submit proof of being actively licensed in a state which has requirements that are substantially equivalent to or more stringent than those of this state at the time applicant was orginally[1] licensed. Applicants must establish their other state licensure by requesting the licensing authority of the other state provide to the Board a statement which indicates the current status of the applicant's license as of the date of statement, the expiration date of the other state license, and the basis for issuing the other state license in effect at the time applicant was licensed including the state's laws and rules and examination requirements; and

(2) Meet the requirements of Sections 457.105(2)(a) and (d), F.S.; and

(3) Meet the minimal requirements set forth in subsections 64B1 – 4.001(4), (5) and (6), F.A.C.

Chapter 64B1 – 4. Qualifications for Examination and Licensure

64B1 – 4.001. Acupuncture Program Requirements.

In order to be certified to take the licensure examination or to be eligible for licensure by endorsement, the applicant must establish that he/she has met the following minimal requirements.

(1) Applicants who were not enrolled as students prior to August 1, 1997, and completed their education after July 31, 2001, must have completed a core curriculum comparable to that of the Accreditation Commission for Acupuncture and Oriental Medicine (ACAOM) master's level program in oriental medicine, or a masters level program in acupuncture with a certificate in herbology, with a minimum of 2,700 hours of supervised instruction.

(2) Applicants who were not enrolled as students prior to August 1, 1997, and completed their education prior to July 31, 2001, must have completed 60 college credits from an accredited postsecondary institution prior to completion of a 3-year course of study in acupuncture and oriental medicine with a minimum of 2,025 hours of supervised instruction.

(3) Applicants who were enrolled as students in a program prior to August 1, 1997, must have completed at least 900 hours of supervised instruction in traditional oriental acupuncture and at least 600 hours of supervised clinical experience. All applicants under this provision must have started classes no later than February 1, 1998.

(4) All applicants must have 60 hours study in injection therapy, to include:

(a) History and development of acupuncture injection therapy;

(b) Differential diagnosis;

(c) Definitions, concepts, and pathophysiology;

(d) The nature, function, channels entered, and contraindications of herbal, homeopathic, and nutritional injectables;

(e) Diseases amenable to treatment with acupuncture injection therapy and the injectables appropriate to treat them;

(f) Identification of appropriate points for treatment, including palpatory diagnosis;

(g) A review of anatomy and referral zones;

(h) Universal precautions including management of blood borne pathogens and biohazardous waste;

(i) Procedures for injections, including preparing the injectables, contraindications and precautions;

(j) 10 hours of clinical practice on a patient or patients; and

(k) Administration techniques and equipment needed.

If the 60 hours of study in injection therapy are not documented on the official transcript submitted, a certificate from a board approved provider must be submitted to verify completion.

(5) All applicants must successfully complete 15 hours of supervised instruction in universal precautions and 20 hours of supervised instruction in Florida Statutes and Rules, including Chapters 456 and 457, F.S., and this rule chapter. If either of these areas are not documented on the official transcript submitted, a certificate from a board approved provider must be submitted to verify completion.

(6) Applicants must have completed an eight hour program or its equivalent that incorporates the safe and beneficial use of laboratory test and imaging findings in the practice of acupuncture and oriental medicine. If an 8 hour program is not documented on the official transcript submitted, a certificate from a board approved provider must be submitted to verify completion.

64B1 – 4.0011. Documentation Necessary for Licensure Application.

A properly completed application shall be submitted on Department of Health Form Application for Acupuncture License, DH – MQA 1116, 06/2020, adopted and incorporated herein by reference as this Board's application and available on the web at http://www.flrules. org/Gateway/reference.asp? No = Ref – 12187, or https://floridaacupuncture. gov/resources/. To complete the application attach the appropriate fees and supporting documents and submit it to the address listed on the instructions.

64B1 – 4.0012. English Proficiency Requirement for Licensure.

(1) Applicants who have passed the national written examination in any language other than English shall demonstrate their ability to communicate in English by earning a passing score on either the Test of English as a Foreign Language examination (hereinafter TOEFL) or the Test of Spoken English examination (hereinafter TSE), as administered by the Educational Testing Services. As used throughout this section, a passing score for the TOEFL is defined as a scaled score of 500 or greater for paper; 173 or greater for computer; or 61 or greater for internet. A passing score for the TSE is defined as a scaled score of 50 or greater. It shall be the individual responsibility of such applicants to apply for and schedule either the TOEFL examination or the TSE examination, and to obtain their official score report from the testing services prior to applying for licensure. These applicants shall submit a copy of their official score report with their application.

(2) Applicants applying for licensure by examination who indicate on their application that they wish to take the national written examination for licensure in Florida in any language other than English shall also at the time of their application submit a copy of their official score report indicating that they have passed either the TOEFL examination or the TSE.

64B1 – 4.0015. Supervised Instruction Defined.

For the purposes of rule 64B1 – 4.001, F.A.C., the Board defines "supervised instruction" as follows:

（1）"Supervised instruction" means a planned and supervised instruction of students during which students function in a hands-on capacity with acupuncture patients.

（2）During the first 200 hours of supervised instruction, the student must observe the supervisor/instructor diagnose and treat patients.

（3）During the second 200 hours of supervised instruction, the student must be under the direct supervision of the supervisor/instructor. Direct supervision shall mean that the supervisor/instructor is present in the same room as the student for all hands-on experience.

（4）During the remaining hours of supervised instruction, the student must be under the direct or indirect supervision of the supervisor/instructor. Indirect supervision shall mean that the supervisor/instructor is physically present on the premises, so that the supervisor/instructor is immediately available to the student when needed.

（5）During the remaining hours of supervised instruction, the student must diagnose and treat a minimum of 30 different patients.

（6）For applicants who enroll on or after July 31, 2001, during supervised instruction, the student must observe and use the findings of laboratory test and imaging findings in the course of patient treatment.

64B1 – 4.004.   Herbal Therapies.

Herbal therapy means the use, prescription, recommendation, and administration of herbal therapy/phytotherapy which consists of plant, animal, and/or mineral substances and shall include all homeopathic preparations to promote, maintain and restore health and to prevent disease.

64B1 – 4.005.   Oriental Massage.

Oriental massage includes traditional Chinese and modern oriental medical techniques which shall include: manual and mechanical stimulation of points, meridians, channels, collaterals, and ah-shi points; all forms of oriental bodywork including acupressure, amma, anmo, guasha, hara, niusha, reiki, reflexology, shiatsu, tuina, traction and counter traction, vibration, and other neuro-muscular, physical and physio-therapeutic techniques used in acupuncture and oriental medicine for the promotion, maintenance, and restoration of health and the prevention of disease.

64B1 – 4.006.   Qi Gong.

Qi Gong means the Chinese system of energy cultivation which uses posture, movement, exercises, breathing, meditation, visualization, and conscious intent to move, cleanse, or purify Qi to promote, maintain and restore health and to prevent disease.

64B1 – 4.007.   Electroacupuncture.

Electroacupuncture means the stimulation of points, meridians, channels, collaterals, and ah-shi points with or without needles with: the administration and/or prescription of percutaneous and transcutaneous electrical nerve and tissue stimulation; and/or the use of microcurrent; low volt; high volt; interferential current; galvanic current; and acupunctoscope.

64B1 – 4.008. Adjunctive Therapies.

Adjunctive therapies shall include the stimulation of acupuncture points, ah-shi points, auricular points, channels, collaterals, meridians, and microsystems with the use of: air; aromatherapy; color; cryotherapy; electric moxibustion; homeopathy; hyperthermia; ion pumping cords; iridology; kirlian photography; laser acupuncture; lifestyle counseling; magnet therapy; paraffin; photonic stimulation; recommendation of breathing techniques; therapeutic exercises and daily activities; sound including sonopuncture; traction; water; thermal therapy; and other adjunctive therapies and diagnostic techniques of traditional Chinese medical concepts and modern oriental medical techniques as set forth in rule 64B1 – 4.010, F.A.C.

64B1 – 4.009. Dietary Guidelines.

Dietary guidelines shall include nutritional counseling as used in acupuncture and oriental medicine and the administration, prescription, and/or recommendation of nutritional supplements to promote, maintain, and restore health and to prevent disease.

64B1 – 4.010. Traditional Chinese Medical Concepts, Modern Oriental Medical Techniques.

Traditional Chinese medical concepts and modern oriental medical techniques shall include acupuncture diagnosis and treatment to prevent or correct malady, illness, injury, pain, addictions, other conditions, disorders, and dysfunction of the human body; to harmonize the flow of Qi or vital force; to balance the energy and functions of a patient; and to promote, maintain, and restore health; for pain management and palliative care; for acupuncture anesthesia; and to prevent disease by the use or administration of: stimulation to acupuncture points, ah-shi points, auricular points, channels, collaterals, meridians, and microsystems which shall include the use of: akabane; allergy elimination techniques; breathing; cold; color; correspondence; cupping; dietary guidelines; electricity; electroacupuncture; electrodermal screening (EDS); exercise; eight principles; five element; four levels; hara; heat; herbal therapy consisting of plant, animal, and/or mineral substances; infrared and other forms of light; inquiring of history; jing-luo; listening; moxibustion; needles; NAET; observation; oriental massage-manual and mechanical methods; palpation; physiognomy; point micro-bleeding therapy; pulses; qi; xue and jin-ye; ryodoraku; san-jiao; six stages; smelling; tongue; tai qi; qi gong; wulun-baguo; yin-yang; zang-fu; Ayurvedic, Chinese, Japanese, Korean, Mongolian, Vietnamese, and other east Asian acupuncture and oriental medical concepts and treatment techniques; French acupuncture; German acupuncture including electroacupuncture and diagnosis; and, the use of laboratory test and imaging findings.

64B1 – 4.011. Diagnostic Techniques.

Diagnostic techniques which assist in acupuncture diagnosis, corroboration and monitoring of an acupuncture treatment plan or in making a determination to refer a patient to other health care providers shall include: traditional Chinese medical concepts and modern oriental medical techniques, recommendation of home diagnostic screening; physical examination; use of laboratory test findings; use of imaging films, reports, or test findings; office screening of hair, saliva and urine; muscle response testing; palpation; reflex; range of motion; sensory testing; thermography; trigger points; vital signs; first-aid; hygiene; and sanitation.

64B1 - 4.012. Acupoint Injection Therapies.

Effective March 1, 2002, adjunctive therapies shall include acupoint injection therapy which shall mean the injection of herbs, homeopathics, and other nutritional supplements in the form of sterile substances into acupuncture points by means of hypodermic needles but not intravenous therapy to promote, maintain, and restore health; for pain management and palliative care; for acupuncture anesthesia; and to prevent disease.

Chapter 64B1 - 6. Continuing Education

64B1 - 6.002. Definitions.

(1) "Approved" means acceptable to the Florida Board of Acupuncture.

(2) "Board" means Florida Board of Acupuncture.

(3) "Committee" means Committee on Continuing Education of the Board.

(4) "Contact Person" means one who is responsible for filing provider approval applications and insures compliance with these rules, maintains complete rosters of participants, and is knowledgeable about the provider's program(s).

(5) "Correspondence Program" means an approved program offered by mail with a defined course of study to be completed by the participant for which an evaluation of performance is made and a rating of satisfactory or unsatisfactory completion of the course is given by the provider.

(6) "Credit Hour" means a minimum of 50 minutes and a maximum of 60 minutes of class time. One-half (1/2) credit hour means a minimum of 25 minutes and a maximum of 30 minutes of class time.

(7) "Department" means the Department of Health.

(8) "Participant" means an acupuncturist who attends a program presented by a provider in order to achieve the stated objectives of the program.

(9) "Program" means a planned educational experience dealing with a specific content based on the stated objectives.

(10) "Provider" means the individual, organization or institution conducting the continuing education program.

64B1 - 6.005. Standards for Approval of Continuing Education Credit.

(1) A continuing education program must contribute to the advancement, extension or enhancement of the licensee's skills and knowledge related to the practice of acupuncture and oriental medicine. Programs should concern the history and theory of acupuncture, acupuncture

diagnosis and treatment techniques, techniques of adjunctive therapies, acupuncturist-patient communication and professional ethics. All continuing education courses are subject to evaluation and approval by the Board to determine that the continuing education course meets the criteria established by the Board which has final determination as to the number of hours of acceptable credit that will be awarded for each program.

(2) Each program offered for continuing education credit must be presented or taught by a person who at a minimum holds a bachelor's degree from an accredited college or university or a post-secondary education institution licensed by the State of Florida, with a major in the subject matter to be presented; or has graduated from a school of acupuncture, or has completed a tutorial program which has a curriculum equivalent to the requirements in this state and was approved by a state licensing authority, a nationally recognized acupuncture/oriental medicine association or a substantially equivalent accrediting body, and has completed three (3) years of professional experience in the licensed practice of acupuncture; and has a minimum of two (2) years teaching experience in the subject matter to be presented, or has taught the same program for which approval is sought a minimum of three (3) times in the past two (2) years before a professional convention, professional group or at any acupuncture school, or has completed specialized training in the subject matter of the program and has a minimum of two (2) years of practical experience in the subject.

(3) In order to meet the continuing education requirements, the continuing education program submitted by the licensee must meet the criteria established by the Board.

(4) No credit will be given for programs which are primarily devoted to administrative or business management aspects of acupuncture practice.

(5) To receive credit for programs on HIV/AIDS at the licensee's first renewal, the program must be, at a minimum, three (3) hours in length and must address the areas mandated in Section 456.033, F.S. The Board accepts HIV/AIDS programs presented or conducted by the Department of Health and programs approved by other professional regulatory boards for the health professions.

(6) Continuing education programs related to biomedical sciences shall be designed to provide course content on the clinical relevance of such programs while advancing, extending or enhancing the licensee's skills and knowledge in biomedical sciences.

64B1 – 6.006. Requirements for the Provider.

Each provider shall:

(1) Register with CE Broker through CEbroker.com, and pay the appropriate provider registration fee direct to CE Broker. The provider registration fee is non-refundable and shall be paid within each biennium upon the earliest of the following events that occurs during the biennium:

(a) When the provider submits a new program or programs for Board approval, or

(b) When the provider provides a continuing education program to Chapter 457, F.S., licensees for licensure renewal credit.

(2) Insure that the continuing education program(s) presented by the provider complies with these rules.

(3) Maintain a complete, alphabetized, legible roster of participants for a period of 3 years following each program presentation.

(4) Maintain a "sign-in" sheet and a "sign-out" sheet with the signatures of participants.

(5) Provide each participant with a certificate certifying that the participant has successfully completed the program. The certificate shall not be issued until completion of the program and shall contain the provider's name, title of program, date of program, location, and number of credit hours.

(6) Notify the Board of any significant changes relative to the maintenance of standards as set forth in these rules.

(7) Ensure that no person receives credit for the same program more than once.

(8) Notify the Board of any change in the presenters or instructors of any approved program, and demonstrate the new instructor meets the criteria set forth in subsection 64B1 - 6.005(2), F.A.C.

(9) Designate a contact person who assumes responsibility for each program, and who is knowledgeable about each program. The contact person shall notify the Board of any significant changes in programs or a lapse in the maintenance of standards.

(10) In a correspondence continuing education program, each provider is responsible for obtaining from each certificateholder a signed statement which states that the participant did in fact read the material, performed the exercises and took the examination personally.

(11) There shall be adequate personnel to assist with administrative matters and personnel with competencies outside content areas in cases when the method of delivery requires technical or other special expertise.

(12) Providers shall maintain records of individual offerings for inspection; records shall include subject matter, objectives, faculty qualifications, evaluation mechanisms, credit hours and rosters of participants.

64B1 - 6.008. Process for Program Approval.

(1) In order to receive Board approval of one or more programs for which continuing education credit is awarded within a biennium to an acupuncture licensee a provider shall submit an application for approval Form DOH/AP006, Continuing Education Program Approval, which is hereby incorporated by reference and will be effective 7 - 26 - 04, copies of which may be obtained from the Board office shall be submitted to the Board Office for program approval.

(2) The following courses, that meet the criteria for approval under this section, are approved by the Board:

(a) Organized courses of study sponsored by a national or state acupuncture and/or oriental medicine organization.

(b) Organized courses of study sponsored by an accredited acupuncture and/or oriental medicine school.

(3) The Board retains the right and authority to audit and/or monitor programs given by any provider. The Board will reject individual programs offered by a provider if the provider has disseminated any false or misleading information in connection with the continuing education program, or if the program provider has failed to conform to and abide by the rules of the Board.

(4) If approved, the provider may identify the program as "approved by the Florida Board of Acupuncture for Purposes of Continuing Education Credit" in any flyer or other advertisement.

64B1 – 6.009. Teaching Time for Continuing Education Credit.

(1) Those persons who teach at programs approved for continuing education credit may claim 3 hours of continuing education credit for each hour of lecture, not to exceed nine hours of continuing education credit per biennium.

(2) No continuing education credit shall be granted to a school faculty member merely as credit for his regular teaching assignments.

64B1 – 6.010. Repealed

Chapter 64B1 – 7. Renewal of License

64B1 – 7.001. Repealed

64B1 – 7.0015. Continuing Education Requirement.

(1) As a condition of the biennial renewal of a license, each licensee shall complete a minimum of 30 credit hours per biennium of continuing education that meets the requirements of Section 457.107, F.S. and Rule 64B1 – 6.005, F.A.C., which shall include:

(a) At least five hours of continuing education credit in Biomedical Sciences as set forth in Rule 64B1 – 6.005, F.A.C.;

(b) Three hours of continuing education credit on HIV/AIDS that meets the requirements of Section 456.033(2), F.S. and subsection 64B1 – 6.005(5), F.A.C. (initial renewal only);

(c) Two hours of continuing education credit on prevention of medical errors that meets the requirements of Section 456.013(7), F.S.; and,

(d) Two hours of continuing education credit on Chapters 456 and 457, F.S. and the rules promulgated by this board. Each licensee may satisfy this requirement by attending a complete board meeting at which another licensee is disciplined, or by providing an expert opinion, without compensation, in a standard of care disciplinary case or by serving as a member of the probable cause panel.

(2) For the first renewal period after initial licensure, the licensee is exempt from the

continuing education requirements of Rule 64B1 – 7.0015, F. A. C., except for the continuing education hours mandated for medical errors and the 3-hour HIV/AIDS course.

(3) Credit hours are not retroactive or cumulative. All credit hours must be earned within the biennium for which they are claimed.

64B1 – 7.002.　Requirements for Reactivation of an Inactive License.

(1) An inactive license shall be reactivated upon payment of the reactivation fee set forth in subsection 64B1 – 2.001 (9), F. A. C., and demonstration that the licensee completed the continuing education requirements as set forth in rule 64B1 – 7.0015, F.A.C., for each biennium in which the license was inactive.

(2) However, any licensee whose license has been inactive for more than two consecutive biennial licensure cycles and who has not practiced for two out of the previous four years in another jurisdiction shall be required to appear before the Board and establish the ability to practice with the care and skill sufficient to protect the health, safety, and welfare of the public. At the time of such appearance, the licensee must:

(a) Show compliance with subsection (1), above;

(b) Account for any activities related to the practice of acupuncture in this or any other jurisdiction during the period that the license was inactive and establish an absence of malpractice or disciplinary actions pending in any jurisdiction;

(c) Prove compliance with the financial responsibility requirements of section 456.048, F.S., and rule 64B1 – 12.001, F.A.C.;

(d) Prove compliance with section 456.033, F.S., and rule 64B1 – 7.0015, F.A.C.

(3) The Department shall not reactivate the certificate of any certificate holder who has:

(a) Committed any act or offense in this or any other jurisdiction which would constitute the basis for disciplining a certificate holder pursuant to section 457.109, F.S.

(b) Failed to comply with the financial responsibility requirements of section 456.048, F.S., and rule 64B1 – 12.001, F.A.C.

(c) Failed to comply with the provisions of section 456.033, F. S., and rule 64B1 – 7.0015, F.A.C.

64B1 – 7.0025.　Reactivation of Retired License.

A licensee may reactivate a retired status license subject to the following requirements:

(1) Payment of the reactivation fee, which shall be the same amount as the renewal fee for an active status licensee under these rules for each biennial licensure period in which the licensee was in retired status;

(2) Demonstrating satisfaction of the continuing education requirements of Rule 64B1 – 7.0015, F.A.C., for each licensure biennial period in which the licensee was in retired status.

64B1 – 7.004.　Notice to the Agency of Mailing Address and Place of Practice of Licensee.

(1) It shall be the duty of each licensee to provide written notification to the Department of

the licensee's current mailing address and place of practice. For purposes of this rule, "place of practice" shall mean the address of the primary physical location where the certificateholder practices acupuncture.

(2) Any time that the current mailing address or place of practice of any licensee changes, written notification of the change shall be provided to the Department within 10 days of the change. Written notice should be sent to the following address: Board of Acupuncture, 4052 Bald Cypress Way, Bin C – 06, Tallahassee, Florida 32399 – 3256. Electronic notification to MQA.Acupuncture@flhealth.gov, is acceptable, however, it is the responsibility of the licensee to ensure that the electronic notification was received by the Department.

Chapter 64B1 – 8.   Infection Control

64B1 – 8.001.   Definitions.

(1) Needles: solid filiform instruments used in the practice of acupuncture. This includes, but is not limited to, dermal needles, plum blossom needles, press needles, prismatic needles and disposable lancets. Pursuant to Section 457.1085, F.S., all acupuncture needles that are to be used on a patient must be sterile and disposable, and each needle may be used only once.

(2) Sterilization: kills all microbial life, including all bacterial spores, for instruments which enter tissue. Sterilization is accomplished by subjecting clean items to steam under pressure (autoclaving), or to dry heat.

64B1 – 8.002.   Monitoring Sterilization and Infection Control.

(1) Sterilization of equipment other than acupuncture needles, when the equipment has penetrated tissue or has been exposed to blood, shall be accomplished by proper autoclaving according to the instructions of the manufacturer of the autoclave.

(2) (a) A sterilization indicator shall be used with each autoclaving to monitor the sterilization procedure.

(b) Strips must indicate both exposure to steam and 250°F.

(3) All sterilized items must be stored and handled in a manner which maintains sterility.

(4) Each acupuncture office utilizing autoclave sterilization techniques shall post the sterilization procedures and shall maintain documentation of all autoclave service.

(5) It shall be the responsibility of the Acupuncturist to insure that personnel responsible for performing sterilization procedures pursuant to this rule shall be adequately trained.

(6) The procedures and equipment used for sterilization must have their efficacy tested periodically. Adequacy of steam under pressure (e.g., autoclave) must have its efficacy verified by appropriate biological monitoring at least once every 40 hours (2400 minutes) of use or at least once every thirty days, whichever comes first.

64B1 – 8.003.   Office Hygiene.

An acupuncture office shall be maintained in a safe and sanitary manner.

64B1－8.004.　Disposal of Biomedical Waste.

Biomedical waste must be managed pursuant to the provisions of chapter 64E－16, F.A.C., effective December 2, 2015, which is hereby incorporated by reference and can be obtained from http://www.flrules.org/Gateway/reference.asp?No=Ref－10517.

64B1－8.005.　Infection Control Training.

Prior to commencement of clinical training, every approved course of study and tutorial program shall provide training in clean needle technique and universal precautions for preventing the transmission of bloodborn pathogens and other infectious diseases, including, for example, HIV/AIDS, hepatitis, staphylococcus, and tuberculosis.

64B1－8.006.　Laboratory Test and Imaging Results Education.

During didactic and clinical training, and as part of continuing education, the Board of Acupuncture requires courses of study as to the safe and beneficial use of laboratory tests and imaging findings in the practice of acupuncture and oriental medicine.

Chapter 64B1－9.　Discipline

64B1－9.001.　Disciplinary Guidelines.

(1) When the Board finds any person has committed any of the acts set forth in Section 456.072(1) or 457.109(1), F.S., or a telehealth provider registered under Section 456.47(4), F.S., it shall issue a final order imposing appropriate penalties as recommended in the following disciplinary guidelines. The language identifying offenses below is descriptive only. The full language of each statutory provision cited must be consulted to determine the conduct included.

(a) Attempting to obtain, obtaining, or renewing a license to practice acupuncture by: bribery, or fraudulent misrepresentations, or through an error of the Department or Board.

(Sections 457.109(1)(a), 456.072(1)(h), F.S.)

1. Error of the Department or Board

	MINIMUM	MAXIMUM
FIRST OFFENSE	Letter of Concern, or laws and rules continuing education	$1,000 fine
SUBSEQUENT OFFENSES	Laws and rules continuing education	$1,000 fine
Telehealth Registrants		
FIRST OFFENSE	Suspension and a corrective action plan	Revocation
ADDITIONAL OFFENSES	Revocation	

2. Bribery or fraudulent misrepresentation

	MINIMUM	MAXIMUM
FIRST OFFENSE	Reprimand and $10,000 fine	$10,000 fine and Revocation
SUBSEQUENT OFFENSES	Reprimand and $10,000 fine	$10,000 fine and Revocation
Telehealth Registrants		
FIRST OFFENSE	Revocation	
ADDITIONAL OFFENSES	Revocation	

(b) Having a license to practice acupuncture revoked, suspended, or otherwise acted against, including the denial of licensure, by the licensing authority of another state, territory, or country. (Sections 457.109(1)(b), 456.072(1)(f), F.S.)

	MINIMUM	MAXIMUM
FIRST OFFENSE	Letter of Concern	Suspension and/or fine and/or continuing education
SUBSEQUENT OFFENSES	$500 fine and suspension and/or continuing education	Revocation
Telehealth Registrants		
FIRST OFFENSE	Letter of Concern	Suspension and corrective action plan
ADDITIONAL OFFENSES	One year suspension and corrective action plan	Revocation

(c) Being convicted or found guilty of, or entering a plea of nolo contendre to, regardless of adjudication, of a crime in any jurisdiction which relates to the practice of acupuncture or to the ability to practice acupuncture. (Sections 457.109(1)(c), 456.072(1)(c), F.S.)

	MINIMUM	MAXIMUM
FIRST OFFENSE	Letter of Concern	Suspension and/or fine and/or continuing education
SUBSEQUENT OFFENSES	Suspension and/or fine and/or continuing education	Revocation

	MINIMUM	MAXIMUM
Telehealth Registrants		
FIRST OFFENSE	Suspension and a corrective action plan	Revocation
ADDITIONAL OFFENSES	One to two year suspension	Revocation

(d) False, deceptive, or misleading advertising or advertising which claims that acupuncture is useful in curing any disease.

(Section 457.109(1)(d), F.S.)

	MINIMUM	MAXIMUM
FIRST OFFENSE	Letter of Concern	$1,000 fine
SUBSEQUENT OFFENSES	Suspension and/or fine and/or continuing education	Revocation
Telehealth Registrants		
FIRST OFFENSE	Letter of Concern	Reprimand
ADDITIONAL OFFENSES	Suspension and a corrective action plan	Revocation

(e) Advertising, practicing, or attempting to practice under a name other than one's own. (Section 457.109(1)(e), F.S.)

	MINIMUM	MAXIMUM
FIRST OFFENSE	Letter of Concern	$1,000 fine
SUBSEQUENT OFFENSES	Suspension and/or fine and/or continuing education	Revocation
Telehealth Registrants		
FIRST OFFENSE	Letter of Concern	Reprimand
ADDITIONAL OFFENSES	Suspension and a corrective action plan	Revocation

(f) Failing to report to the Department any person who the licensee knows is in violation of this chapter or of the rules of the Department or Board.

(Sections 457.109(1)(f), 456.072(1)(i), F.S.)

	MINIMUM	MAXIMUM
FIRST OFFENSE	Letter of Concern	$500 fine
SUBSEQUENT OFFENSES	Suspension and/or fine and/or continuing education	Revocation
Telehealth Registrants		
FIRST OFFENSE	Letter of Concern	Reprimand
ADDITIONAL OFFENSES	Suspension and a corrective action plan	Revocatio

(g) Aiding, assisting, procuring, employing, or advising any unlicensed person to practice acupuncture contrary to Chapter 457 or 456, F.S., or to a rule of the Department or Board. (Sections 457.109(1)(g), 456.072(1)(j), F.S.)

	MINIMUM	MAXIMUM
FIRST OFFENSE	Reprimand and $500 fine and continuing education	$5,000 fine and or suspension
SUBSEQUENT OFFENSES	$5,000 fine and/or suspension	Revocation
Telehealth Registrants		
FIRST OFFENSE	Reprimand	Revocation
ADDITIONAL OFFENSES	Suspension and a corrective action plan	Revocation

(h) Failing to perform any statutory or legal obligation placed upon a licensed acupuncturist. (Sections 457.109(1)(h), 456.072(1)(k), F.S.)

	MINIMUM	MAXIMUM
FIRST OFFENSE	Letter of Concern and $500 fine	Suspension and $1,000 fine
SUBSEQUENT OFFENSES	Suspension and $1,000 fine	Revocation
Telehealth Registrant		
FIRST OFFENSE	Reprimand	Suspension and a corrective action plan
ADDITIONAL OFFENSES	Suspension and a corrective action plan	Revocation

(i) Making or filing a report, signed in the capacity of a licensed acupuncturist, which the licensee knows to be false, intentionally or negligently failing to file a report or record required by state or federal law, willfully impeding or obstructing such filing or inducing another person to do so.

(Sections 457.109(1)(i), 456.072(1)(l), F.S.)

	MINIMUM	MAXIMUM
FIRST OFFENS	Letter of Concern and $500 fine	$5,000 and or suspension
SUBSEQUENT OFFENSES	$5,000 fine and continuing education	Revocation
Telehealth Registrants		
FIRST OFFENSE	Reprimand	Revocation
ADDITIONAL OFFENSES	suspension and a corrective action plan	Revocation

(j) Exercising influence within a patient-acupuncturist relationship for purposes of engaging a patient in sexual activity, or engaging or attempting to engage a patient in sexual activity.

(Sections 457.109(1)(j), 456.072(1)(v), F.S.)

	MINIMUM	MAXIMUM
FIRST OFFENSE	Reprimand and 500 fine	$10,000 fine, suspension and or Revocation
SUBSEQUENT OFFENSES	$5,000 fine and suspension	Revocation
Telehealth Registrants		
FIRST OFFENSE	Suspension and a corrective action plan	Revocation
ADDITIONAL OFFENSES	Revocation	

(k) Making misleading, deceptive, untrue, or fraudulent representations in or related to the practice of acupuncture or employing a trick or scheme in the practice of acupuncture when such scheme or trick fails to conform to the generally prevailing standards of treatment in the community.

(Section 457.109(1)(k), F.S.)

	MINIMU	MAXIMUM
FIRST OFFENSE	Reprimand and $10,000 fine	$10,000 fine and revocation
SUBSEQUENT OFFENSES	Reprimand and $10,000 fine	$10,000 fine and revocation

	MINIMU	MAXIMUM
Telehealth Registrants		
FIRST OFFENSE	Letter of Concern	Reprimand
ADDITIONAL OFFENSES	Suspension and a corrective action plan	Revocation

(1) Soliciting patients, either personally or through an agent, through the use of fraud, intimidation, undue influence, or a form of overreaching or vexatious conduct.

(Sections 457.109(1)(1), 456.072(1)(y), F.S.)

	MINIMUM	MAXIMUM
FIRST OFFENSE	Reprimand and $10,000 fine	$10,000 fine, suspension and or revocation
SUBSEQUENT OFFENSES	Reprimand and $10,000 fine	$10,000 fine, suspension and or revocation
Telehealth Registrants		
FIRST OFFENSE	Reprimand	Suspension and a corrective action plan
ADDITIONAL OFFENSES	Reprimand	Revocation

(m) Failing to keep written medical records which are consistent with the standard of care in acupuncture.

(Section 457.109(1)(m), F.S.)

	MINIMUM	MAXIMUM
FIRST OFFENSE	Letter of Concern and continuing education in documentation	Reprimand and $1,000 fine
SUBSEQUENT OFFENSES	Reprimand and $1,000 fine	Probation and or suspension
Telehealth Registrants		
FIRST OFFENSES	Reprimand	Suspension and a corrective action plan
ADDITIONAL OFFENSES	Suspension and a corrective action plan	Revocation

（n）Exercising influence on the patient to exploit the patient for the financial gain of the licensee or of a third party.

（Sections 457.109（1）（n），456.072（1）（n），F.S.）

	MINIMUM	MAXIMUM
FIRST OFFENSE	Reprimand and $1,000 fine	Suspension and/or $10,000 fine
SUBSEQUENT OFFENSES	$2,000 fine and suspension	Revocation
Telehealth Registrants		
FIRST OFFENSE	Reprimand	Suspension and a corrective action plan
ADDITIONAL OFFENSES	Reprimand	Revocation

（o）Being unable to practice acupuncture with reasonable skill and safety to patients by reason of illness, use of alcohol, drugs, narcotics, chemicals, or any other type of material or as a result of any mental or physical condition.

（Sections 457.109（1）（o），456.072（1）（z），F.S.）

	MINIMUM	MAXIMUM
FIRST OFFENSE	Suspension until such time as the licensee can provide Board's satisfaction to demonstrate ability to practice with reasonable skill and safety	Revocation
SUBSEQUENT OFFENSES	Suspension until such time as the licensee can provide Board's satisfaction to demonstrate ability to practice with reasonable skill and safety	Revocation
Telehealth Registrants		
FIRST OFFENSE	Suspension and a corrective action plan	Revocation
ADDITIONAL OFFENSES	Suspension and a corrective action plan	Revocation

（p）Gross or repeated malpractice or the failure to practice acupuncture with that level of care, skill, and treatment which is recognized by a reasonably prudent, similar acupuncturist as being acceptable under similar conditions and circumstances.

（Section 457.109（1）（p），F.S.）

	MINIMUM	MAXIMUM
FIRST OFFENSE	Letter of Concern and continuing education	$1,000 fine, suspension and continuing education
SUBSEQUENT OFFENSES	Probation or suspension and/or $5,000 fine	Revocation
Telehealth Registrants		
FIRST OFFENSE	Reprimand	Suspension and corrective action plan
ADDITIONAL OFFENSES	Suspension and a corrective action plan	Revocation

(q) Practicing or offering to practice beyond the scope permitted by law or accepting and performing professional responsibilities which the licensee knows or has reason to know that he or she is not competent to perform.

(Sections 457.109(1)(q), 456.072(1)(o), F.S.)

	MINIMUM	MAXIMUM
FIRST OFFENSE	Letter of Concern and continuing education	$1,000 fine, suspension and continuing education
SUBSEQUENT OFFENSES	Probation or suspension and/or $2,000 fine	Revocation
Telehealth Registrants		
FIRST OFFENSE	Reprimand	Suspension and a corrective action plan
ADDITIONAL OFFENSES	Suspension and a corrective action plan	Revocation

(r) Delegating or contracting for professional responsibilities by a person when the licensee delegating or contracting for such responsibilities knows or has reason to know that such person is not qualified by training, experience, or licensure to perform them.

(Sections 457.109(1)(r), 456.072(1)(p), F.S.)

	MINIMUM	MAXIMUM
FIRST OFFENSE	Letter of Concern and continuing education	$1,000 fine, suspension and CE
SUBSEQUENT OFFENSES	Probation or suspension and/or $2,000 fine	Revocation
Telehealth Registrants		

	MINIMUM	MAXIMUM
FIRST OFFENSE	Reprimand	Suspension and a corrective action plan
ADDITIONAL OFFENSES	Suspension and a correction action plan	Revocation

（s）Violating any provision of Chapter 457 or 456, F.S., a rule of the Board or Department, or a lawful order of the Board previously entered in a disciplinary hearing or failing to comply with a lawfully issued subpoena of the department.

（Sections 457.109（1）（s）, 456.072（1）（q）, F.S.）

	MINIMUM	MAXIMUM
FIRST OFFENSE	Letter of Concern and $500 fine	Suspension
SUBSEQUENT OFFENSES	$500 fine and suspension	Revocation
Telehealth Registrants		
FIRST OFFENSE	Reprimand	Revocation
ADDITIONAL OFFENSES	Suspension and a corrective action plan	Revocation

（t）Conspiring with another to commit an act, or committing an act, which would tend to coerce, intimidate, or preclude another licensee from lawfully advertising his or her services.

（Section 457.109（1）（t）, F.S.）

	MINIMUM	MAXIMUM
FIRST OFFENSE	Letter of Concern	$1,000 fine
SUBSEQUENT OFFENSES	$1,000 fine and suspension	Revocation
Telehealth Registrants		
FIRST OFFENSE	Letter of Concern	Reprimand
ADDITIONAL OFFENSES	Suspension and a corrective action plan	Revocation

（u）Fraud or deceit or gross negligence, incompetence, or misconduct in the operation of a course of study.

1. Gross negligence, incompetence, or misconduct：

（Section 457.109（1）（u）, F.S.）

	MINIMUM	MAXIMUM
FIRST OFFENSE	Reprimand and $2,000 fine	$10,000 fine and probation or suspension
SUBSEQUENT OFFENSES	Suspension and $2,000 fine	$10,000 fine and revocation
Telehealth Registrants		
FIRST OFFENS	Suspension and a corrective action plan	Revocation
ADDITIONAL OFFENSES	Revocation	

2. Fraud or deceit:

	MINIMUM	MAXIMUM
FIRST OFFENSE	Reprimand and $10,000 fine	$10,000 fine and Revocation
SUBSEQUENT OFFENSES	Reprimand and $10,000 fin	$10,000 fine and Revocation
Telehealth Registrants		
FIRST OFFENSE	Suspension and a corrective action plan	Revocation
ADDITIONAL OFFENSES	Suspension	Revocation

(v) Failing to comply with state, county, or municipal regulations or reporting requirements, relating to public health and the control of contagious and infectious diseases.
(Section 457.109(1)(v), F.S.)

	MINIMUM	MAXIMUM
FIRST OFFENSE	Reprimand and $500 fine and continuing education	Reprimand and $1,000 and continuing education
SUBSEQUENT OFFENSES	Reprimand and $1,000 and continuing education	Reprimand and $5,000 and continuing education
Telehealth Registrants		
FIRST OFFENSE	Reprimand	Suspension and a corrective action plan
ADDITIONAL OFFENSES	Suspension and a corrective action plan	Revocation

(w) Failing to comply with any rule of the Board relating to health and safety, including, but not limited to, the sterilization of needles and equipment and the disposal of potentially infectious materials.

(Sections 457.072(1)(w), 456.072(1)(b), F.S.)

	MINIMUM	MAXIMUM
FIRST OFFENSE	Reprimand and $500 fine and continuing education	Reprimand and $1,000 and continuing education
SUBSEQUENT OFFENSES	Reprimand and $1,000 and continuing education	Reprimand and $5,000 and continuing education
Telehealth Registrants		
FIRST OFFENSE	Reprimand	Suspension and a corrective action plan
ADDITIONAL OFFENSES	Suspension and a correction action plan	Revocation

(x) Failing to comply with continuing education requirements, including requirements for HIV/AIDS education.

(Sections 457.109(1)(x), 456.072(1)(b), and (e), F.S.)

	MINIMU	MAXIMUM
FIRST OFFENSE	Suspension until continuing education completed	$1,000 and suspension until continuing education completed
SUBSEQUENT OFFENSES	Suspension until continuing education completed	Revocation
Telehealth Registrants		
FIRST OFFENSE	Letter of Concern	Reprimand
ADDITIONAL OFFENSES	Suspension and a corrective action plan	Suspension and a corrective action plan

(y) Having been found liable in a civil proceeding for knowingly filing a false report or complaint with the department against another licensee.

(Section 456.072(1)(g), F.S.)

	MINIMUM	MAXIMUM
FIRST OFFENSE	Reprimand and $500 fine	Suspension and $1,000 fine
SUBSEQUENT OFFENSES	Suspension and $2,000 fine	Revocation

	MINIMUM	MAXIMUM
Telehealth Registrants		
FIRST OFFENSE	Reprimand	Suspension
ADDITIONAL OFFENSES	Suspension	Revocation

(z) Improperly interfering with an investigation or inspection authorized by statute, or with any disciplinary proceeding.

(Section 456.072(1)(r), F.S.)

	MINIMUM	MAXIMUM
FIRST OFFENSE	Letter of Concern	$1,000 fine and/or suspension
SUBSEQUENT OFFENSES	$2,000 fine and suspension	Revocation
Telehealth Registrants		
FIRST OFFENSE	Letter of Concern	Reprimand
ADDITIONAL OFFENSES	Suspension and a corrective action plan	Suspension and a corrective action plan

(aa) Failing to report to the Board in writing with 30 days after the licensee has been convicted or found guilty of, or entered a pleas of nolo contendere to, regardless of adjudication, a crime in any jurisdiction.

(Section 456.072(1)(x), F.S.)

	MINIMUM	MAXIMUM
FIRST OFFENSE	Letter of Concern	$2,000 fine and CE's
SUBSEQUENT OFFENSES	Reprimand and $500 fine	$2,000 fine and CE
Telehealth Registrants		
FIRST OFFENSE	Letter of Concern	Reprimand
ADDITIONAL OFFENSES	Suspension and a corrective action plan	Revocation

(bb) Using information about people involved in a motor vehicle accident which has been derived from accident reports made by law enforcement officers or persons involved in accidents pursuant to Section 316.066, F.S., or using information published in a newspaper or other news publication or through a radio or television broadcast that has used information gained from such reports, for the purposes of solicitation of the people involved in such accidents.

(Section 456.072(1)(y), F.S.)

	MINIMUM	MAXIMUM
FIRST OFFENSE	Reprimand and $500 fine	Suspension
SUBSEQUENT OFFENSES	Reprimand and $1,000 fine	Revocation
Telehealth Registrants		
FIRST OFFENSE	Suspension and a corrective action plan	Suspension and a corrective action plan
ADDITIONAL OFFENSES	Suspension and a corrective action plan	Revocation

(cc) Being convicted of, or entering a plea of guilty or nolo contendere to, any misdemeanor or felony, regardless of adjudication, under 18 U.S.C. s. 669, ss. 285 – 287, s. 371, s. 1001, s. 1035, s. 1341, s. 1343, s. 1347, s. 1349, or s. 1518, or 42 U.S.C. ss. 1320a – 7b, relating to the Medicaid program.

(Section 456.072(1)(ii), F.S.)

	MINIMUM	MAXIMUM
FIRST OFFENSE	Reprimand and $10,000 fine	Revocation
SUBSEQUENT OFFENSES	Reprimand and $10,000 fine	Revocation
Telehealth Registrants		
FIRST OFFENSE	Revocation	
ADDITIONAL OFFENSES	Revocation	

(dd) Failing to comply with, failing to successfully complete or or being terminated from an impaired practitioner treatment program.

(Section 456.072(1)(hh), F.S.)

	MINIMUM	MAXIMUM
FIRST OFFENSE	Suspension	Revocation
SUBSEQUENT OFFENSES	Suspension	Revocation

续 表

	MINIMUM	MAXIMUM
Telehealth Registrants		
FIRST OFFENSE	Suspension and corrective action plan	Suspension and corrective action plan
ADDITIONAL OFFENSES	Suspension and corrective action plan	Revocation

(ee) Failing to remit the sum owed to the State for an overpayment from the Medicaid Program pursuant to a final order, judgment, or Stipulation or settlement. Section 456.072(1) (jj), F.S.

(Section 456.072(1)(jj), F.S.)

	MINIMUM	MAXIMUM
FIRST OFFENSE	Suspension until complied	Revocation
SUBSEQUENT OFFENSES	Suspension until complied	Revocation
Telehealth Registrants		
FIRST OFFENSE	Suspension and a corrective action plan	Revocation
ADDITIONAL OFFENSES	Suspension and a corrective action plan	Revocation

(ff) Being terminated from the state Medicaid Program pursuant to Section 409.913, F.S., any other state Medicaid program, or the federal Medicare program, unless eligibility to participate in the program from which the practitioner was terminated has been restored. Section 456.072(1)(kk), F.S.

(Section 456.072(1)(kk), F.S.)

	MINIMUM	MAXIMUM
FIRST OFFENSE	Revocation	Revocation
Telehealth Registrants		
FIRST OFFENSE	Revocation	
ADDITIONAL OFFENSES	Revocation	

(gg) Being convicted of, or entering a plea of guilty or nolo contendere to, any misdemeanor or felony, regardless of adjudication, a crime in any jurisdiction which related to health care fraud. Section 456.072(1)(ll), F.S.

（Section 456.072(1)(ll), F.S.）

	MINIMUM	MAXIMUM
FIRST OFFENSE	$10,000 fine	$10,000 fine and/or suspension or revocation
SUBSEQUENT OFFENSES	$10,000 fine	$10,000 fine and revocation
Telehealth Registrants		
FIRST OFFENSE	Revocation	
ADDITIONAL OFFENSEs	Revocation	

（hh）Willfully failing to comply with Section 627.64194 or 641.513, F.S., with such frequency as to indicate a general business practice.

（Section 456.072(1)(oo), F.S.）

	MINIMUM	MAXIMUM
FIRST OFFENSE	Reprimand and $1,000 fine	$4,000.00 fine and suspension
SUBSEQUENT OFFENSES	$5,000 fine and probation	$10,000 fine and revocation
Telehealth Registrants		
FIRST OFFENSE	Suspension and a corrective action plan	Revocation
ADDITIONAL OFFENSES	Suspension and a corrective action plan	Revocation

（ii）Providing information, including written documentation, indicating that a person has a disability or supporting a person's need for an emotional support animal under Section 760.27, F.S., without personal knowledge of the person's disability or disability-related need for the specific emotional support animal.

（Section 456.072(1)(pp), F.S.）

	MINIMUM	MAXIMUM
FIRST OFFENSE	Reprimand and $1,000 fine	Suspension and $4,000 fine
SUBSEQUENT OFFENSES	Suspension and $8,000 fine	Revocation
Telehealth Registrants		

	MINIMUM	MAXIMUM
FIRST OFFENSE	Suspension and a corrective action plan	Revocation
ADDITIONAL OFFENSES	Suspension and a corrective action plan	Revocation

（jj）Except as otherwise provided by law, failure to comply with the parental consent requirements of Section 1014.06, F.S. (Section 456.072(1)(rr), F.S.)

	MINIMUM	MAXIMUM
FIRST OFFENSE	Reprimand and $1,000 fine.	Reprimand and $2,000 fine
SUBSEQUENT OFFENSES	Suspension and $2,500 fine.	Revocation
Telehealth Registrants		
FIRST OFFENSE	Reprimand	Suspension and corrective action plan
ADDITIONAL OFFENSES	Suspension and corrective action plan	Revocation

（kk）Being convicted or found guilty of, entering a plea of guilty or nolo contendere to, regardless of adjudication, or committing or attempting, soliciting, or conspiring to commit an act that would constitute a violation of any of the offenses listed in Section 456.074(5), F.S. or similar offense in another jurisdiction. (Section 456.072(1)(ss), F.S.)

	MINIMUM	MAXIMUM
FIRST OFFENSE	Revocation	NA
SUBSEQUENT OFFENSES	NA	NA
Telehealth Registrants		
FIRST OFFENSE	Revocation	NA
ADDITIONAL OFFENSES	NA	NA

（2）Based upon consideration of the following factors, the Board may impose disciplinary action other than those penalties recommended above：

（a）The danger to the public；

（b）The number of repetitions of offenses, other than an adjudicated offense for which the licensee is presently being penalized;

(c) The length of time since date of violation;

(d) The number of complaints filed against the licensee;

(e) The length of time the licensee has practiced acupuncture;

(f) The actual damage, physical or otherwise, to a patient;

(g) The deterrent effect of the penalty imposed;

(h) The effect of the penalty upon the licensee's livelihood;

(i) Any efforts for rehabilitation;

(j) The actual knowledge of the licensee pertaining to the violation;

(k) Attempts by the licensee to correct or stop a violation or refusal of a licensee to correct or stop a violation;

(l) Any action relating to discipline or denial of a certificate or license in another state including, findings of guilt or innocence, standards applied, penalties imposed and penalties served.

(3) Violations and Range of Penalties. In imposing discipline upon applicants and licensees, in proceedings pursuant to Sections 120.57(1) and (2), F.S., the Board shall act in accordance with the disciplinary guidelines and shall impose a penalty within the range corresponding to the violations. Any of the above penalties may may include continuing education. For applicants, any and all offenses listed herein are sufficient for refusal to certify an application for licensure. In addition to the penalty imposed, the Board shall recover the costs of investigation and prosecution of the case. Additionally, if the Board makes a finding of pecuniary benefit or self-gain related to the violation, then the Board shall require refunds of fees billed and collected from the patient or a third party on behalf of the patient.

(4) The provisions of subsections (1) through (4), above, shall not be construed as to prohibit civil action or criminal prosecution as provided in Section 457.116 or 456.072, F.S., and the provision of subsections (1) through (4), above, shall not be construed so as to limit the ability of the Board to enter into binding stipulations with accused parties as per Section 120.57(4), F.S.

(5) Telehealth guidelines.

(a) The range of disciplinary action for registered out-of-state telehealth providers shall be, in ascending order of severity, Letter of Concern, reprimand, suspension, and Revocation.

(b) A suspension may be for a definite term or may be accompanied by a corrective action plan established by the Board.

(c) A suspension for a definite term may be terminated early only upon aproval[1] of the Board. A suspension accompanied by a corrective action plan may be terminated upon successful compliance with the corrective action plan or as otherwise determined by the Board.

(d) A "corrective action plan" must accompany a suspension and must include rehabilitative provisions established by the Board which are narrowly tailored to address the conduct which resulted in the underlying disciplinary violations. In order to satisfy a corrective action plan, the Registrant must provide proof of successful completion of all terms to the Board. A corrective action plan may follow a suspension for a definate term. Nothing in this provision shall be interpreted as restricting the Board's ability to impose a suspension for a definite term absent, or accompanied by a correction action plan.

64B1 – 9.002.   Citations.

(1) Definitions. As used in this rule:

(a) "Citation" means an instrument which meets the requirements set forth in Section 456.077, F.S., and which is served upon a subject for the purpose of assessing a penalty in an amount established by this rule;

(b) "Subject" means the licensee, applicant, person, partnership, corporation, or other entity alleged to have committed a violation designated in this rule.

(2) In lieu of the disciplinary procedures contained in Section 456.073, F.S., the department is hereby authorized to dispose of any violation designated herein by issuing a citation to the subject within six months after the filing of the complaint which is the basis for the citation.

(3) The Board hereby designates the following violations as citation violations which shall result in a penalty of $500.00:

(a) Violation of Section 457.109(1)(d) or (e), F.S.;

(b) Violation of Rule 64B1 – 10.002, F.A.C.;

(c) Failure to renew license with proper continuing education credit.

64B1 – 9.003.   Notice of Noncompliance.

(1) Definitions.

(a) "Notice of noncompliance" is a notification by the department issued to a certificateholder as a first response to minor violations of Board rules, which is not accompanied by a fine or other disciplinary penalty.

(b) "Minor violation" refers to a violation of a Board rule that does not result in economic or physical harm to a person or adversely affect the public health, safety, or welfare or create a significant threat of such harm.

(2) The Board designates the following as minor violations for which a notice of noncompliance may be issued for the first violation of failure to provide written notice of a licensee's current mailing address and place of practice in violation of Rule 64B1 – 7.004, F.A.C.

64B1 – 9.004.   Probable Cause Determination.

(1) The determination as to whether probable cause exists to believe that a violation of the provisions of Chapter 456 or 457, F.S., or of the rules promulgated thereunder has occurred, shall be made by a majority vote of a probable cause panel of the Board.

(2) The probable cause panel shall be composed of membership authorized under Section 456.073, F.S., and may include one former board member whose term of service shall not

exceed one year, unless reappointed by the Board Chairperson.

(3) The probable cause panel shall be selected by the Chairperson of the Board.

(4) The probable cause panel shall meet at such times as called by the Board Chairperson or the Board Executive Director.

(5) The presiding officer of the panel shall be selected by the Board Chairperson.

64B1 - 9.006. Mediation.

(1) "Mediation" means a process whereby a mediator is appointed by the Department to encourage and facilitate resolution of a legally sufficient complaint. It is an informal and non-adversarial process with the objective of assisting the parties or the complainant and the subject of a complaint to reach a mutually acceptable agreement.

(2) The Board finds that mediation is an acceptable method of dispute resolution for the first alleged violation of failure to conspicuously identify the licensee by name in an advertisement, in violation of Rule 64B1 - 9.007, F.A.C.

64B1 - 9.007. Advertising.

(1) Advertising by persons licensed or certified under chapter 457, F.S., is permitted so long as the information disseminated is in no way false, deceptive, or misleading and so long as the information does not claim that acupuncture is useful in curing any disease. Any advertisement or advertising shall be deemed false, deceptive, or misleading if it:

(a) Contains a misrepresentation of facts, or

(b) Makes only a partial disclosure of relevant facts; or

(c) Creates false or unjustified expectations of beneficial assistance, or

(d) Contains any representations or claims, as to which the person making the claims does not intend to perform, or

(e) Contains any other representation, statement, or claim which misleads or deceives, or

(f) Fails to conspicuously identify the licensee by name in the advertisement.

(2) As used in the rules of this board, the terms "advertisement" and "advertising" shall mean any statements, oral or written, disseminated to or before the public or any portion thereof, with the intent of furthering the purpose, either directly or indirectly, of selling professional services, or offering to perform professional services, or inducing members of the public to enter into any obligation relating to such professional services.

(3) It shall not be considered false, deceptive, or misleading for any persons licensed or certified under chapter 457, F.S., to use the following initials or terms:

(a) L.Ac.;

(b) R.Ac.;

(c) A.P.;

(d) D.O.M.;

(e) Licensed Acupuncturist;

(f) Registered Acupuncturist;

(g) Acupuncture Physician; and,

(h) Doctor of Oriental Medicine.

(4) Any licensee who advertises through an agent or through a referral service shall be held responsible for the content of such advertising and shall ensure that the advertising complies with this rule and chapter 457, F.S.

Chapter 64B1 – 10. Acupuncture Medical Records

64B1 – 10.001. Content and Retention of Medical Records.

(1) Acupuncturists are required to maintain written medical records justifying the course of treatment of each patient. These records must include for each patient at least the following:

(a) Patient's Medical History;

(b) Acupuncture Diagnostic Impressions;

(c) Points Used and/or Treatment Procedures Administered at Each Visit;

(d) Acupuncturists' Recommendations;

(e) Patient Progress Notes;

(f) Laboratory test results when appropriate and medically necessary; and,

(g) Imaging films, reports or test results when appropriate and medically necessary.

(2) All medical records must be maintained by the acupuncturist for a period of five (5) years from the date of the last entry to the record.

64B1 – 10.002. Medical Records of an Acupuncturist Who Dies, Terminates His Practice, or Relocates; Retention; Time Limitations.

(1) The executor, administrator, personal representative or survivor of a deceased acupuncturist licensed pursuant to Chapter 457, F.S., shall retain medical records in existence upon the death of the acupuncturist concerning any patient of the acupuncturist for at least a period of two (2) years from the date of the death of the acupuncturist.

(2) Within one (1) month from the date of death of the acupuncturist, the executor, administrator, personal representative or survivor of the deceased acupuncturist shall cause to be published in the newspaper of greatest general circulation in the county where the acupuncturist maintained his office, a notice indicating to the patients of the deceased acupuncturist that the acupuncturist's medical records are available to the patients or their duly constituted representative from a person at a certain location.

(3) At the conclusion of a 24 month period of time from the date of the acupuncturist's death, or thereafter, the executor, administrator, personal representative, or survivor shall cause to be published once during each week for four (4) consecutive weeks, in the newspaper of greatest general circulation in the county where the acupuncturist maintained his office, a notice indicating to the patients of the deceased acupuncturist that the acupuncturist's medical records

will be disposed of or destroyed one (1) month or later from the last day of the fourth week of publication.

(4) An acupuncturist licensed pursuant to Chapter 457, F.S., who terminates his practice or relocates and is no longer available to his patients shall ensure that the medical records which pertain to his patients are retained for at least two (2) years following such termination of practice or relocation.

(5) An acupuncturist licensed pursuant to Chapter 457, F.S., who terminates his practice or relocates and is no longer available to his patients and who does not transfer his practice to another acupuncturist or physician shall provide written notice of such termination or relocation by U.S. Mail to all patients who have received treatment within the sixty (60) days prior to the termination or relocation and who require active, ongoing treatment. The notice shall inform the patients that the acupuncturist's medical records are available to the patients or their duly constituted representative from a specific person at a certain location.

(6) In all other cases, at least sixty (60) days prior to the date of an acupuncturist's termination of practice or relocation, the acupuncturist shall cause to be published once during each week for four (4) consecutive weeks, in the newspaper of greatest general circulation in the county where the acupuncturist maintains his office, a notice indicating to the patients of such acupuncturist that the acupuncturist's medical records are available to the patients or their duly constituted representative from a specific person at a certain location.

(7) At the conclusion of a two (2) year period of time from the date of the acupuncturist's termination of practice or relocation, or thereafter, the acupuncturist shall cause to be published once during each week for four (4) consecutive weeks, in the newspaper of greatest general circulation in the county where the acupuncturist maintained his office, a notice indicating to the patients of the acupuncturist that the acupuncturist's medical records will be disposed of or destroyed one (1) month or later from the last day of the fourth week of publication.

Chapter 64B1 – 12. Financial Responsibility

64B1 – 12.001. Financial Responsibility.

As a prerequisite for licensure or license renewal every acupuncturist is required to maintain medical malpractice insurance or provide proof of financial responsibility as set forth herein:

(1) Obtaining and maintaining professional liability coverage in an amount not less than $10,000 per claim, with a minimum annual aggregate of not less than $30,000, from an authorized insurer as defined under Section 624.09, F.S., from a surplus lines insurer as defined under Section 626.914(2), F.S., from a risk retention group as defined under Section 627.942, F.S., from the Joint Underwriting Association established under Section 627.351(4), F.S., or through a plan of self-insurance as provided in Section 627.357, F.S.

(2) Obtaining and maintaining an unexpired, irrevocable letter of credit, established pursuant

to Chapter 675, Florida Statutes in an amount not less than $10,000 per claim, with a minimum aggregate availability of credit of not less than $30,000. The letter of credit shall be payable to the acupuncturist as beneficiary upon presentment of a final judgment indicating liability and awarding damages to be paid by the acupuncturist or upon presentment of a settlement agreement signed by all parties to such agreement when such final judgment or settlement is a result of a claim arising out of the rendering of, or the failure to render, acupuncture services. Such letter of credit shall be nonassignable and nontransferable. Such letter of credit shall be issued by any bank or savings association organized and existing under the laws of the State of Florida or any bank or savings association organized under the laws of the United States that has its principal place of business in this state or has a branch office which is authorized under the laws of this state or of the United States to receive deposits in this state.

(3) Obtaining and maintaining a surety bond in an amount not less than $10,000 per claim, with a minimum annual aggregate of not less than $30,000 written by a company licensed to do business in this state and rated A + by Best's.

(4) Upon application to the Board, the following licensees shall be exempted from meeting the requirements of this rule:

(a) Any acupuncturist who practices exclusively as an officer, employee or agent of the federal government or of the State of Florida or its agencies or subdivision. For purposes of this rule, an agent of the State of Florida, its agencies or its subdivisions is a person who is eligible for coverage under any self insurance or insurance program authorized by the provisions of Section 768.28(14), F.S., or who is a volunteer under Section 110.501(1), F.S.

(b) Any person whose license has become inactive under Chapter 457, F.S., and who is not practicing in this state. Any person applying for reactivation of a license must show either that such licensee maintained tail insurance coverage which provided liability coverage for incidents that occurred on or after October 1, 1993, or the initial date of licensure in this state, whichever is later, and incidents that occurred before the date on which the license became inactive; or such licensee must submit an affidavit stating that such licensee has no unsatisfied medical malpractice judgments or settlements at the time of application for reactivation.

(c) Any person licensed or certified under Chapter 457, F.S., who practices only in conjunction with his/her teaching duties at an accredited school. Such person may engage in the practice of acupuncture to the extent that such practice is incidental to and a necessary part of duties in connection with the teaching position in the school.

(d) Any person holding an active license under Chapter 457, F.S., who is not practicing in this state. If such person initiates or resumes practice in this state, he/she must notify the Board of such activity.

(e) Any person who can demonstrate to the Board that he/she has no malpractice exposure in the State of Florida.

KENTUCKY

KENTUCKY REVISED STATUTES ANNOTATED

311.671   Applicability of KRS 311.671 to 311.686

In order to protect the life, health, and safety of the public, any person practicing or offering to practice as an acupuncturist shall be licensed as provided in KRS 311.671 to 311.686. It shall be unlawful for any person not licensed under KRS 311.671 to 311.686 to practice acupuncture in this state, or to use any title, sign, card, or device to indicate that he or she is an acupuncturist. The provisions of KRS 311.671 to 311.686 are not intended to limit, preclude, or otherwise interfere with the practice of other health-care providers, working in any setting and certified or licensed by appropriate agencies or committees of the Commonwealth of Kentucky, whose practices and training may include elements of the same nature as the practice of a licensed acupuncturist.

311.672   Definitions for 311.671 to 311.686

In KRS 311.671 to 311.686, the following words and phrases shall have the meanings given to them, unless the context clearly indicates otherwise:

(1) "Acupuncturist" means an individual licensed to practice acupuncture by the board;

(2) "Board" means the State Board of Medical Licensure;

(3) "Committee" means the Acupuncture Advisory Committee under the State Board of Medical Licensure;

(4) "Licensure" means licensure by the board to practice acupuncture; and

(5) "Practice of acupuncture" means the insertion of acupuncture needles, with or without accompanying electrical or thermal stimulation, at certain acupuncture points or meridians on the surface of the human body for purposes of changing the flow of energy in the body and may include acupressure, cupping, moxibustion, or dermal friction. The practice of acupuncture shall not include laser acupuncture, osteopathic manipulative treatment, chiropractic adjustments, physical therapy, or surgery.

LRC NOTES

Legislative Research Commission Note (7 – 12 – 06): 2006 Ky. Acts ch. 249, sec. 2, subsec. (3), read: "Council" means the Acupuncture Advisory Council under the State Board of Medical Licensure." However, 2006 Ky. Acts ch. 249, sec. 3, created the Acupuncture Advisory Committee, not the Acupuncture Advisory Council. The Reviser of Statutes has changed the references to "Council" to "Committee" in codifying this statute, under the authority of KRS 7.136(1)(h).

311.673 Administration regulations; Acupuncture Advisory Committee; membership; meetings; duties

(1) The board shall promulgate administrative regulations in accordance with KRS Chapter 13A relating to the licensure and regulation, including temporary licensure, of acupuncturists. Regulation of acupuncture includes continuing education requirements and fee schedules.

(2) The board shall establish an eight (8) member Acupuncture Advisory Committee that shall review and make recommendations to the board regarding matters relating to acupuncturists that come before the board, including but not limited to:

(a) Applications for acupuncturist licensure;

(b) Licensure renewal requirements;

(c) Fees;

(d) Applicable standards of practice for acupuncture practitioners;

(e) Continuing education requirements;

(f) Rotating appointment of committee members;

(g) Disciplinary actions, at the request of a panel of the board; and

(h) Promulgation and revision of administrative regulations.

(3) Members of the Acupuncturist Advisory Committee shall be appointed by the board for four (4) year terms, on a rotating basis to provide for continuity, and shall consist of:

(a) One (1) member of the board;

(b) Two (2) physicians licensed by the board whose practices include the use of acupuncture;

(c) One (1) member of the public who is not associated with or financially interested in the practice of acupuncture; and

(d) Four (4) acupuncture practitioners licensed by the board.

(4) The chairperson and secretary of the committee shall be elected by a majority vote of the committee members annually. The president shall be responsible for presiding over meetings that shall be held on a regular basis, but no less than two (2) times each calendar year. Additional meetings may be held each calendar year at the call of the chairperson or by the written request

of at least three (3) committee members. The secretary shall keep a record of the minutes of the committee's meetings. Five (5) members of the committee shall constitute a quorum to conduct business.

(5) Members shall receive reimbursement for expenditures relating to attendance at committee meetings consistent with state policies for reimbursement of travel expenses for state employees.

(6) The board may remove any member on the member's request or for poor attendance at committee meetings, neglect of duties, or malfeasance in office.

311.674 Licensure as an acupuncturist; approval and denial of applications; renewal; reciprocity

(1) To be licensed by the board as an acupuncturist, an applicant shall:

(a) Submit an application approved by the board, with all sections completed, with the required fee;

(b) Be of good character and reputation, if in accordance with KRS Chapter 335B;

(c) Have achieved a passing score on the acupuncture examination administered by the National Commission for Certification of Acupuncture and Oriental Medicine; and

(d) Have graduated from a course of training of at least one thousand eight hundred (1,800) hours, including three hundred (300) clinical hours, that is approved by the Accreditation Commission for Acupuncture and Oriental Medicine.

All provisions of this subsection, including graduation from an approved course of training as specified in paragraph (d) of this subsection, must be met by all applicants before initial licensure as an acupuncturist may be granted.

(2) An acupuncturist who is legally authorized to practice acupuncture in another state and who is presently in good standing in that other state may be licensed by endorsement from the state of his or her credentialing if that state has standards substantially equivalent to those of this Commonwealth.

(3) The board may request any reasonable information from the applicant and from collateral sources that is necessary for the board to make an informed decision. The applicant will execute any necessary waiver or release so that the board may obtain necessary information from collateral sources. An application will be considered completed when the applicant has fully answered all sections of the approved application and the board has received all necessary additional information from the applicant and collateral sources.

(4) An acupuncturist's license shall be renewed every two (2) years upon fulfillment of the following requirements:

(a) The applicant has submitted a renewal application approved by the board within the time specified, with all sections completed, with the required fee; and

(b) The applicant is of good character and reputation.

(5) The board shall notify each applicant in writing of the action it takes on an application

within one hundred twenty (120) days following the board's receipt of a completed application.

(6) Notwithstanding any of the requirements for licensure established in this section, and after providing the applicant with reasonable notice of its intended action and after providing a reasonable opportunity to be heard, the board may deny licensure to an applicant without a prior evidentiary hearing upon a finding that the applicant has violated any provision of this section or is otherwise unfit to practice. If the board denies an application, it shall notify the applicant of the grounds on which the denial is based. Orders denying a license may be appealed pursuant to KRS 311.593.

LRC NOTES

Legislative Research Commission Note (7-12-06): For the sake of clarity and under the authority of KRS 7.136(1)(c), the Reviser of Statutes has further divided subsection (1) of 2006 Ky. Acts. ch. 249, sec. 4.

311.675 Temporary licensure as an acupuncturist; notification upon cancellation of temporary license

(1) Whenever, in the opinion of the executive director based upon verified information contained in the application, an applicant for a license to practice as an acupuncturist is eligible under the applicable provisions of KRS 311.671 to 311.686, the executive director may issue to the applicant, on behalf of the board, a temporary license which shall entitle the holder to practice as an acupuncturist for a maximum of six (6) months from the date of issuance unless the temporary license is canceled by the executive director. The executive director may cancel the temporary license at any time without a hearing, for reasons deemed sufficient with appropriate consultation with the board, and the executive director shall cancel the temporary license immediately upon direction by the board or upon the board's denial of the application for a license. The temporary license shall not be renewable.

(2) The executive director shall present to the board the application for licensure made by the holder of the temporary license. If the board issues a regular license to the holder of a temporary license, the fee paid in connection with the temporary license shall be applied to the regular license fee.

(3) If the executive director cancels a temporary license, he or she shall promptly notify, by United States certified mail, the holder of the temporary license at the last known address on file with the board. The temporary license shall be terminated and of no further force or effect three (3) days after the date the notice was sent by certified mail.

311.676 Requirements for use of designation and display of license; prohibited activities; penalties

(1) An acupuncture practitioner shall use the designation "licensed acupuncturist" or "L.

Ac." following his or her name in all advertisements, professional literature, and billings used in connection with his or her practice.

(2) The license issued by the board shall be conspicuously displayed in the licensed acupuncture practitioner's place of business.

(3) A person who is not licensed under KRS 311.671 to 311.686 shall not use any terms, words, abbreviations, letters, or insignia that indicate or imply that he or she is engaged in the practice of acupuncture.

(4) Any person who violates this section shall be guilty of a Class A misdemeanor.

311.677 Persons and activities not regulated by KRS 311.671 to 311.686

The provisions of KRS 311.671 to 311.686 shall not apply to:

(1) Persons licensed, certified, or registered under any other provision of the Kentucky Revised Statutes and does not prohibit them from rendering services consistent with the laws regulating their professional practices and the ethics of their professions;

(2) Student interns or trainees pursuing a program of studies in an institution approved by the board for teaching the practice of acupuncture, if the person is designated an acupuncture intern or student in training and his or her activities are performed under supervision and constitute a part of the supervised program of study;

(3) Activities of visiting acupuncturists who are legally qualified to perform acupuncture in another state in performing their duties as teachers at a board-approved institution or board-approved workshop or tutorial. As used in this subsection, "duties" means classroom instruction and demonstration of relevant techniques. It does not include the provision of any services to a patient in exchange for a fee; or

(4) Activities, services, and use of title on the part of a person as part of their employment by the federal government.

311.678 Required disclosure to patients; informed consent

An acupuncturist shall obtain informed consent from each patient in a manner consistent with the acceptable and prevailing standards of practice within this Commonwealth and, at a minimum, the acupuncturist shall disclose to the patient the following written information prior to or during the patient's initial visit:

(1) The acupuncturist's qualifications, including his or her education, license information, and the definition and scope of the practice of acupuncture in the Commonwealth; and

(2) Possible outcomes of the treatment to be given, including any pain, bruising, infection, needle sickness, or other side effects that may occur.

311.679 Reporting and recordkeeping requirements

(1) An acupuncturist shall comply with all applicable state and municipal reporting requirements imposed on health-care professionals regarding public health.

(2) An acupuncturist shall maintain a record for each patient treated, in a manner consistent

with the acceptable and prevailing standards of practice within the Commonwealth. At a minimum, the record for each patient shall include:

(a) A signed copy of the information disclosed by the acupuncturist to the patient under KRS 311.678;

(b) Evidence that the acupuncturist has conducted or overseen an interview concerning the patient's medical history and current physical condition;

(c) Evidence of the acupuncturist having conducted a traditional acupuncture examination;

(d) A record of the treatment, including the acupuncture points treated; and

(e) The evaluation and instructions given.

311.680 Written plan governing consultation with patients and medical emergencies; treatment of patients with serious disorders or conditions; administrative regulations

(1) Every licensed acupuncturist shall develop a written plan for consultation, emergency transfer, and referral to appropriate health-care facilities or to other health-care practitioners operating within the scope of their authorized practices, which meets the requirements contained in administrative regulations promulgated by the board. The written plan shall be filed with the board and maintained at the acupuncturist's practice location and updated as appropriate to meet current regulatory requirements.

(2) If, in the course of conducting an interview regarding the patient's medical history, the patient discloses that he or she suffers from one (1) of the potentially serious disorders or conditions listed in subsection (3) of this section, the acupuncturist shall verify that the patient is currently under the care of a physician and consult with the treating physician before providing acupuncture treatment. If the patient refuses to provide a medical history or disclose information regarding any of the conditions listed below, acupuncture treatment shall not be provided.

(3) For purposes of this section, "potentially serious disorder or condition" means:

(a) Hypertension and cardiac conditions;

(b) Acute, severe abdominal pain;

(c) Undiagnosed neurological changes;

(d) Unexplained weight loss or gain in excess of fifteen percent (15%) of the patient's body weight in less than a three (3) month period;

(e) Suspected fracture or dislocation;

(f) Suspected systemic infections;

(g) Serious hemorrhagic disorder;

(h) Acute respiratory distress without a previous history;

(i) Pregnancy;

(j) Diabetes; or

(k) Cancer.

311.681 Renewal of license; grace period; termination, suspension, revocation, and reinstatement of license

（1）Any person licensed as an acupuncturist shall renew his or her license every two（2）years. He or she shall pay to the board a renewal fee established by the board in administrative regulations. The fee shall be paid on or before June 1 of the year in which the license expires. A license that is not renewed within sixty（60）days after June 1 shall expire for failure to renew in a timely manner.

（2）The board shall notify the licensed acupuncturist of the renewal date at the acupuncturist's last known address. The notice shall include an application and notice of renewal fees. The licensed acupuncturist's failure to receive the renewal notice shall not be considered an excuse to waive a late-payment fee.

（3）A sixty（60）day grace period shall be allowed after June 1 of each year, during which the acupuncturist may continue to practice. The acupuncturist may renew his or her license upon payment of the renewal fee and a late-renewal fee as established by the board in administrative regulation.

（4）Any license not renewed by the end of the grace period shall terminate, and the acupuncturist shall no longer be eligible to practice acupuncture in the Commonwealth. An individual with a terminated license may have his or her license reinstated upon payment of the renewal fee and a reinstatement fee as established by the board in administrative regulations. A person who applies for reinstatement shall not be required to take an examination as a condition of reinstatement if the person's reinstatement application is made within five（5）years of the date of termination.

（5）A suspended license shall expire and terminate if not renewed. Renewal of a suspended license shall not entitle the licensed practitioner to practice until the suspension has ended or the right to practice has been restored by the board.

（6）A revoked license shall terminate and may not be renewed. If a revoked license is reinstated, the licensed practitioner shall pay the renewal fee and the reinstatement fee under subsections（1）and（4）of this section.

（7）If a person fails to reinstate his or her license within five（5）years of its termination, the license shall not be renewed, restored, reissued, or reinstated. The person shall obtain a new license under the conditions established in KRS 311.674.

311.682 Continuing education requirements

（1）The board shall, by administrative regulation, prescribe continuing education requirements not to exceed thirty（30）hours biennially, as a condition for renewal of a license. All education programs that contribute to the advancement, extension, or enhancement of professional skills and knowledge related to the practice of acupuncture, whether conducted by a nonprofit or profit-making entity, are eligible for approval. The continuing professional education requirements must be in acupuncture or oriental medicine subjects, including but not limited to anatomy, biological sciences, adjunctive therapies, sanitation and sterilization, emergency protocols, and diseases.

(2) The board shall have the authority to set a fee for each continuing education provider.

(3) The licensed practitioner shall retain in his or her records the certificates of completion of continuing professional education requirements to prove compliance with this section.

(4) All national and state acupuncture and oriental medicine organizations and acupuncture and oriental medicine schools are approved to provide continuing professional education in accordance with this section.

LRC NOTES

Legislative Research Commission Note (7 – 12 – 06): For the sake of clarity and under the authority of KRS 7.136(1)(c), the Reviser of Statutes has divided 2006 Ky. Acts. ch. 249, sec. 12, into subsections.

311.683 Application for license of inactive status; reactivation

(1) A person licensed under KRS 311.674 and 311.675 may apply for inactive status upon submitting an application and paying an inactive-status fee.

(2) An inactive license may be reactivated upon application to the board. If a license has been inactive for more than five (5) consecutive years, the licensed practitioner shall apply for a new license and shall meet all the requirements in existence for a license under KRS 311.674 and 311.675. That application for licensure shall require:

(a) Evidence of the license holder's payment of an inactive-status fee; and

(b) Payment of the initial licensure fee.

311.684 Revocation of certificate; written admonishment; other disciplinary proceedings

(1) The board may:

(a) Revoke a license;

(b) Suspend a license for a period not to exceed five (5) years;

(c) Deny an application for a license;

(d) Decline to renew a license;

(e) Indefinitely restrict or limit a license;

(f) Issue a fine of up to two thousand dollars ($2,000) per violation and/or the costs of the proceedings;

(g) Place a license on probation for a period not to exceed five (5) years;

(h) Reprimand the acupuncturist; or

(i) Impose any combination of such sanctions, upon proof that the acupuncturist has:

1. Knowingly made or presented or caused to be made or presented any false, fraudulent,

or forged statement, writing, certificate, diploma, or other document relating to an application for licensure;

2. Practiced, aided, or abetted in the practice of fraud, forgery, deception, collusion, or conspiracy relating to an examination for licensure;

3. Entered a guilty or nolo contendere plea, or been convicted, by any court within or without the Commonwealth of Kentucky, of committing an act which is or would be a felony under the laws of the Commonwealth of Kentucky or of the United States;

4. Entered a guilty or nolo contendere plea, or been convicted, by any court within or without the Commonwealth of Kentucky, of any misdemeanor offense which has dishonesty as a fundamental and necessary element, including but not limited to crimes involving theft, embezzlement, false swearing, perjury, fraud, or misrepresentation;

5. Become addicted to, or is an abuser of, alcohol, drugs, or any illegal substance;

6. Developed a physical or mental disability or other condition that presents a danger in continuing to practice acupuncture to patients, the public, or other health-care personnel;

7. Knowingly made, caused to be made, or aided or abetted in the making of a false statement in any document executed in connection with the practice of acupuncture;

8. Aided, assisted, or abetted the unlawful practice of medicine or acupuncture;

9. Willfully violated a confidential communication;

10. Performed the services of an acupuncturist in an unprofessional, incompetent, or grossly or chronically negligent manner;

11. Been removed, suspended, expelled, or placed on probation by any health-care facility or professional society for unprofessional conduct, incompetence, negligence, or violation of any provision of this section;

12. Violated any applicable provision of a statute or administrative regulation relating to acupuncture practice;

13. Violated any term of a final order or agreed order issued by the board; or

14. Failed to complete the required number of hours of approved continuing education.

(2) All disciplinary proceedings against an acupuncturist shall be conducted in accordance with KRS 311.591, 311.592, 311.593, 311.599, and KRS Chapter 13B and related administrative regulations promulgated under KRS Chapter 311.

(3) (a) The board may issue a written admonishment to the licensed acupuncturist when, in the judgment of the board:

1. An alleged violation is not of a serious nature; and

2. The evidence presented to the board after the investigation, including an appropriate opportunity for the licensed acupuncturist to respond, provides a clear indication that the alleged violation did in fact occur.

(b) A copy of the admonishment shall be placed in the permanent file of the licensed acupuncturist.

(c) The licensed acupuncturist shall have the right to file a response to the admonishment within thirty (30) days of its receipt and to have the response placed in the permanent licensure file.

(d) The licensed acupuncturist may alternatively, within thirty (30) days of the admonishment's receipt, file a request for a hearing with the board.

(e) Upon receipt of a request for a hearing, the board shall set aside the written admonishment and set the matter for a hearing under the provisions of KRS Chapter 13B.

(4) At any time during the investigative or hearing processes, the board may enter into an agreed order or accept an assurance of voluntary compliance with the licensed acupuncturist which effectively deals with the complaint.

(5) The board may, upon the agreement of the aggrieved party, use mediation to handle disciplinary matters. The board may appoint any member or members of the board, any staff member, or any other person or combination thereof to serve in the mediation process.

(6) The board may reconsider, modify, or reverse its disciplinary actions.

LRC NOTES

Legislative Research Commission Note (7-12-06): For the sake of clarity and under the authority of KRS 7.136(1)(c), the Reviser of Statutes has divided 2006 Ky. Acts ch. 249, sec. 14(1) into paragraphs and subparagraphs.

311.685   Hearing required before imposition of sanctions; right to hearing and appeal; petition for reissuance of revoked license; probation; decisions of board not subject to judicial review

(1) The board, before suspending, revoking, imposing probationary or supervisory conditions upon a licensed acupuncturist, imposing an administrative fine, issuing a written reprimand, or any combination of these actions regarding any licensed acupuncturist under KRS 311.671 to 311.686, shall set the matter for a hearing under the provisions of KRS Chapter 13B.

(2) After denying an application under KRS 311.671 to 311.686 or issuing a written admonishment, the board, at the request of the aggrieved party, shall grant a hearing under the provisions of KRS Chapter 13B.

(3) Except for final orders denying an initial application or renewal for licensure or final orders issued pursuant to KRS 13B.125(3), all final orders of the board affecting an acupuncturist's license shall become effective thirty (30) days after notice is given to the license holder unless otherwise agreed; however, the board's panels may provide that a final order be effective immediately when, in the panel's opinion, based upon sufficient reasonable cause, the health, welfare, and safety of patients or the general public would be endangered by delay.

（4）Any acupuncturist who is aggrieved by a final order of the board denying an initial or renewal application for licensure or rendering disciplinary action against a license holder may seek judicial review of the order by filing a petition with the Circuit Court of the county in which the board's offices are located in accordance with KRS Chapter 13B. Decisions of the board's panels relating to petitions for reinstatement of revoked licenses are not final orders for purposes of this statute, and are not subject to judicial review.

（5）The court shall not award injunctive relief against the board without providing the board with the reasonable opportunity to be heard.

（6）An acupuncturist whose license has been revoked may, after five（5）years from the effective date of the revocation order, petition the board to reissue the license to again practice acupuncture in the Commonwealth of Kentucky.

（7）The board shall not be required to issue a new license, and a decision of the board not to reissue a license shall not be subject to judicial review. A license shall not be reissued following a petition under subsection（6）of this section unless the former license holder satisfies the board that he or she is presently of good moral character and qualified both physically and mentally to resume the practice of acupuncture without undue risk or danger to patients or the public.

（8）In the event the board reissues a revoked license under the circumstances as described in this section, the reissued license shall be under probation for a period of not less than two（2）years nor more than five（5）years with conditions fixed by the board, including a condition that any violation of the remaining conditions of probation shall result in automatic revocation of the license.

311.686　Emergency order suspending, limiting, or restricting license; complaint and hearing; procedural rules for hearing; emergency order invalid after issuance of final order

（1）At any time when an inquiry panel established under KRS 311.591 has probable cause to believe that an acupuncturist has violated the terms of an agreed order as defined in KRS 311.550（19）, or violated the terms of a disciplinary order, or that an acupuncturist's practice constitutes a danger to the health, welfare, or safety of patients or the general public, the inquiry panel may issue an emergency order in accordance with KRS 13B.125 suspending, limiting, or restricting the acupuncturist's license.

（2）For the purposes of a hearing conducted under KRS 311.592 on an emergency order issued under this section, the findings of fact in the emergency order shall constitute a rebuttable presumption of substantial evidence of a violation of law that constitutes immediate danger to the health, welfare, or safety of patients or the general public. For the purposes of this hearing only, hearsay shall be admissible and may serve as a basis of the board's findings.

（3）An emergency order as described in subsection（1）of this section shall not be issued unless grounds exist for the issuance of a complaint. The inquiry panel shall issue a complaint prior to the date of the emergency hearing or the emergency order shall become void.

(4) An emergency order suspending, limiting, or restricting a license shall not be maintained after a final order as defined in KRS 311. 550 (20) is served on the charged acupuncturist pursuant to the proceeding on the complaint. An appeal of an emergency order shall not prejudice the board from proceeding with the complaint.

LOUISIANA

LOUISIANA STATUTES ANNOTATED

§ 1356. Definitions

As used in this Part the following definitions apply:

(1) "Acupuncture" means treatment by means of mechanical, thermal or electrical stimulation effected by the insertion of needles at a point or combination of points on the surface of the body predetermined on the basis of the theory of the physiological interrelationship of body organs with an associated point or combination of points, or the application of heat or electrical stimulation to such point or points, for the purpose of inducing anesthesia, relieving pain, or healing diseases, disorders and dysfunctions of the body, or achieving a therapeutic or prophylactic effect with respect thereto.

(2) "Acupuncture detoxification", also known as acu detox, means the treatment by means of the insertion of acupuncture needles in a combination of points on the ear.

(3) "Acupuncture detoxification specialist", known as an A.D.S., means an individual certified to practice acupuncture detoxification.

(4) "Board" means the Louisiana State Board of Medical Examiners.

(5) "Licensed acupuncturist" means an individual other than a physician who is certified by the board to practice acupuncture pursuant to the provisions of R.S. 37: 1358.

(6) "NADA" means the National Acupuncture Detoxification Association.

(7) "Physician" means an individual licensed to practice medicine in Louisiana.

(8) "Physician acupuncturist" means a physician certified by the board to practice acupuncture pursuant to the provisions of R.S. 37: 1357.

(9) Repealed by Acts 2016, No. 550, § 2.

§ 1357. Physician acupuncturists

The board shall certify as a physician acupuncturist a physician licensed to practice medicine in Louisiana who has successfully completed either of the following:

(1) Six months' training in acupuncture in a school or clinic approved by the board.

(2) Three hundred credit hours of continuing medical education in acupuncture designated as category one continuing medical education hours by the American Medical Association.

§ 1357.1. Practice of acupuncture detoxification; certification; promulgation of rules; public health emergency

A. The board shall certify as an acupuncture detoxification specialist an individual who works under the general supervision of a physician licensed by the board to practice in the state or a licensed acupuncturist certified by the board to practice in the state and has successfully completed the following:

(1) NADA training by a registered NADA trainer.

(2) NADA certification.

(3) Registration with the board.

B. Pursuant to the provisions of this Section, the board shall promulgate rules and regulations in collaboration with its Integrative and Complementary Medicine Committee that it deems necessary to regulate the certification of acupuncture detoxification specialists and the practice of acupuncture detoxification in the state. Such rules and regulations shall include but not be limited to the following:

(1) Provisions regarding the adoption of fees.

(2) Provisions regarding the action to deny, suspend, revoke, or place on probation individuals who act beyond the scope of practice or engage in unprofessional conduct.

(3) Provisions regarding the general supervision of acupuncture detoxification specialists.

C. Acupuncture detoxification specialists from other states who are certified by NADA shall be allowed to practice acupuncture detoxification in Louisiana during a public health emergency and for such periods thereafter as the Louisiana Department of Health deems the need for emergency services to continue to exist, and under rules and regulations set forth by the board.

§ 1358. Licensed acupuncturists

The board shall certify as a licensed acupuncturist an individual who meets both of the following:

(1) Holds active status with the National Certification Commission for Acupuncture and Oriental Medicine.

(2) Has successfully passed the certification examination, including the Biomedicine portion of the examination, given by the National Certification Commission for Acupuncture and Oriental Medicine.

§ 1359. Annual report by board to legislature

The board shall report annually to the legislature concerning the status of acupuncture practice in the state.

§ 1360. Powers and duties of the Louisiana State Board of Medical Examiners

In addition to the powers and duties established in R. S. 37: 1270, the Louisiana State Board of Medical Examiners may do any of the following:

(1) Adopt, revise, and enforce rules and regulations that it deems necessary to ensure the competency of applicants, the protection of the public, and the proper administration of this Part in accordance with the Administrative Procedure Act.

(2) Approve the license of duly qualified applicants and deny, suspend, revoke, or place on probation any licensee who acts beyond the scope of practice or engages in unprofessional conduct.

(3) Conduct hearings on charges calling for the denial, suspension, or revocation of or the refusal to renew a license.

(4) Adopt fees under its authority pursuant to R.S. 37: 1281, for the purpose of administering the provisions of this Part.

(5) Establish an advisory committee on acupuncture to provide such assistance as the board may deem necessary or request in the administration of this Part.

LOUISIANA ADMINISTRATIVE CODE

Subchapter A General Provisions

§ 2101. Scope of Chapter

A. The rules of this Chapter govern the certification of physician acupuncturists and licensed acupuncturists to practice acupuncture and of acupuncture detoxification specialists to practice acupuncture detoxification in the state of Louisiana.

§ 2103. Definitions

A. As used in this Chapter and Chapter 51, the following terms shall have the meanings specified.

Acupuncture Practice Act or *Act* — R. S. 37: 1356 – 1360, as hereafter amended or supplemented.

Acupuncture — treatment by means of mechanical, thermal, or electrical stimulation effected by the insertion of needles at a point or combination of points on the surface of the body predetermined on the basis of the theory of the physiological interrelationship of body organs with an associated point or combination of points, or the application of heat or electrical stimulation to such point or points, for the purpose of inducing anesthesia, relieving pain, or healing diseases, disorders, and dysfunctions of the body, or achieving a therapeutic or prophylactic effect with respect thereto.

Acupuncture Detoxification (acu detox) — the treatment by means of insertion of acupuncture needles in a combination of points on the ear in accordance with NADA protocol. The performance of acupuncture detoxification constitutes a subcategory of the practice of acupuncture.

Acupuncture Detoxification Specialist (ADS) — an individual who possesses current certification, duly issued by the board, to practice acupuncture detoxification under the supervision of a physician or licensed acupuncturist.

Applicant — a person who has applied to the board for certification as a physician acupuncturist, licensed acupuncturist or acupuncture detoxification specialist in the state of Louisiana.

Application — a request directed to and received by the board, in a format approved by the board, for certification to perform or practice acupuncture or acupuncture detoxification in the state of Louisiana, together with all information, certificates, documents, and other materials required by the board to be submitted with such forms.

Board — the Louisiana State Board of Medical Examiners.

Certification — the board's official recognition of an individual's current certificate, duly issued by the board, evidencing the board's certification of such individual under the law.

General Supervision — as used in this Chapter and Chapter 51, shall mean responsible oversight of the services rendered by an acupuncture detoxification specialist as specified in § 5106.B of these rules.

Good Moral Character — as applied to an applicant, means that:

a. the applicant, if a physician, has not, prior to or during the pendency of an application to the board, been guilty of any act, omission, condition, or circumstance which would provide legal cause under R.S. 37: 1285 for the denial, suspension, or revocation of medical licensure;

b. the applicant has not, prior to or during the pendency of an application to the board, been culpable of any act, omission, condition, or circumstance which would provide cause under § 5113 of these rules for the suspension or revocation of certification as a physician acupuncturist, licensed acupuncturist, or acupuncture detoxification specialist;

c. the applicant has not, prior to or in connection with his application, made any representation to the board, knowingly or unknowingly, which is in fact false or misleading as to a material fact or omits to state any fact or matter that is material to the application; or

d. the applicant has not made any representation or failed to make a representation or engaged in any act or omission which is false, deceptive, fraudulent, or misleading in achieving or obtaining any of the qualifications for certification required by this Chapter.

Licensed Acupuncturist (LAc) — an individual, other than a physician possessing a current license, duly issued by the board to practice acupuncture in this state.

NADA — the National Acupuncture Detoxification Association.

Physician Acupuncturist — a physician possessing current certification, duly issued by the board, to practice acupuncture.

Primary Practice Site — the location at which a physician, licensed acupuncturist or acupuncture detoxification specialist spends the majority of time in the exercise of the privileges conferred by licensure or certification issued by the board.

Proposed Supervising Licensed Acupuncturist — a licensed acupuncturist who has submitted to the board an application for approval as a supervising acupuncturist.

Proposed Supervising Physician — a physician who has submitted to the board an application for approval as a supervising physician.

Supervising Licensed Acupuncturist — a licensed acupuncturist registered with the board under this Chapter to provide supervision to an acupuncture detoxification specialist.

Supervising Physician — a physician registered with the board under this Chapter to supervise an acupuncture detoxification specialist.

Universal Precautions — a set of precautions developed by the United States Center for Disease Control (CDC) that are designed to prevent transmission of human immunodeficiency virus (HIV), hepatitis B virus (HBV) and other blood borne pathogens when providing first aid or health care. Under universal precautions blood and certain bodily fluids of all patients are considered potentially infectious for HIV, HBV and other blood borne pathogens.

B. Masculine terms wheresoever used in this Chapter shall also be deemed to include the feminine.

Subchapter B. Physician Acupuncturist Certification

§ 2105.   Scope of Subchapter

A. The rules of this Subchapter prescribe the qualifications and procedures requisite to certification as a physician acupuncturist in the state of Louisiana.

§ 2107.   Qualifications for Certification as Physician Acupuncturist

A. To be eligible for certification as a physician acupuncturist, an applicant shall:

1. be a physician possessing a current, unrestricted license to practice medicine in the state of Louisiana duly issued by the board;

2. be of good moral character as defined by § 2103.A; and

3. have successfully completed:

a. not less than six months of training in acupuncture in a school or clinic approved by the board pursuant to §§ 2118 – 2121 of this Chapter; or

b. not less than 300 credit hours of continuing medical education in acupuncture designated as category one continuing medical education hours by the American Medical Association.

B. The burden of satisfying the board as to the qualifications and eligibility of the applicant for certification shall be upon the applicant. An applicant shall not be deemed to possess such qualifications unless the applicant demonstrates and evidences such qualifications in the manner prescribed by, and to the satisfaction of, the board.

§ 2109. Application Procedure for Physician Acupuncturist

A. Application for certification as a physician acupuncturist shall be made in a format approved by the board.

B. An application for certification under this Chapter shall include:

1. proof, documented in a form satisfactory to the board, that the applicant possesses the qualifications set forth in this Chapter; and

2. such other information and documentation as the board may require to evidence qualification for certification.

C. All documentation submitted in a language other than English shall be accompanied by a translation into English certified by a translator other than the applicant who shall attest to the accuracy of such translation under penalty of perjury.

D. The board may refuse to consider any application which is not complete in every detail, including submission of every document required by the application form. The board may, in its discretion, require a more detailed or complete response to any request for information set forth in the application form as a condition to consideration of an application.

E. Each application submitted to the board shall be accompanied by the applicable fee, as provided in Chapter 1 of these rules.

Subchapter C. Licensed Acupuncturist and Acupuncture Detoxification Specialist Certification; Qualifications for Referral and Supervising Physicians and Licensed Acupuncturists

§ 2111. Scope of Subchapter

A. The rules of this Subchapter prescribe the qualifications and procedures requisite to licensure as a licensed acupuncturist, certification as an acupuncture detoxification specialist, and those of a supervising physician and supervising licensed acupuncturist in the state of Louisiana.

§ 2113. Qualifications for Licensure as a Licensed Acupuncturist

A. To be eligible for a license as a licensed acupuncturist, an applicant:

1. shall be at least 21 years of age;

2. shall be of good moral character as defined by § 2103.A;

3. shall have successfully completed a four-year course of instruction in a high school or its equivalent;

4. shall be a citizen of the United States or possess valid and current legal authority to reside and work in the United States duly issued by the United States Citizenship and Immigration Services (USCIS) of the United States, Department of Homeland Security, under and pursuant to the Immigration and Nationality Act (66 Stat. 163) and the commissioner's regulations

thereunder (8 CFR);

5. shall meet both of the following:

a. hold active status with the National Certification Commission for Acupuncture and Oriental Medicine; and

b. have successfully passed the certification examination, including the biomedicine portion of the examination, given by the National Certification Commission for Acupuncture and Oriental Medicine or its successor.

6. shall affirm that he or she shall establish and maintain a relationship with a physician, as defined in § 5106.A of these rules, at all times while engaged in the practice of acupuncture.

B. The burden of satisfying the board as to the qualifications and eligibility of the applicant shall be upon the applicant, who shall demonstrate and evidence such qualifications in the manner prescribed by and to the satisfaction of the board.

§ 2114. Qualifications for Certification as an Acupuncture Detoxification Specialist; Qualifications for Registration of Supervising Physician or Supervising Licensed Acupuncturist

A. To be eligible for certification as an acupuncture detoxification specialist, an applicant:

1. shall be at least 21 years of age;

2. shall be of good moral character as defined by § 2103.A of this Chapter;

3. shall have successfully completed a four-year course of instruction in a high school or its equivalent;

4. shall be a citizen of the United States or possess valid and current legal authority to reside and work in the United States duly issued by the United States Citizenship and Immigration Services (USCIS) of the United States, Department of Homeland Security, under and pursuant to the Immigration and Nationality Act (66 Stat. 163) and the commissioner's regulations thereunder (8 CFR);

5. shall have:

a. successfully completed NADA training by a registered NADA trainer; and

b. current certification by the NADA to perform acupuncture detoxification; and

6. shall affirm that he or she shall only provide acu detox under the general supervision of a physician or a licensed acupuncturist, as defined in § 5106.B of these rules.

B. Prior to undertaking the supervision of an acupuncture detoxification specialist a physician shall be registered with the board. To be eligible for registration to supervise an ADS a proposed supervising physician shall, as of the date of the application:

1. possess a current, unrestricted license to practice medicine in the state of Louisiana; and

2. not currently be enrolled in any postgraduate residency training.

C. Prior to undertaking the supervision of an acupuncture detoxification specialist a licensed acupuncturist shall be registered with the board. To be eligible for registration to supervise an ADS a proposed supervising LAc shall, as of the date of the application:

1. possess a current, unrestricted license to practice as a LAc; and

2. have held certification or licensure by the board to practice as a LAc in this state for at least two years immediately preceding the date of application.

D. The burden of satisfying the board as to the qualifications and eligibility of the applicant acupuncture detoxification specialist, proposed supervising physician or proposed supervising licensed acupuncturist shall be upon the applicant, proposed supervising physician or proposed supervising licensed acupuncturist, who shall demonstrate and evidence such qualifications in the manner prescribed by and to the satisfaction of the board.

§ 2115.   Application Procedure for Licensed Acupuncturist

A. Application for certification as a licensed acupuncturist shall be made in a format approved by the board.

B. An application under this Subchapter shall include:

1. proof, documented in a form satisfactory to the board that the applicant possesses the qualifications set forth in this Chapter;

2. attestation by the applicant certifying the truthfulness and authenticity of all information, representations, and documents contained in or submitted with the completed application; and

3. such other information and documentation as the board may require.

C. All documentation submitted in a language other than English shall be accompanied by a translation into English certified by a translator other than the applicant who shall attest to the accuracy of such translation under penalty of perjury.

D. The board may reject or refuse to consider any application which is not complete in every detail, including submission of every document required by the application form. The board may in its discretion require a more detailed or complete response to any request for information set forth in the application form as a condition to consideration of an application.

E. Each application submitted to the board shall be accompanied by the applicable fee, as provided in Chapter 1 of these rules.

F. Upon submission of a completed application, together with the documents required thereby, and the payment of the application fee, the applicant shall be required to appear before the board or its designee if the board has questions concerning the applicant's qualifications.

§ 2116.   Application Procedure for Acupuncture Detoxification Specialist

A. Application for certification as an ADS shall be made in a format approved by the board and shall include notification of intent to practice in a format approved by the board, signed by a proposed supervising physician or proposed supervising licensed acupuncturist who is registered with or has applied for registration to the board as a supervising physician or supervising licensed acupuncturist.

B. Application for certification and approval under this Subchapter shall include:

1. proof, documented in a form satisfactory to the board that the applicant possesses the

qualifications set forth in of this Chapter;

2. attestation by the applicant certifying that the requirements of § 5106.B of these rules shall be followed in the exercise of the privileges conferred by certification under this Part;

3. attestation by the applicant certifying the truthfulness and authenticity of all information, representations, and documents contained in or submitted with the completed application; and

4. such other information and documentation as the board may require.

C. All documentation submitted in a language other than English shall be accompanied by a translation into English certified by a translator other than the applicant who shall attest to the accuracy of such translation under penalty of perjury.

D. The board may reject or refuse to consider any application which is not complete in every detail, including submission of every document required by the application. The board may in its discretion require a more detailed or complete response to any request for information set forth in the application form as a condition to consideration of an application.

E. Each application submitted to the board shall be accompanied by the applicable fee, as provided in Chapter 1 of these rules.

§ 2117. Application Procedure for Registration of Supervising Physician or Supervising Licensed Acupuncturist

A. Application for registration of a supervising physician or supervising LAc for an acupuncture detoxification specialist, shall be made in a format approved by the board, include proof satisfactory to the board that the applicant possesses the qualifications set forth in this Chapter, and contain such other information and documentation as the board may require.

B. The board may reject or refuse to consider any application which is not complete in every detail, including submission of every document required by the application. The board may in its discretion require a more detailed or complete response to any request for information set forth in the application form as a condition to consideration of an application.

C. A separate fee shall not be assessed for registration or approval of a supervising physician or supervising LAc for an ADS.

Subchapter D. Board Approval of Acupuncture Schools and Colleges

§ 2118. Scope of Subchapter

A. The rules of this Subchapter provide the method and procedures by which acupuncture schools and colleges are approved by the board.

§ 2119. Applicability of Approval

A. As provided in this Chapter the successful completion of formal training in acupuncture from a school or college approved by the board is among the alternative qualifications requisite to certification as a physician acupuncturist or licensed acupuncturist. This qualification will be deemed to be satisfied if the school or college in which the applicant received training in acupuncture was approved by the board as of the date on which the applicant completed such training.

§ 2121. Approval of Acupuncture Schools or Colleges

A. A school or college providing training in acupuncture which is currently accredited by the Accreditation Commission for Acupuncture and Oriental Medicine (ACAOM), or its predecessor, the National Accreditation Commission for Schools and Colleges of Acupuncture and Oriental Medicine (NACSCAOM), shall concurrently be deemed approved by the board.

B. A school or college providing training in acupuncture which has been accorded candidacy status by ACAOM, or its predecessor, NACSCAOM, shall concurrently be deemed conditionally approved by the board, provided that board approval shall be automatically withdrawn if accreditation is not awarded by ACAOM within three years of the date on which candidacy status was recognized.

C. The board may approve additional schools or programs providing training in acupuncture upon the request of an applicant or application by any such school or program and upon the submission to the board of documentation that such school or program provides training in acupuncture under standards substantially equivalent to those prescribed by ACAOM for accreditation.

Subchapter E. Certification, License Issuance, Approval of Registration of Supervising Physician or Supervising Licensed Acupuncturist, Termination, Renewal, Reinstatement

§ 2125. Issuance of Certification and Licensure, Approval of Registration

A. If the qualifications, requirements, and procedures specified by this Chapter for a physician acupuncturist are met to the satisfaction of the board, the board shall certify the applicant as a physician acupuncturist.

B. If the qualifications, requirements, and procedures specified by this Chapter for a licensed acupuncturist are met to the satisfaction of the board, the board shall certify the applicant as a licensed acupuncturist.

C. If the qualifications, requirements, and procedures specified by this Chapter for an acupuncture detoxification specialist are met to the satisfaction of the board, the board shall certify the applicant as an ADS. Issuance of certification to an applicant under this Chapter shall constitute approval of registration of the proposed supervising physician or proposed supervising licensed acupuncturist.

D. Although a physician or licensed acupuncturist must notify the board each time he or she intends to undertake the general supervision of an acupuncture detoxification specialist, registration with the board is only required once. Notification of supervision of a new or additional ADSs by a registered supervising physician or LAc shall be deemed given to the board upon the ADS's filing with the board of a notice of intent to practice in accordance with § 2127.F of this Chapter.

E. The board shall maintain a list of physicians and LAcs who are registered to supervise an ADS. Each registered physician, registered LAc and ADS is responsible for updating the board within 15 days should any of the information required and submitted change after a physician or LAc has been registered to supervise an ADS.

§ 2127. Expiration and Termination of Certification and Licensure; Modification

A. Every certification and license issued by the board under this Chapter shall expire, and become null, void, and to no effect on the last day of the year in which it was issued.

B. The timely submission of an application for renewal of certification or licensure, as provided by § 2129 of this Chapter, shall operate to continue the expiring certification or license in full force and effect pending issuance or denial of renewal.

C. Licensure as a licensed acupuncturist whether an initial license or renewal thereof, shall terminate and become void, null and to no effect on and as of any day that the licensed acupuncturist's license expires for failure to timely renew.

D. Except as provided in Subsection F of this Section, certification as an acupuncture detoxification specialist, whether an initial certificate or renewal thereof, shall terminate and become void, null and to no effect on and as of any day that:

1. the supervising physician or supervising licensed acupuncturist no longer possesses a current, unrestricted license to practice as a physician or as a LAc in the state of Louisiana;

2. the supervising physician or supervising acupuncturist, whether voluntarily or involuntarily, ceases the active practice of medicine or practice as a LAc;

3. the relationship between the ADS and the supervising physician or the supervising LAc is terminated; or

4. the ADS's certification expires for failure to timely renew.

E. Certification shall not terminate upon termination of a relationship between a supervising physician or supervising LAc and ADS provided that:

1. the ADS currently has a supervisory relationship with another supervising physician or supervising LAc; alternatively, the ADS ceases to practice until such time as notification is provided to the board, in a format approved by the board, that he or she has entered into a supervisory relationship with a new supervising physician or supervising LAc who satisfies the qualifications, requirements and procedures of this Chapter. Such notification shall be deemed effective as of the date received by the board, subject to final approval at the next board meeting; and

2. the ADS notifies the board of any changes in or additions to his supervising physicians or

supervising LAcs within 15 days of the date of such change or addition.

§ 2129. Renewal of Certification and Licensure; Verification of Registration

A. Every certificate or license issued by the board under this Chapter shall be renewed annually on or before the last day of the year in which it was issued by submitting to the board a properly completed application for renewal, in a format specified by the board, together with evidence of the completion of 15 hours of accredited continuing professional education and the renewal fee prescribed in Chapter 1 of these rules.

B. Renewal applications and instructions may be obtained from the board's web page or upon personal or written request to the board.

C. Each registered supervising physician and supervising licensed acupuncturist shall annually verify the accuracy of registration information on file with the board in a format approved by the board.

§ 2130. Reinstatement of Expired License

A. A license that has expired as a result of non-renewal for less than two years from the date of expiration, may be reinstated by the board subject to the conditions and procedures hereinafter provided.

B. An application for reinstatement shall be submitted in a format approved by the board and be accompanied by:

1. a statistical affidavit in a form provided by the board;

2. a recent photograph of the applicant;

3. such other information and documentation as is referred to or specified in this Chapter or as the board may require to evidence qualification for licensure; and

4. the renewal fee and delinquent fee, set forth in Chapter 1 of these rules, for each year during which the license was expired.

a. if the application is made less than one year from the date of expiration, the penalty shall be equal to the renewal fee of the license;

b. if the application is made more than one but less than two years from the date of expiration, the penalty shall be equal to twice the renewal fee of the license.

C. An individual whose license has lapsed and expired for a period in excess of two years shall not be eligible for reinstatement consideration but may apply to the board for an initial license pursuant to the applicable rules of this Chapter.

D. A request for reinstatement may be denied by virtue of the existence of any grounds for denial of licensure as provided by the Act or these rules.

E. The burden of satisfying the board as to the qualifications and eligibility of the applicant for reinstatement of the license as a licensed acupuncturist shall be on the applicant. An applicant shall not be deemed to possess such qualifications unless the applicant demonstrates and evidences such qualifications in a manner prescribed by and to the satisfaction of the board.

Subchapter F.   Restricted Licensure, Permits

§ 2131.   Emergency Temporary Permit

A. Acupuncture Detoxification Specialist. The board may issue an emergency temporary permit to an acupuncture detoxification specialist, valid for a period of not more than 60 days, to provide voluntary, gratuitous acu detox services in this state during a public health emergency and for such periods thereafter as the Louisiana Department of Health ("LDH") shall deem the need for emergency services to continue to exist, at sites specified by LDH or approved by the board. Application for such permit shall be made in accordance with §412 of this Part and include notification of intent to practice under a supervising physician or supervising LAc in a manner approved by the board.

B. Services performed by an ADS issued a permit under this Section shall be limited to acu detox, approved by and performed under the general supervision of the supervising physician or supervising LAc. All services shall be documented by the ADS and available for review by the supervising physician or supervising LAc.

C. Licensed Acupuncturist. The board may issue an emergency temporary permit to a licensed acupuncturist to provide voluntary, gratuitous acupuncture services in this state during a public health emergency, and for such periods thereafter as LDH shall deem the need for emergency services to continue to exist, in accordance with §412 of this Part.

Subchapter G.   Acupuncture Advisory Committee

§ 2139.   Scope of Subchapter

A. To assist the board on matters relative to acupuncture, an acupuncture advisory committee is hereby constituted, to be composed and appointed and to have such duties and responsibilities as hereinafter provided.

§ 2141.   Constitution, Function and Responsibilities of Advisory Committee

A. The board shall constitute and appoint an acupuncture advisory committee which shall be organized and function in accordance with the provisions of this Subchapter.

B. Composition. The committee shall be comprised of five members selected by the board, four of whom shall be licensed acupuncturists and one of whom shall be a physician acupuncturist. All members of the advisory committee will be licensed by the board and practice and reside in this state.

C. Insofar as possible or practical, in its appointment of members to the advisory committee the board shall maintain geographic diversity so as to provide representative membership on the advisory committee by individuals residing in various areas of the state.

D. Term of Service. Each member of the committee shall serve for a term of four years, or until a successor is appointed and shall be eligible for reappointment. Committee members serve at the pleasure of the board. Committee members may be reappointed to two additional terms of four years.

E. Functions of the Committee. The committee will provide the board with recommendations relating to:

1. applications for licensure;

2. educational requirements for licensure;

3. changes in related statutes and rules;

4. perform such other functions and provide such additional advice and recommendations as may be requested by the board.

F. Committee Meetings. The committee shall meet at least once each calendar year, or more frequently as may be deemed necessary by a quorum of the committee or by the board. Three members of the committee constitute a quorum. The committee shall elect from among its members a chair. The chair shall call, designate the date, time, and place of, and preside at all meetings of the committee. The chair shall record or cause to be recorded accurate and complete written minutes of all meetings of the committee and shall cause copies of the same to be provided to the board.

G. Confidentiality. In discharging the functions authorized under this Section, the committee and the individual members thereof shall, when acting within the scope of such authority, be deemed agents of the board. Committee members are prohibited from communicating, disclosing, or in any way releasing to anyone other than the board, any confidential information or documents obtained when acting as the agents of the board without first obtaining the written authorization of the board.

Subchapter H.   Continuing Education

§ 2149.   Scope of Subchapter

A. The rules of this Subchapter provide standards for the continuing professional education required for annual renewal of a license to practice as a licensed acupuncturist, and prescribe procedures applicable to satisfaction and documentation thereof.

§ 2151.   Continuing Education Requirement

A. To be eligible for annual license renewal a licensed acupuncturist shall evidence and document in a format specified by the board the successful completion of 15 hours of approved continuing professional education.

§ 2153.   Qualifying Programs and Activities

A. To be acceptable as qualified continuing professional education under these rules, an activity or program must have significant intellectual or practical content, dealing primarily with matters related to acupuncture, and its primary objective must be to maintain or increase the participant's competence as an acupuncturist.

§ 2155.　Approval of Program Sponsors

A. Any education program, course, seminar or activity accredited by the National Certification Commission for Acupuncture and Oriental Medicine or its successor or recognized by the United States Department of Education shall be deemed approved by the board for purposes of qualifying as an approved continuing professional education.

§ 2157.　Documentation Procedure

A. A format or method specified by the board for documenting and certifying completion of continuing professional education shall be completed by licensees and returned with or as part of an annual renewal application.

B. Any continuing professional education activities not approved by the board pursuant to these rules shall be referred to the advisory committee for its evaluation and recommendations. If the committee determines that a continuing education activity does not qualify for recognition by the board or does not qualify for the number of continuing education units claimed by the applicant, the board shall give notice of such determination to the applicant for renewal. The board's decision with respect to approval and recognition of any such activity shall be final.

§ 2159.　Failure to Satisfy Continuing Education Requirements

A. An applicant for license renewal who fails to evidence satisfaction of the continuing professional education requirements shall be given written notice of such failure by the board. The license of the applicant shall remain in full force and effect for a period of 60 days following the mailing of such notice, following which it shall be deemed expired, unrenewed, and subject to revocation without further notice, unless the applicant shall have, within such 60 days, furnished the board satisfactory evidence, by affidavit, that:

1. applicant has satisfied the applicable continuing professional education requirements; or

2. applicant's failure to satisfy the continuing professional education requirements was occasioned by disability, illness, or other good cause as may be determined by the board.

B. The license of a licensed acupuncturist whose license has expired by nonrenewal or been revoked for failure to satisfy the continuing education requirements of these rules may be reinstated by the board within the time and in accordance with the procedures for reinstatement provided by these rules.

§ 2161.　Waiver of Requirements

A. The board may, in its discretion, waive all or part of the continuing professional education required by these rules in favor of a licensed acupuncturist who makes written request for such waiver and evidences to the satisfaction of the board a permanent physical disability, illness, financial hardship, or other similar extenuating circumstances precluding the satisfaction of the continuing professional education requirements.

MISSISSIPPI

ANNOTATED MISSISSIPPI CODE

§ 73 – 71 – 1. Short title

This chapter shall be known and may be cited as the "Acupuncture Practice Act." Whenever a reference is made to the Acupuncture Practice Act by the provisions of any statute, it is to be construed as referring to the provisions of this chapter.

§ 73 – 71 – 3. Legislative purpose and intent

(1) In its concern with the need to eliminate the fundamental causes of illness and with the need to treat the whole person, the Legislature intends to establish in this chapter a framework for the practice of the art and science of acupuncture.

(2) The purposes of this chapter are to encourage the effective utilization of the skills relative to practitioners of acupuncture by citizens desiring their services; to remove the existing legal constraints that unnecessarily hinder the effective provision of health care services; and to subject individuals practicing acupuncture to regulation and control as a primary and independent health care profession.

§ 73 – 71 – 5. Definitions

As used in this chapter, unless the context otherwise requires, the following terms shall have the following meanings:

(a) "Accredited college of acupuncture" means any college, school or division of a university or college that offers the degree of Master of Science in Oriental Medicine (MSOM) or its equivalent and that is accredited by the Accreditation Commission of Acupuncture and Oriental Medicine (ACAOM).

(b) "Acupuncturist" means a person who has received a professional degree from a college of acupuncture and Oriental medicine.

(c) "Acupuncturist-patient relationship" means that the acupuncturist has assumed the responsibility for making clinical judgments regarding the health of the patient and the need for medical treatment, and the patient has agreed to follow the acupuncturist's instructions.

(d) "Acupuncture practitioner" means a practitioner licensed under this chapter to practice the techniques of acupuncture in this state and includes the term "acupuncturist."

(e) "Advisory council" means the Mississippi Council of Advisors in Acupuncture established in this chapter.

(f) "Board" means the State Board of Medical Licensure established in Section 73 - 43 - 1 et seq.

(g) "Complementary and integrative therapies" means a heterogeneous group of preventive, diagnostic and therapeutic philosophies and practices, which at the time they are performed may differ from current scientific knowledge, or whose theoretical basis and techniques may diverge from western medicine routinely taught in accredited medical colleges, or both. These therapies include, but are not limited to, acupuncture, acutherapy and acupressure.

(h) "Impaired practitioner" means a practitioner who is unable to practice acupuncture with reasonable skill and safety because of a physical or mental disability as evidenced by a written determination from a competent authority or written consent based on clinical evidence, including deterioration of mental capacity, loss of motor skills, or abuse of drugs or alcohol of sufficient degree to diminish the person's ability to deliver competent patient care.

(i) "Informed consent" means the acupuncture practitioner has informed the patient, in a manner that would be understood by a reasonable person, of the diagnostic and treatment options, risk assessment and prognosis and has provided the patient with an estimate of the charges for treatment to be rendered and the patient has consented to the recommended treatment.

(j) "NCCAOM" means the National Certification Commission for Acupuncture and Oriental Medicine.

(k) "Physician" means a doctor of medicine or osteopathy who is legally authorized to practice medicine in the State of Mississippi.

(l) "Practice of acupuncture" means:

(i) To treat, correct, change, alleviate or prevent disease, illness, pain, deformity, defect, injury or other physical or mental conditions by the techniques of acupuncture, including:

1. The administering or applying of an apparatus or other therapeutic technique as defined in this chapter; or

2. The using of complementary and integrative therapies as defined in this chapter; or

3. The rendering of advice or recommendation by any means including telephonic and other electronic communications with regard to any of the above.

(ii) To represent, directly or indirectly, publicly or privately, an ability and willingness to do an act described in this paragraph.

(iii) To use any title, words, abbreviation or letters in a manner or under circumstances that induce the belief that the person using them is qualified to do any act described in this paragraph.

(m) "Techniques of acupuncture" includes acupuncture, moxibustion or heating modalities, cupping, magnets, ion pumping cords, electroacupuncture including electrodermal assessment, application of cold packs, dietary, nutritional and lifestyle counseling, manual therapy (Tui Na), massage, breathing and exercise techniques, the administration of any herb and nutritional supplement and meridian therapy. The terms used in this paragraph are defined as follows:

(i) "Acupuncture" means the insertion and manipulation of needles to the body, and the use of Oriental medicine and other modalities and procedures at specific locations on the body, for the prevention or correction of any disease, illness, injury, pain or other condition.

(ii) "Cupping" means the heating of air or mechanical creation of suction in a cup, application to specific locations on the body to induce local vasodialation and mechanical expansion of underlying tissue.

(iii) "Ion pumping cords" means the application of wires containing diodes to acupuncture needles that have been placed on the body.

(iv) "Magnets" means the application of magnets to specific locations on the body.

(v) "Electroacupuncture including electrodermal assessment" means the use of electronic biofeedback, and electrostimulation instruments.

(vi) "Cold packs" means the application of cold packs and ice to specific locations on the body to reduce heat conditions or inflammation in surface tissues of the body.

(vii) "Dietary, nutritional and lifestyle counseling" means in depth patient interviews and counseling to determine whether poor dietary, lifestyle or nutritional practices are a factor in a patient's illness and to educate toward a healthier lifestyle.

(viii) "Manual therapy (Tui Na) and massage" means mobilization of skeletal and soft tissues.

(ix) "Breathing and exercise techniques" means the use of Qi Gong and other techniques of therapeutic breathing and exercise.

(x) "Administration of herbal and botanical substances" means the administration of herbs of animal, vegetable or mineral origin for health maintenance and the treatment of effects of disease.

(xi) "Vitamin, mineral or nutritional supplement" means a nutritional substance, including a concentrate or extract of such a substance.

(xii) "Devices for meridian therapy" means all assessment and/or treatment devices for use with acupuncture meridians.

§ 73 – 71 – 7. **Practice requirements; evaluation by physician; exceptions; informed consent; practitioner information; diagnosis not to be made**

All of the following shall apply to an acupuncture practitioner who is licensed to practice in Mississippi:

（a）Except as otherwise provided in paragraph （c）, the practitioner may perform acupuncture on a patient only if the patient was evaluated by a physician, as appropriate, for the condition being treated within six （6） months before the date that acupuncture is performed. The State Board of Medical Licensure, with advice from the Mississippi Council of Advisors in Acupuncture, may by rule modify the scope of the evaluation under this paragraph or the period during which treatment must begin under this paragraph.

（b）The practitioner must obtain a written statement signed by the patient on a form prescribed by the State Board of Medical Licensure stating that the patient has been evaluated by a physician within the prescribed time. The form must contain a clear statement that the patient should be evaluated by a physician for the condition being treated by the practitioner.

（c）Notwithstanding the provisions of paragraph （a）, a practitioner may, without an evaluation from a physician, perform acupuncture on a patient for:

（i）Smoking addiction;

（ii）Weight loss; or

（iii）Substance abuse, to the extent permitted by regulations adopted by the State Board of Medical Licensure, with advice from the Mississippi Council of Advisors in Acupuncture.

（d）Before treating a patient, the practitioner shall advise the patient that acupuncture is not a substitute for conventional medical diagnosis and treatment and shall obtain the informed consent of the patient.

（e）On initially meeting a patient in person, the practitioner shall provide in writing the practitioner's name, business address, and business telephone number, and information on acupuncture, including the techniques that are used.

（f）While treating a patient, the practitioner shall not make a diagnosis. If a patient's condition is not improving or a patient requires emergency medical treatment, the practitioner shall consult promptly with a physician.

§ 73 - 71 - 9.　Repealed by Laws 2017, Ch. 391 （S.B. No. 2214）, § 2, eff. July 1, 2017

§ 73 - 71 - 11.　Mississippi Council of Advisors in Acupuncture; creation; membership; quorum; compensation; reports

（1）There is hereby established the Mississippi Council of Advisors in Acupuncture to aid the State Board of Medical Licensure in administering the provisions of this chapter.

（2）The council shall consist of three （3） persons appointed by the Executive Director of the State Medical Licensure Board to be selected from a list of six （6） nominees of the Mississippi Oriental Medicine Association. Members of the council shall either be acupuncture practitioners who are not medical, osteopathic or chiropractic doctors or surgeons, or medical doctors who are registered to practice acupuncture or qualify as an acupuncture practitioner.

（3）The initial members of the council shall be appointed by the Governor for staggered terms as follows: one (1) member shall be appointed for a term ending on July 1, 2011, and two (2) members shall be appointed for terms ending on July 1, 2012. After the expiration of the initial terms, each successor member shall be appointed for a term of three (3) years. A vacancy shall be filled by appointment by the Governor for the remainder of the unexpired term. Council members shall serve until their successors have been appointed and qualified.

(4) No council member shall serve more than two (2) consecutive full terms, and any member failing to attend three (3) consecutive meetings after proper notice has been given by the council shall automatically be removed as a council member, unless excused for reasons set forth in council regulations.

(5) The Governor may remove any member from the council for neglect of any duty required by law, for incompetence, for improper or unprofessional conduct as defined by board regulations, for conflict of interest, or for any reason that would justify the suspension or revocation of his or her license to practice acupuncture.

(6) A majority of the members of the council shall constitute a quorum to conduct business. It shall require an affirmative vote of a majority of those members present at a meeting to take any action or pass any motion. The council shall, not later than September 1, 2009, and annually thereafter in the month of July, hold a meeting and elect from its membership a chairman and vice chairman. The council shall meet at any other times as it deems necessary or advisable by the chairman, a majority of its members, or the Governor. Reasonable notice of all meetings shall be given in the manner prescribed by the Open Meetings Law (Section 25-3-41 et seq.). Members of the council are not liable to civil action for any act performed in good faith in the execution of duties as a council member.

(7) Members of the council shall be reimbursed for expenses and mileage as provided in Section 25-3-41, but shall receive no other compensation, perquisite or allowance for service on the council.

(8) The council shall report annually to the Legislature statistics regarding the number of licensees, results of the licensing examinations, and violations investigated during the previous year.

§ 73-71-13. State Board of Medical Licensure; regulatory authority and responsibilities

(1) The State Board of Medical Licensure is hereby empowered, authorized and directed to adopt, amend, promulgate and enforce such rules, regulations and standards governing the practice of acupuncture as may be necessary to further the accomplishment of the purpose of this chapter, and in so doing shall utilize as the basis thereof the corresponding recommendations of the advisory council.

(2) The board's authority and responsibility include the following:

(a) Grant, deny, renew, restrict, suspend or revoke licenses to practice acupuncture in accordance with the provisions of this chapter or other applicable state law;

(b) Examine by established protocol the qualifications and fitness of applicants for a license to practice acupuncture in this state;

(c) Conduct investigations of suspected violations of this chapter to determine whether there are sufficient grounds to initiate disciplinary proceedings;

(d) Inspect premises and equipment, on a triennial basis and assess an inspection fee in the amount of One Hundred Dollars ($100.00) per inspection and an additional fee of Fifty Dollars ($50.00) for each licensed acupuncturist employed by the inspected establishment;

(e) Hold hearings on all matters properly brought before the board, to administer oaths, receive evidence, make necessary determinations and enter orders consistent with the findings. The board may require by subpoena the attendance and testimony of witnesses and the production of papers, records or other documentary evidence and commission depositions. The board may designate one or more of its members to serve as its hearing officer. The board shall adopt rules and regulations for hearings before the board and the rules shall afford any person appearing before the board the safeguards of procedural due process. Formal rules of evidence shall not apply;

(f) Contract with independent consultants or other appropriate agencies to administer examinations for licensure, according to the provisions of this chapter, and establish a fee for such examination not to exceed Five Hundred Dollars ($500.00);

(g) Establish and publish a schedule of fees for annual licensing, certification and renewal not to exceed Four Hundred Dollars ($400.00) annually; and

(h) Keep and maintain accurate records of all board business in accordance with state law.

The powers enumerated in this section are granted for the purpose of enabling the board to supervise effectively the practice of acupuncture and are to be construed liberally to accomplish this objective.

§ 73 – 71 – 15.　Unlicensed practice of acupuncture prohibited

Unless licensed as an acupuncture practitioner under this chapter, or exempt from licensure under the provisions of this chapter, no person shall practice or hold himself or herself out as practicing or engaging in the practice of acupuncture, either for compensation or gratuitously.

§ 73 – 71 – 17.　Effect of licensure; construction of chapter

(1) An acupuncture practitioner license authorizes the holder to engage in the practice of acupuncture.

(2) This chapter shall not be construed to limit, interfere with, or prevent any other class of licensed health care professionals from practicing within the scope of their licenses as defined by each profession's state licensing statute.

(3) This chapter shall not be construed to make unlawful the activities of persons involved in research performed under the auspices of a federal or state regulated research institution.

(4) The practice and techniques of acupuncture shall not include the practice of physical therapy as defined in the Mississippi Physical Therapy Practice Law, Title 73, Chapter 23 of the Mississippi Code of 1972.

§ 73 – 71 – 19. License requirements; education; examination

(1) No person shall be licensed to practice acupuncture unless he or she has passed an examination and/or has been found to have the necessary qualifications as prescribed in the regulations adopted by the board.

(2) Before any applicant is eligible for an examination or qualification, he or she shall furnish satisfactory proof that he or she:

(a) Is a citizen or permanent resident of the United States;

(b) Has demonstrated proficiency in the English language;

(c) Is at least twenty-one (21) years of age;

(d) Is of good moral character;

(e) Has completed a program of acupuncture and has received a certificate or diploma from an institute approved by the board, according to the provisions of this chapter;

(f) Has completed a clinical internship training as approved by the board; and

(g) Has received training in cardiopulmonary resuscitation (CPR).

(3) The board may hold an examination at least once a year, and all applicants shall be notified in writing of the date and time of all examinations. The board may use a NCCAOM examination if it deems that national examination to be sufficient to qualify a practitioner for licensure in this state. In no case shall the state's own examination be less rigorous than the nationally recognized examination.

(4) In addition to the written examination, if the nationally recognized examination does not provide a suitable practical examination comparable to board standards, the board shall examine each applicant in the practical application of Oriental medical diagnostic and treatment techniques in a manner and by methods that reveal the applicant's skill and knowledge.

(5) The board shall require all qualified applicants to be examined in the following subjects:

(a) Anatomy and physiology;

(b) Pathology;

(c) Diagnosis;

(d) Hygiene, sanitation and sterilization techniques;

(e) All major acupuncture principles, practices and techniques; and

(f) Clean Needle Technique Exam.

(6) To assist the board in conducting its licensure investigation, all applicants shall undergo a fingerprint-based criminal history records check of the Mississippi central criminal database and the Federal Bureau of Investigation criminal history database. Each applicant shall submit a full set of the applicant's fingerprints in a form and manner prescribed by the board, which shall be

forwarded to the Mississippi Department of Public Safety (department) and the Federal Bureau of Investigation Identification Division for this purpose. Any and all state or national criminal history records information obtained by the board that is not already a matter of public record shall be deemed nonpublic and confidential information restricted to the exclusive use of the board, its members, officers, investigators, agents and attorneys in evaluating the applicant's eligibility or disqualification for licensure, and shall be exempt from the Mississippi Public Records Act of 1983. Except when introduced into evidence in a hearing before the board to determine licensure, no such information or records related thereto shall, except with the written consent of the applicant or by order of a court of competent jurisdiction, be released or otherwise disclosed by the board to any other person or agency. The board shall provide to the department the fingerprints of the applicant, any additional information that may be required by the department, and a form signed by the applicant consenting to the check of the criminal records and to the use of the fingerprints and other identifying information required by the state or national repositories. The board shall charge and collect from the applicant, in addition to all other applicable fees and costs, such amount as may be incurred by the board in requesting and obtaining state and national criminal history records information on the applicant.

(7) The board shall issue a license to every applicant whose application has been filed with and approved by the board and who has paid the required fees and who either:

(a) Has passed the board's written examination and practical examination, with a score of not less than seventy percent (70%) on each examination; or

(b) Has achieved a passing score on a board approved nationally recognized examination, which examination includes a written and practical portion, as determined by the board; or

(c) Has received certification from a board approved national certification process; or

(d) Has achieved a passing score on a board approved nationally recognized written examination and has passed the board's practical examination with a score of not less than seventy percent (70%).

(8) The board shall keep a record of all examinations held, together with the names and addresses of all persons taking examinations, and the examination results. Within forty-five (45) days after the examination, the board shall give written notice of the results of the examination to each applicant.

§ 73 - 71 - 21.　License reciprocity

The board may, at its discretion, issue a license without examination to an acupuncture practitioner who has been licensed, certified or otherwise formally legally recognized as an acupuncturist or acupuncture practitioner in any state or territory if all three (3) of the following conditions are met to its satisfaction:

(a) The applicant meets the requirements of practice in the state or territory in which the applicant is licensed, certified, or registered as an acupuncturist or acupuncture practitioner;

(b) The requirements for practice in the state or territory in which the applicant is licensed, certified or registered as an acupuncturist or acupuncture practitioner are at least as stringent as those of this state; and

(c) The state or territory in which the applicant is licensed, certified or legally recognized as an acupuncturist or acupuncture practitioner permits an acupuncture practitioner licensed in this state to practice acupuncture or acupuncture in that jurisdiction by credentials examination.

The issuance of a license by reciprocity to a military-trained applicant, military spouse or person who establishes residence in this state shall be subject to the provisions of Section 73 – 50 – 1 or 73 – 50 – 2, as applicable.

§ 73 – 71 – 23. Continuing education requirements

(1) The board shall establish, by regulation, mandatory continuing education requirements for acupuncture practitioners licensed in this state, including the following:

(a) Each person licensed under this chapter, whether or not residing within the state, shall complete thirty (30) hours of continuing education within each biennial renewal period, except during the initial biennial renewal period; and

(b) Each person not obtaining the required number of hours of continuing education may have his or her license renewed for just cause, as determined by the board, so long as the board requires that the deficient hours of continuing education, and all unpaid fees, are made up during the following renewal period in addition to the current continuing education requirements for the renewal period. If any acupuncture practitioner fails to make up the deficient hours and complete the later renewal period, or fails to make up any unpaid fees, then his or her license shall not be renewed until all fees are paid and all of the required hours are completed and documented to the board.

(2) The board shall establish by regulation education standards and record keeping requirements for continuing education providers. A provider of continuing education courses shall apply to the board for approval to offer continuing education courses for credit toward this requirement on a form developed by the board, shall pay a fee covering the cost of approval and for monitoring of the provider by the board. Institutions, associations and individuals providing continuing education shall maintain records of attendance, including sign-in sheets, for a period of three (3) years.

§ 73 – 71 – 25. Institutes of acupuncture; standards for board approval

(1) The board shall establish standards for approval of schools and colleges offering education and training in the practice of acupuncture.

(2) Before approval of an institute of acupuncture, the board shall determine that the institute meets standards of professional education. These standards shall provide that the institute:

(a) Require, as a prerequisite to graduation, a program of study of at least two thousand five hundred (2,500) hours;

（b）Meet the minimum requirements of a board approved national accrediting body；

（c）Require participation in a carefully supervised clinical or internship program；and

（d）Confer a certificate，diploma or degree in acupuncture only after personal attendance in classes and clinics.

§ 73 – 71 – 27. Grandfather provision；unqualified practice prohibited；liability insurance requirement

（1）Any acupuncturist validly licensed，certified or registered under prior law of this state shall be deemed as licensed under the provisions of this chapter.

（2）All acupuncturists licensed under this section shall not accept or perform professional responsibilities that the licensee knows or has reason to know that the person is not qualified by training，experience or certification to perform. Violation of this section shall subject the licensee to the revocation or suspension of his or her license. The board shall make regulations on those requirements and shall grant previously licensed，certified or registered acupuncturists qualification on a case-by-case basis.

（3）The board shall require each licensee to obtain and maintain an adequate amount of professional liability insurance and provide proof of that insurance to the board.

§ 73 – 71 – 29. Reporting and record keeping requirements

（1）Persons licensed under this chapter shall be subject to the following reporting requirements：

（a）All morbidity，mortality，infectious disease，abuse and neglect reporting requirements of this state；

（b）Reporting completion of the required continuing education study to the board with his or her license renewal；

（c）Notification of the board in writing of any change of address within thirty（30）days of the change；

（d）Notification of the board in writing of termination or temporary closing of the licensee's practice if the cessation of business is expected to be over ninety（90）days，or otherwise limit access to patient records. The licensee shall notify the board upon resuming practice；and

（e）Posting his or her license in a conspicuous location in his or her place of practice at all times.

（2）Persons licensed under this chapter shall be subject to the following record keeping requirements：

（a）Maintenance of accurate records of each patient that he or she treats. The records shall include the name of the patient，medical history，subjective symptoms，objective findings and treatment rendered；

（b）Maintenance of patient records for a period of seven（7）years；and

（c）Maintenance of documents proving completion of required continuing education study for a period of three（3）years.

§ 73 - 71 - 31.   Health and sanitation requirements

(1) Acupuncture practitioners shall comply with all applicable public health laws of this state.

(2) Sanitation practices shall include:

(a) Hands shall be washed with soap and water or other disinfectant between treatment of different patients;

(b) Skin in the area of penetration shall be swabbed with alcohol or other germicidal solution before inserting needles;

(c) Needles and other equipment used in the practice of acupuncture shall be sterilized before using;

(d) Needles and other hazardous waste shall be disposed of in a manner prescribed by law; and

(e) Other sanitation practices shall be observed to insure health and safety of patients, as prescribed by the board.

§ 73 - 71 - 33.   Grounds for disciplinary action

The following acts constitute grounds for which the board may initiate disciplinary actions:

(a) Attempting to obtain, or renewing a license to practice acupuncture by bribery or misinterpretation;

(b) Having a license to practice acupuncture revoked, suspended, or otherwise acted against, including the denial of licensure by the licensing authority of another state or territory for reasons that would preclude licensure in this state;

(c) Being convicted or found guilty, regardless of adjudication, in any jurisdiction of a felony, or a crime of moral turpitude, or a crime that directly relates to acupuncture. For the purposes of this paragraph, a plea of guilty or a plea of nolo contendere accepted by the court shall be considered as a conviction;

(d) Advertising, practicing, or attempting to practice under a name other than one's own;

(e) The use of advertising or solicitation that is false or misleading;

(f) Aiding, assisting, procuring, employing or advertising an unlicensed person to practice acupuncture contrary to this chapter or a rule of the board;

(g) Failing to perform any statutory or legal obligation placed upon an acupuncture practitioner;

(h) Making or filing a report that the licensee knows to be false, intentionally or negligently failing to file a report required by state or federal law, willfully impeding or obstructing that filing or inducing another person to do so. Those reports shall include only those that are signed in the capacity of an acupuncture practitioner;

(i) Exercising coercion, intimidation or undue influence in entering into sexual relations with a patient, or continuing the patient-practitioner relationship with a patient with whom the licensee has sexual relations, if those sexual relations cause the licensee to perform services incompetently. This paragraph shall not apply to sexual relations between acupuncture practitioners and their spouses;

(j) Making deceptive, untrue or fraudulent misrepresentations in the practice of acupuncture;

(k) Soliciting patients, either personally or through an agent, through the use of fraud, intimidation or undue influence, or a form of overreaching conduct;

(l) Failing to keep written medical records justifying the course of treatment of the patient;

(m) Exercising undue influence on the patient to exploit the patient for financial gain of the licensee or of a third party;

(n) Being unable to practice acupuncture with reasonable skill and safety to patients by reason of illness or intemperate use of alcohol, drugs, narcotics, chemicals, or any other type of material or as a result of any mental or physical condition;

(o) Malpractice or the failure to practice acupuncture to that level of care, skill and treatment that is recognized by a reasonably prudent similar practitioner of acupuncture as being acceptable under similar conditions and circumstances;

(p) Practicing or offering to practice beyond the scope permitted by law or accepting or performing professional responsibilities that the licensee knows or has reason to know that he or she is not qualified by training, experience or certification to perform;

(q) Delegating professional responsibilities to a person when the licensee delegating those responsibilities knows, or has reason to know, that the person is not qualified by training, experience or licensure to perform them;

(r) Violating any provision of this chapter, a rule of the board, or a lawful order of the board previously entered in a disciplinary hearing or failing to comply with a lawfully issued subpoena of the board;

(s) Conspiring with another to commit an act, or committing an act, that coerces, intimidates or precludes another licensee from lawfully advertising or providing his or her services;

(t) Fraud or deceit, or gross negligence, incompetence or misconduct in the operation of a course of study;

(u) Failing to comply with state, county or municipal regulations or reporting requirements relating to public health and the control of contagious and infectious disease;

(v) Failing to comply with any rule of the board relating to health and safety, including, but not limited to, sterilization of equipment and the disposal of potentially infectious materials;

(w) Incompetence, gross negligence or other malpractice in the practice of acupuncture;

(x) Aiding the unlawful practice of acupuncture;

(y) Fraud or dishonesty in the application or reporting of any test for disease;

(z) Failure to report, as required by law, or making false or misleading report of, any contagious or infectious disease;

(aa) Failure to keep accurate patient records; or

(bb) Failure to permit the board or its agents to enter and inspect acupuncture premises and equipment as set by rules promulgated by the board.

§ 73 – 71 – 35. Disciplinary proceedings; penalties; mental or physical examination; reinstatement

(1) Disciplinary proceedings under this chapter shall be conducted in the same manner as other disciplinary proceedings are conducted by the State Board of Medical Licensure.

(2) When the board finds any person guilty of any of the acts set forth in Section 73 – 71 – 33, it may then enter an order imposing one or more of the following penalties:

(a) Refusal to certify to the board an application for licensure;

(b) Revocation or suspension of a license;

(c) Restriction of practice;

(d) Imposition of an administrative fine not to exceed One Thousand Dollars ($1,000.00) for each count or separate offense;

(e) Issuance of a reprimand;

(f) Placement of the acupuncture practitioner on probation for a period of time and subject to the conditions as the board may specify.

(3) In enforcing this chapter, upon finding of the board that probable cause exists to believe that the licensee is unable to serve as an acupuncture practitioner because of committing any of the acts set forth in Section 73 – 71 – 33 or any of the crimes set forth in Section 73 – 71 – 37, the board shall have to issue an order to compel the licensee to submit to a mental or physical examination by a physician designated by the board. If the licensee refuses to comply with the order, the board's order directing the examination may be enforced by filing a petition for enforcement in any court of competent jurisdiction. The licensee against whom the petition is filed shall not be named or identified by initials in any public court record or document, and the proceedings shall be closed to the public unless the licensee stipulates otherwise. The board shall be entitled to the summary procedure provided in applicable state law. An acupuncture practitioner affected under this subsection shall at reasonable intervals be afforded an opportunity to demonstrate that he or she can resume the competent practice of acupuncture with reasonable skill and safety of the patients. In any proceeding under this subsection, neither the record of proceedings nor the orders entered by the board shall be used against the acupuncture practitioner in any other proceeding.

(4) The board shall not reinstate the license of an acupuncture practitioner, or cause a license to be issued to a person it has deemed to be unqualified, until such time as the board is satisfied that he or she has complied with all the terms and conditions set forth in the final order and that he or she is capable of safely engaging in the practice of acupuncture.

§ 73 – 71 – 37. Unlawful acts; penalties

(1) It is unlawful for any person to:

（a）Hold himself or herself out as an acupuncture practitioner unless licensed as provided in this chapter;

（b）Practice acupuncture, or attempt to practice acupuncture, without an active license or as otherwise permitted by board rule established under the authority of this chapter;

（c）Obtain, or attempt to obtain, a license to practice acupuncture by fraud or misrepresentation; or

（d）Permit an employed person to engage in the practice of acupuncture unless the person holds an active license as a practitioner of acupuncture, except as provided by this chapter.

（2）Any person who violates any provision of this section is guilty of a misdemeanor and, upon conviction, shall be punished by a fine of not more than One Thousand Dollars（ $1,000.00）, or by imprisonment in the county jail for not more than six（6）months, or both.

§ 73 – 71 – 39.　Program for impaired acupuncturists; good faith reporting requirement

（1）The board shall establish a program of care, counseling or treatment for impaired acupuncturists.

（2）The program of care, counseling or treatment shall include a written schedule of organized treatment, care, counseling, activities or education satisfactory to the board designed for the purposes of restoring an impaired person to a condition by which the impaired person can practice acupuncture with reasonable skill and safety of a sufficient degree to deliver competent patient care.

（3）All persons authorized to practice by the board shall report in good faith any acupuncturist they reasonably believe to be an impaired practitioner as defined in Section 73 – 71 – 5.

§ 73 – 71 – 41.　Disclosure of privileged information; conditions; immunity; waiver

（1）No licensed acupuncturist shall disclose any information concerning the licensed acupuncturist's care of a patient except on written authorization or by waiver by the licensed acupuncturist's patient or by court order, by subpoena, or as otherwise provided in this section.

（2）Any licensed acupuncturist releasing information under written authorization or other waiver by the patient or under court order, by subpoena, or as otherwise provided by this section shall not be liable to the patient or any other person.

（3）The privilege provided by this section shall be waived to the extent that the licensed acupuncturist's patient places the licensed acupuncturist's care and treatment of the patient or the nature and extent of injuries to the patient at issue in any civil criminal proceeding.

§ 73 – 71 – 43.　Licensed renewal fee and continuing education required

Each licensee shall be required to pay biennial license renewal fees and meet continuing education requirements as provided in this chapter.

§ 73 – 71 – 45.　License renewal; time limit; new license requirements

（1）A license that has expired may be renewed at any time within ninety（90）days after its expiration upon filing of an application for renewal on a form provided by the board and payment of the renewal fee in effect on the last regular renewal date. If the license is not renewed within ninety (90) days after its expiration, the acupuncture practitioner, as a condition precedent to renewal, shall pay the renewal fees plus a late fee to be set by the board.

(2) A person who fails to renew his or her license within four (4) years after its expiration may not renew that license, and it may not be restored, reissued or reinstated after that time; but that person may apply for and obtain a new license if he or she meets the following requirements:

(a) Takes and passes a suitable examination, or demonstrates continued practice and continuing education acceptable to the board; and

(b) Pays all fees that would be required if an initial application for licensure were being made.

§ 73 – 71 – 47.　Inactive license status; reinstatement requirements

At any time while a license is valid, or expired but not lapsed, the licensee may request that his or her license be placed on inactive status. While on inactive status, the licensee is not subject to fees or continuing education requirements. As a condition of reinstatement, the licensee must satisfy the following requirements:

(a) Demonstrate that he or she has not committed any acts or crimes constituting grounds for denial of licensure under any provisions of this chapter;

(b) Pay fees to reactivate status as designated by the board;

(c) Meet continuing education requirements equivalent to those that would have been met in the preceding two (2) years; and

(d) Establish to the satisfaction of the board that, with due regard for the public interest, he or she is qualified to practice as an acupuncture practitioner.

§ 73 – 71 – 49.　Suspended and revoked licenses

(1) A suspended license is subject to expiration and shall be renewed as provided in this chapter, but while the license remains suspended, and until it is reinstated, the renewal does not entitle the practice of acupuncture, or any other activity or conduct in violation of the order of the board by which the license was suspended.

(2) A revoked license is subject to expiration as provided in this chapter but it may not be renewed. If it is reinstated after its expiration, the former licensee, as a condition of reinstatement, shall pay a reinstatement fee in an amount equal to the renewal fee in effect on the last regular renewal fee date, if any, accrued at the time of its expiration.

§ 73 – 71 – 51.　Fees

(1) The board may charge reasonable fees for the following:

(a) Initial application fee for licensing;

(b) Written and practical examination not including the cost of the nationally recognized examination;

（c）Biennial licensing renewal for acupuncture practitioners;

（d）Late renewal more than thirty（30）days, but not later than one（1）year, after expiration of a license, which late fee is in addition to any other fees;

（e）Reciprocal licensing fee;

（f）Annual continuing education provider registration fee; and

（g）Any and all fees to cover reasonable and necessary administrative expenses as established by the Council of Advisors in Acupuncture.

（2）All fees shall be set forth in regulations duly adopted by the board.

（3）All fees and other funds collected under this chapter shall be deposited into the special fund of the State Board of Medical Licensure.

§ 73‑71‑53. **Repealed by Laws 2017, Ch. 391（S.B. No. 2214）, § 3, eff. July 1, 2017**

MISSISSIPPI ADMINISTRATIVE CODE

Pt. 2625, R. 1.1. Scope.

The following rules pertain to acupuncture practitioners performing the technique of acupuncture. Except as otherwise provided below, the practitioner may perform acupuncture on a patient only if the patient was evaluated by a physician, as appropriate, for the condition being treated within six（6）months before the date that acupuncture is performed. The Board with advice from the Mississippi Council of Advisors in Acupuncture, may by rule modify the scope of the evaluation under this paragraph or the period during which treatment must begin under this paragraph.

The practitioner must obtain a written statement signed by the patient on a form prescribed by the Board stating that the patient has been evaluated by a physician within the prescribed time. The form must contain a clear statement that the patient should be evaluated by a physician for the condition being treated by the practitioner.

A practitioner may, without an evaluation from a physician, perform acupuncture on a patient for:

A. smoking addiction;

B. weight loss; or

C. substance abuse, to the extent permitted by the Board, with advice from the Mississippi Council of Advisors in Acupuncture.

While treating a patient, the practitioner shall not make a medical diagnosis, but may provide pattern differentiation according to Traditional Chinese Medicine. If a patient's condition is not improving or a patient requires emergency medical treatment, the practitioner shall consult promptly with a physician.

Acupuncture may be performed in the state of Mississippi by a physician licensed to practice medicine and adequately trained in the art and science of acupuncture. Adequately trained will be defined as a minimum of 200 hours of AMA or AOA approved Category I CME in the field of acupuncture. Such licensed individuals wishing to utilize acupuncture in their practice may do so provided that any and all portions of the acupuncture treatment are performed by the person so licensed and no surrogate is authorized in this state to serve in his or her stead. The practice of acupuncture by a physician should follow the same quality of standard that the physician, or any other physician in his or her community, would render in delivering any other medical treatment. The applicable standard of care shall include all elements of a doctor-patient relationship. The elements of this valid relationship are:

A. verify that the person requesting the medical treatment is in fact who they claim to be;

B. conduct an appropriate examination of the patient that meets the applicable standard of care and is sufficient to justify the differential diagnosis and proposed therapies;

C. establish a differential diagnosis through the use of accepted medical practices, i.e., a patient history, mental status exam, physical exam and appropriate diagnostic and laboratory testing;

D. discuss with the patient the diagnosis, risks and benefits of various treatment options and obtain informed consent;

E. insure the availability of appropriate follow-up care including use of traditional medicine; and

F. maintain a complete medical record.

The Board of Medical Licensure must have on file copies of required CME prior to any Mississippi licensed physician being approved to provide treatment by acupuncture. Licensees approved by the Mississippi State Board of Medical Licensure to practice acupuncture prior to January 2011 shall not be required to meet the aforementioned CME requirements.

Pt. 2625, R. 1.2. Definitions.

For the purpose of Part 2625, Chapter 1 only, the following terms have the meanings indicated:

A. "Board" means the Mississippi State Board of Medical Licensure.

B. "Council" means the Mississippi Council of Advisors in Acupuncture.

C. "NCCAOM" means the National Certification Commission for Acupuncture and Oriental Medicine.

D. "ACAOM" means the Accreditation Commission of Acupuncture and Oriental Medicine.

E. "CCAOM" means the Council of Colleges of Acupuncture and Oriental Medicine.

Pt. 2625, R. 1.3. Qualifications for Licensure.

On or after July 1, 2009, applicants for acupuncture licensure must meet the following requirements：

A. Satisfy the Board that he or she is at least twenty-one（21）years of age and of good moral character.

B. Satisfy the Board that he or she is a citizen or permanent resident of the United States of America.

C. Submit an application for license on a form supplied by the Board, completed in every detail with a recent photograph（wallet-size/passport type）attached. A Polaroid or informal snapshot will not be accepted.

D. Pay the appropriate fee as determined by the Board.

E. Present a certified copy of birth certificate or valid and current passport.

F. Submit proof of legal change of name if applicable（notarized or certified copy of marriage or other legal proceeding）.

G. Provide information on registration or licensure in all other states where the applicant is or has been registered or licensed as an acupuncturist.

H. Provide favorable references from two（2）acupuncturists licensed in the United States with whom the applicant has worked or trained.

I. Provide proof, directly from the institution, of successful completion of an educational program for acupuncturists that are in candidacy status or accredited by ACAOM, NCCAOM or its predecessor or successor agency that is at least three（3）years in duration and includes a supervised clinical internship to ensure that applicants with an education outside the US are recognized because of the NCCAOM review process for foreign applicants.

J. Pass the certification examinations administered by the NCCAOM and have current NCCAOM Diplomate status in Acupuncture or Oriental Medicine that is consistent with one of the following：

1. If taken before June 1, 2004, pass the Comprehensive Written Exam（CWE）, the Clean Needle Technique portion（CNTP）, and the Practical Examination of Point Location Skills（PEPLS）.

2. If taken on or after June 1, 2004, and before January 1, 2007, pass the NCCAOM Foundations of Oriental Medicine Module, Acupuncture Module, Point Location Module and Biomedicine Module.

3. If taken on or after January 1, 2007, pass the NCCAOM Foundations of Oriental Medicine Module, Acupuncture Module with Point Location Module, and the Biomedicine Module.

K. If applicant is a graduate of an international educational program, provide proof that the applicant is able to communicate in English as demonstrated by one of the following：

1. Passage of the NCCAOM examination taken in English.

2. Passage of the TOEFL（Test of English as a Foreign Language）with a score of 560 or higher on the paper based test or with a score of 220 or higher on the computer based test.

3. Passage of the TSE (Test of Spoken English) with a score of 50 or higher.

4. Passage of the TOEIC (Test of English for International Communication) with a score of 500 or higher.

L. Provide proof of successful completion of a NCCAOM-approved clean needle technique course sent directly from the course provider to the Board.

M. Provide proof of current cardiopulmonary resuscitation (CPR) certification from either the American Heart Association or the American Red Cross.

N. Provide proof of malpractice insurance with a minimum of $1 million dollars in coverage.

O. Submit fingerprints for state and national criminal history background checks.

Pt. 2625, R. 1.4. Practice Standards.

Before treatment of a patient, the acupuncturist (if not a Mississippi licensed physician) shall be sure that the patient has been evaluated by a licensed physician for the condition to be treated within the last six (6) months. The Board, with advice from the Mississippi Council of Advisors in Acupuncture, may be rule modify the scope of the evaluation under this paragraph or the period during which treatment must begin under this paragraph and shall review the diagnosis for which the patient is receiving treatment.

The acupuncturist shall obtain informed consent from the patient after advising them of potential risks and benefits of acupuncture treatment plan.

The acupuncturist shall obtain a written statement signed by the patient on a form prescribed by the Board stating that the patient has been evaluated by a physician within the prescribed time.

The acupuncturist shall obtain a detailed medical history that would identify contraindications to acupuncture such as a bleeding disorder.

An acupuncture practitioner will use sterilized equipment that has been sterilized according to standards of the Centers for Disease Control and Prevention (CDC).

An acupuncturist shall comply with all applicable state and municipal requirements regarding public health.

Pt. 2625, R. 1.5. Patient Records.

A licensed acupuncturist shall maintain a complete and accurate record of each patient. The record shall be sufficient to demonstrate a valid acupuncturist-patient relationship:

A. verify that the person requesting the medical treatment is in fact who they claim to be;

B. obtain a written statement signed by the patient on a form prescribed by the Board stating that the patient has been evaluated by a physician within the prescribed time;

C. conduct and appropriate examination of the patient that meets the applicable standard of care and is sufficient to justify the differential diagnosis and proposed therapies;

D. establish a differential diagnosis through the use of accepted medical practices, i.e., a patient history, mental status exam, physical exam and appropriate diagnostic and laboratory testing;

E. discuss with the patient the diagnosis, risks and benefits of various treatment options and obtain informed consent;

F. insure the availability of appropriate follow-up care including use of traditional medicine; and

G. maintain a complete medical record.

Patient records must be maintained for a period of seven (7) years from the date of last treatment or longer if required by future statute or regulation.

At patient's request, the acupuncturist shall provide the patient or other authorized person a copy of the acupuncture record. Refer to Administrative Code Part 2635 Chapter 10, Release of Medical Records.

Acupuncturists are subject to a peer review process conducted by the Council.

Pt. 2625, R. 1.6. Supervision.

Before treating a patient, the acupuncturist shall advise the patient that acupuncture is not a substitute for conventional medical diagnosis and treatment and shall obtain the informed consent of the patient.

On initially meeting a patient in person, the acupuncturist shall provide in writing the acupuncturist's name, business address, and business telephone number, and information on acupuncture, including the techniques that are used.

While treating a patient, the acupuncturist shall not make a diagnosis. If a patient's condition is not improving or a patient requires emergency medical treatment, the acupuncturist shall consult promptly with a physician.

Pt. 2625, R. 1.7. Duty to Notify Board of Change of Address.

Any acupuncturist who is licensed to practice as an acupuncturist in this state and changes their practice location or mailing address shall immediately notify the Board in writing of the change. Failure to notify within 30 days could result in disciplinary action.

The Board routinely sends information to licensed acupuncturists. Whether it be by U.S. Mail or electronically, it is important that this information is received by the licensee. The licensure record of the licensee should include a physical practice location, mailing address, email address and telephone number where the Board can correspond with the licensee directly. The Board discourages the use of office personnel's mailing and email addresses as well as telephone numbers. Failure to provide the Board with direct contact information could result in disciplinary action.

Pt. 2625, R. 1.8. Continuing Education.

A. Every acupuncturist must earn or receive not less than thirty (30) hours of acupuncture related continuing education courses as precedent to renewing their license for the next fiscal year. This thirty (30) hours is per two-year cycle. Excess hours may not be carried over to another two-year cycle. *For the purpose of this regulation, the two-year period begins July 1, 2010, and every two years thereafter.* Continuing education courses must be sponsored and/or approved by one of the following organizations:

    1. Mississippi Council of Advisors in Acupuncture

    2. Mississippi Oriental Medicine Association

    3. American Society of Acupuncturists

    4. National Certification Commission for Acupuncture and Oriental Medicine

    5. American Acupuncture Council

    6. American Board of Oriental Reproductive Medicine

B. All persons licensed as acupuncturists must comply with the following continuing education rules as a prerequisite to license renewal.

    1. Acupuncturists receiving their initial license to perform acupuncture in Mississippi after June 30 are exempt from the minimum continuing education requirement for the two-year period following their receiving a license. The thirty (30) hour continuing education certification will be due within the next two-year cycle.

    2. The approved hours of any individual course or activity will not be counted more than once in a two (2) year period toward the required hour total regardless of the number of times the course or activity is attended or completed by any individual.

    3. The Board may waive or otherwise modify the requirements of this rule in cases where there is illness, military service, disability or other undue hardship that prevents a license holder from obtaining the requisite number of continuing education hours. Requests for waivers or modification must be sent in writing to the Executive Director prior to the expiration of the renewal period in which the continuing education is due.

Pt. 2625, R. 1.9. Violations.

Any acupuncturist who falsely attests to completion of the required continuing education may be subject to disciplinary action pursuant to Mississippi Code, Section 73 – 71 – 33 and 73 – 71 – 35.

Any acupuncturist that fails to obtain the required continuing education may be subject to disciplinary action pursuant to Mississippi Code, Section 73 – 71 – 33 and 73 – 71 – 35, and may not be allowed to renew license. If continuing education deficiencies are discovered during an audit of the licensee, the licensee shall be suspended from practice for the longer of (i) a period of 3 months or (ii) until deficiencies are remedied. Any licensee suspended as a result of a continuing education audit may request a hearing for the purpose of appealing the suspension. Suspension as a result of falsified certification of continuing education shall begin upon determination of the false certification and shall not require notice or hearing as described below.

Continuing education obtained as a result of compliance with the terms of the Board Orders in any disciplinary action shall not be credited toward the continuing education required to be obtained in any two (2) year period.

Pt. 2625, R. 1.10. Renewal Schedule.

The license of every person licensed to practice as an acupuncturist in the state of Mississippi shall be renewed annually.

On or before May 1 of every year, the State Board of Medical Licensure shall notify every acupuncturist to whom a license was issued or renewed during the current licensing period of the forthcoming annual renewal of license. The notice shall provide instructions for obtaining and submitting applications for renewal. The applicant shall obtain and complete the application and submit it to the Board in the manner prescribed by the Board in the notice before June 30 with the renewal fee of an amount established by the Board. The payment of the annual license renewal fee shall be optional with all acupuncturists over the age of seventy (70) years. Upon receipt of the application and fee, the Board shall verify the accuracy of the application and issue to applicant a license of renewal for the ensuing one (1) year period, beginning July 1 and expiring June 30 of the succeeding licensure period.

An acupuncturist practicing in Mississippi who allows a license to lapse by failing to renew the license as provided in the foregoing paragraph may be reinstated by the Board on satisfactory explanation for such failure to renew, by completion of a reinstatement form, and upon payment of the renewal fee for the current year. If the license has not been renewed within ninety (90) days after its expiration, the renewal shall be assessed a late fee of $200.

Any acupuncturist who allows a license to lapse shall be notified by the Board within thirty (30) days of such lapse.

Any acupuncturist who fails to renew a license within four (4) years after its expiration may not renew that license. The license will become null and void and the acupuncturist will have to apply for and obtain a new license.

Any person practicing as an acupuncturist during the time a license has lapsed shall be considered an illegal practitioner and shall be subject to Mississippi Code, Section 73 – 71 – 33 and 73 – 71 – 35.

Pt. 2625, R. 1.11. Professional Ethics.

All license holders shall comply with the Code of Ethics adopted by the NCCAOM except to the extent that they conflict with the laws of the State of Mississippi or the rules of the Board. If the NCCAOM Code of Ethics conflicts with state law or rules, the state law or rules govern the matter. Violation of the Code of Ethics or state law or rules may subject a license holder to disciplinary action pursuant to Part 2625, Rule 1.10.

Pt. 2625, R. 1.12. Disciplinary Proceedings.

A. Hearing Procedure and Appeals

No individual shall be denied a license or have a license suspended, revoked or restriction placed thereon, unless the individual licensed as an acupuncturist has been given notice and opportunity to be heard. For the purpose of notice, disciplinary hearings and appeals, the Board hereby adopts and incorporates by reference all provisions of the "Rules of Procedure" now utilized by the Board for those individuals licensed to practice medicine in the state of Mississippi.

B. Reinstatement of License

1. A person whose license to practice as an acupuncturist has been revoked, suspended, or otherwise restricted may petition the Mississippi State Board of Medical Licensure to reinstate their license after a period of one (1) year has elapsed from the date of the revocation or suspension. The procedure for the reinstatement of a license that is suspended for being out of compliance with an order for support, as defined in Section 93 – 11 – 153, shall be governed by Sections 93 – 11 – 157 or 93 – 11 – 163, as the case may be.

2. The petition shall be accompanied by two (2) or more verified recommendations from physicians or acupuncturists licensed by the Board of Medical Licensure to which the petition is addressed and by two (2) or more recommendations from citizens each having personal knowledge of the activities of the petitioner since the disciplinary penalty was imposed and such facts as may be required by the Board of Medical Licensure.

The petition may be heard at the next regular meeting of the Board of Medical Licensure but not earlier than thirty (30) days after the petition was filed. No petition shall be considered while the petitioner is under sentence for any criminal offense, including any period during which he or she is under probation or parole. The hearing may be continued from time to time as the Board of Medical Licensure finds necessary.

3. In determining whether the disciplinary penalty should be set aside and the terms and conditions, if any, which should be imposed if the disciplinary penalty is set aside, the Board of Medical Licensure may investigate and consider all activities of the petitioner since the disciplinary action was taken against him or her, the offense for which he or she was disciplined, their activity during the time their license was in good standing, their general reputation for truth, professional ability and good character; and it may require the petitioner to pass an oral examination.

Pt. 2625, R. 1.13. Impaired Acupuncturists.

Any individual licensed to practice as an acupuncturist, shall be subject to restriction, suspension, or revocation in the case of disability by reason of one or more of the following:

A. mental illness, or

B. physical illness, including but not limited to deterioration through the aging process, or loss of motor skills

C. excessive use or abuse of drugs, including alcohol

If the Board has reasonable cause to believe that an acupuncturist is unable to practice with reasonable skill and safety to patients because of one or more of the conditions described above, referral of the acupuncturist shall be made, and action taken, if any, in the manner as provided in Sections 73 – 25 – 55 through 73 – 25 – 65, including referral to the Mississippi Professionals Health Program, sponsored by the Mississippi State Medical Association.

Pt. 2625, R. 1.14. Use of Professional Titles.

A licensee shall use the title "Acupuncturist" or "Licensed Acupuncturist," "Lic. Ac.," or "L.Ac.," immediately following his/her name on any advertising or other materials visible to the public which pertain to the licensee's practice of acupuncture. Only persons licensed as an acupuncturist may use these titles. A licensee who is also licensed in Mississippi as a physician, dentist, chiropractor, optometrist, podiatrist, and/or veterinarian is exempt from the requirement that the licensee's acupuncture title immediately follow his/her name.

Pt. 2625, R. 1.15. Acupuncture Advertising. Misleading or Deceptive Advertising.

Acupuncturists shall not authorize or use false, misleading, or deceptive advertising, and, in addition, shall not engage in any of the following:

A. Hold themselves out as a physician or surgeon or any combination or derivative of those terms unless also licensed by the Board of Medical Licensure as a physician as defined under the Mississippi Medical Practice Act.

B. Use the terms "board certified." Acupuncturists may use the term "certified" provided the advertising also discloses the complete name of the board which conferred the referenced certification.

C. Use the terms "certified" or any similar words or phrases calculated to convey the same meaning if the advertised certification has expired and has not been renewed at the time the advertising in question was published, broadcast, or otherwise promulgated.

Pt. 2625, R. 1.16. Sale of Goods from Practitioner's Office.

Due to the potential for patient exploitation in the sale of goods, acupuncturists should be mindful of appropriate boundaries with patients, should avoid coercion in the sale of goods in their offices, and should not engage in exclusive distributorship and/or personal branding.

Acupuncturists should make available disclosure information with the sale of any goods in order to inform patients of their financial interests.

Acupuncturists may distribute goods free of charge or at cost in order to make such goods readily available.

Acupuncturists may make available for sale in their offices durable medical goods essential to the patient's care and non-health related goods associated with a charitable organization.

Pt. 2625, R. 1.17. Effective Date of Rules.

The above rules pertaining to the practice of acupuncturists shall become effective October 17, 2009.

Pt. 2625, R. 1.18. Repealed

SOUTH CAROLINA

CODE OF LAWS OF SOUTH CAROLINA
1976 ANNOTATED

§ 40 – 47 – 700.   Citation of article.

This article may be cited as the "Acupuncture Act of South Carolina".

§ 40 – 47 – 705.   Definitions.

For purposes of this article:

(1) "Acupuncture" means a form of health care developed from traditional and modern oriental concepts for health care that employs oriental medical techniques, treatment, and adjunctive therapies for the promotion, maintenance, and restoration of health and the prevention of disease. The practice of acupuncture does not include:

(a) osteopathic medicine and osteopathic manipulative treatment;

(b) "chiropractic" or "chiropractic practice" as defined in Section 40 – 9 – 10; or

(c) "physical therapy" as defined in Section 40 – 45 – 20 or therapies allowed as part of the practice of physical therapy.

(2) "Auricular (ear) detoxification therapy" means the insertion of disposable sterile acupuncture needles into the five auricular acupuncture points stipulated by the National Acupuncture Detoxification Association protocol for the sole purpose of treatment of chemical dependency, detoxification, and substance abuse.

(3) "Board" means the State Board of Medical Examiners.

(4) "Committee" means the Acupuncture Advisory Committee as established by this article as an advisory committee responsible to the board.

(5) "NADA" means the National Acupuncture Detoxification Association.

(6) "NCAAOM" means the National Certification Commission for Acupuncture and Oriental Medicine.

(7) "ACAOM" means Accreditation Commission for Acupuncture and Oriental Medicine.

（8）"Auricular therapy" means the insertion of disposable needles into and limited only to the ear, to treat a limited number of conditions.

§ 40 - 47 - 710.   **Acupuncture Advisory Committee; membership; terms; filling vacancies; removal of members; meeting schedule; officers.**

（A）There is established the Acupuncture Advisory Committee to be composed of five members to be appointed by the Board of Medical Examiners for terms of four years and until their successors are appointed and qualify. Three members must be licensed to practice acupuncture under this article; one of whom has practiced acupuncture for a minimum of three years; one member must be licensed to practice medicine under this chapter and may be an acupuncturist; and one member must be from the State at large. The advisory committee members shall receive mileage, per diem, and subsistence as provided by law for members of state boards, committees, and commissions and have such responsibilities as provided for in this article and as the board may determine.

（B）Vacancies must be filled in the manner of the original appointment for the unexpired portion of the term. The board, after notice and opportunity for hearing, may remove any member of the committee for negligence, neglect of duty, incompetence, revocation or suspension of license, or other dishonorable conduct. No member may serve more than two full four-year terms consecutively but may be eligible for reappointment four years from the date the last full four-year term expired.

（C）The committee shall meet at least two times yearly and at other times as may be necessary. Four members constitute a quorum. At its initial meeting, and at the beginning of each year thereafter, the committee shall elect from its membership a chairman, vice chairman, and secretary to serve for a term of one year.

（D）The committee shall receive and account for all monies under the provisions of this article and shall pay all monies collected to the board for deposit with the State Treasurer as provided for by law.

§ 40 - 47 - 715.   **Powers and duties.**

（A）The committee may:

（1）recommend regulations to the board relating to professional conduct to carry out the provisions of this article including, but not limited to, professional certification and the establishment of ethical standards of practice for persons holding a license to practice as acupuncturists, auricular therapists, and auricular detoxification specialists in this State;

（2）recommend requirements to the board for continuing professional education acupuncturists, auricular therapists, and auricular detoxification specialists to the board;

（3）request and receive the assistance of state educational institutions or other state agencies and recommend to the board information of consumer interest describing the regulatory functions of the advisory committee and the procedures by which consumer complaints are filed with and resolved by the board. The board shall make the information available to the public and appropriate state agencies.

(B) The committee shall:

(1) conduct hearings and keep records and minutes necessary to carry out its functions;

(2) provide notice of all hearings authorized under this article pursuant to the Administrative Procedures Act;

(3) determine the qualifications and make recommendations regarding the issuance of licenses to qualified acupuncturists, auricular therapists, and auricular detoxification specialists;

(4) recommend to the board whether to issue or renew licenses under those conditions prescribed in this article;

(5) keep a record of its proceedings and a register of all licensees, including their names and last known places of employment and residence. The board shall annually compile and make available a list of acupuncturists, auricular therapists, and auricular detoxification specialists authorized to practice in this State. An interested person may obtain a copy of this list upon application to the board and payment of an amount sufficient to cover the cost of printing and mailing;

(6) report annually to the board on duties performed, actions taken, and recommendations made;

(7) hear disciplinary cases and recommend findings of fact, conclusions of law, and sanctions to the board. The board shall conduct a final hearing at which it shall make a final decision;

(8) perform such duties and tasks as may be delegated to the committee by the board.

§ 40 – 47 – 720. License to practice acupuncture; requirements and qualifications; temporary licenses.

(A) Each applicant for a license to practice acupuncture shall:

(1) submit a completed application as prescribed by the board;

(2) submit fees as provided for in Section 40 – 47 – 800;

(3) hold an active certification in acupuncture by the National Commission for the Certification of Acupuncturists and Oriental Medicine;

(4) be of good moral character;

(5) not have pled guilty or nolo contendere to or been convicted of a felony or crime of moral turpitude.

(B) The application must be complete in every detail before it may be approved. When the administrative staff of the board has reviewed the entire application for completeness and correctness, has found the applicant eligible, and the applicant has appeared before the committee or a designated board member, a temporary license may be issued. At the next committee meeting the entire application must be considered, and if qualified, the committee may recommend to the board that a permanent license be issued. If the committee declines to recommend issuance of a permanent license, the committee may extend or withdraw the temporary license.

§ 40 - 47 - 725. Licensing of current acupuncture practitioners.

(A) (1) An acupuncturist who is currently approved by the board to practice acupuncture in this State, who has remained in good standing, and who has successfully completed a nationally recognized clean needle technique course approved by the board must receive initial licensure under this article after submitting:

(a) a completed application as prescribed by the board;

(b) fees as provided for in Section 40 - 47 - 800.

(2) However, a license issued pursuant to subsection (A)(1) is only valid for two years. Thereafter for license renewal, the individual must hold an active certification from the National Commission for the Certification of Acupuncture and Oriental Medicine and satisfy the licensure and renewal requirements prescribed in this article.

(B) An individual who has continuously practiced acupuncture in this State since 1980, who has remained in good standing, must be issued a license and renewal licenses without meeting the requirements of this chapter after submitting:

(1) a completed application as prescribed by the board; and

(2) fees as provided for in Section 40 - 47 - 800.

§ 40 - 47 - 730. Licenses to perform auricular therapy; qualifications; temporary licenses.

(A) An applicant for a license to perform auricular therapy:

(1) must be twenty-one years of age;

(2) shall submit a completed application as prescribed by the medical board;

(3) shall submit fees as provided for in Section 40 - 47 - 800;

(4) shall provide evidence of certification as having been trained to utilize auricular points only, in addition to those utilized by a detoxification specialist;

(5) successful completion of a national certified program approved by the Acupuncture Advisory Committee and the State Board of Medical Examiners;

(6) successful completion of a Clean Needle Technique course approved by the board.

(B) The application must be complete in every detail before it may be approved. When the administrative staff of the board has reviewed the entire application for completeness and correctness, has found the applicant eligible, and the applicant has appeared before the committee or a designated board member, a temporary license may be issued. At the next committee meeting the entire application must be considered, and if qualified, the committee may recommend to the board that a permanent license be issued, if the committee declines to recommend issuance of a permanent license, the committee may extend or withdraw the temporary license.

§ 40 – 47 – 735. **Licenses to perform auricular detoxification therapy; qualifications; temporary licenses.**

(A) An applicant for a license to perform auricular detoxification therapy:

(1) must be at least twenty-one years of age;

(2) shall submit a completed application as prescribed by the board;

(3) shall submit fees as provided for in Section 40 – 47 – 800;

(4) shall have successfully completed a nationally recognized training program in auricular detoxification therapy for the treatment of chemical dependency detoxification and substance abuse, as approved by the board;

(5) shall have successfully completed a nationally recognized clean needle technique course approved by the board.

(B) The application must be complete in every detail before it may be approved. When the administrative staff of the board has reviewed the entire application for completeness and correctness, has found the applicant eligible, and the applicant has appeared before the committee or a designated board member, a temporary license may be issued. At the next committee meeting the entire application must be considered, and if qualified, the committee may recommend to the board that a permanent license be issued. If the committee declines to recommend issuance of a permanent license, the committee may extend or withdraw the temporary license.

§ 40 – 47 – 740. **Licensing of current auricular therapists or auricular detoxification specialists.**

(A) An auricular therapist or an auricular detoxification specialist who is currently approved by the board to practice in this State, who has remained in good standing, and who has successfully completed a nationally recognized clean needle technique course approved by the board must receive initial licensure under this article after submitting:

(1) a completed application as prescribed by the board;

(2) fees as provided for in Section 40 – 47 – 800.

(B) However, a license issued pursuant to subsection (A) is only valid for two years. Thereafter for license renewal the individual must have successfully passed a board-approved nationally recognized training program in auricular therapy or auricular detoxification and satisfy the licensure requirements prescribed in this article.

§ 40 – 47 – 745. **Unauthorized practice; penalty; cease and desist orders and injunctions; privileged communications.**

(A) It is unlawful for a person not licensed under this article to hold himself out as an acupuncturist, auricular therapist, or auricular detoxification specialist. The titles "Licensed Acupuncturist" (L.Ac.) and "Acupuncturist" may only be used by a person licensed to practice acupuncture pursuant to this article. Further, a person licensed to practice auricular therapy or auricular detoxification may not practice acupuncture or hold himself out as an acupuncturist. The title "Auricular Detoxification Specialist" (ADS) may only be used by a person licensed to practice auricular detoxification therapy pursuant to this article. Possession of a license as an auricular therapist or an auricular detoxification specialist does not, by itself, entitle a person to identify himself or herself as an acupuncturist. A person who holds himself out as an acupuncturist, auricular therapist, or auricular detoxification specialist without being licensed pursuant to this article, during a period of suspension, or after his or her license has been revoked by the board is guilty of a misdemeanor and, upon conviction, must be fined not more than three hundred dollars or imprisoned not more than ninety days, or both.

(B) For the purpose of any investigation or proceeding under this article, the board or a person designated by the board may administer oaths and affirmations, subpoena witnesses, take testimony, and require the production for any documents or records which the board considers relevant to the inquiry.

(C) If the board has sufficient evidence that a person is violating a provision of this article, the board, in addition to all other remedies, may order the person to immediately cease and desist from this conduct. The board may apply to an administrative law judge as provided under Article 5, Chapter 23 of Title 1 for an injunction restraining the person from this conduct. An administrative law judge may issue a temporary injunction ex parte and upon notice and full hearing may issue any other order in the matter it considers proper. No bond may be required of the board by an administrative law judge as a condition to the issuance of an injunction or order contemplated by the provisions of this section.

(D) Each communication, whether oral or written, made by or on behalf of a person or firm to the board or a person designated by the board to investigate or otherwise hear matters relating to the revocation, suspension, or other restriction on a license or other discipline of a license holder, whether by way of complaint or testimony, is privileged and exempt from disclosure for any reason except to the extent disclosed in proceedings before the board. No action or proceeding, civil or criminal, may lie against the person or firm for the communication except upon other proof that the communication was made with malice.

(E) No provision of this article may be construed as prohibiting the respondent or his legal counsel from exercising the respondent's constitutional right of due process under the law or prohibiting the respondent from normal access to the charges and evidence filed against him as part of due process under the law.

§ 40 – 47 – 750.　Auricular therapy defined; supervision.

Auricular therapy may take place under the supervision of a licensed acupuncturist or a person licensed to practice medicine under this chapter. A treatment by an auricular therapist is strictly limited to inserting needles into the ear. Inserting needles anywhere else on the body is considered practicing acupuncture without a license.

§ 40 – 47 – 755. Auricular detoxification therapy defined; supervision.

Auricular detoxification therapy may take place under the direct supervision of a licensed acupuncturist or a person licensed to practice medicine under this chapter. A treatment by an auricular detoxification specialist is strictly limited to the five ear-point treatment protocol for detoxification, substance abuse, or chemical dependency as stipulated by NADA.

§ 40 – 47 – 760. Exempted activities.

This article does not apply to:

(1) the practice of acupuncture if it is an integral part of the program of study by students enrolled in an acupuncture education program under the direct clinical supervision of a licensed acupuncturist with at least five years of clinical experience and the program is accredited or is a candidate for accreditation or is actively seeking accreditation from ACAOM;

(2) a person employed as an acupuncturist or an auricular detoxification specialist by the United States Government if these services are provided solely under the direction or control of the United States Government.

§ 40 – 47 – 765. Grounds for revocation, suspension, or denial of license.

Misconduct constituting grounds for revocation, suspension, probation, reprimand, restrictions, or denial of a license must be found when an acupuncturist, auricular therapist, or auricular detoxification specialist:

(1) has knowingly allowed himself or herself to be misrepresented as a medical doctor;

(2) has filed or has had filed on his or her behalf with the board any false, fraudulent, or forged statement or documents;

(3) has performed any work assignment, task, or other activity which is outside the scope of practice of licensure;

(4) misuses alcohol or drugs to such a degree to render him or her unfit to practice;

(5) has been convicted of a felony or a crime involving moral turpitude or drugs;

(6) has sustained any physical or mental disability which renders further practice dangerous to the public;

(7) has engaged in any dishonorable or unethical conduct that is likely to deceive or harm patients;

(8) has used or made any false or fraudulent statement in any document connected with practice or licensure;

(9) has obtained or assisted another person in obtaining fees under dishonorable, false, or fraudulent circumstances;

(10) has violated or conspired with another person to violate any provision of this article;

(11) otherwise demonstrates a lack of the ethical or professional competence required to practice;

(12) has failed to refer to a licensed medical doctor or dentist, as appropriate, a patient

whose medical condition should have been determined to be beyond their scope of practice; or

(13) continues to provide acupuncture, auricular detoxification therapy, or auricular therapy services to any patient who the licensee treats at least one time per month for three consecutive months, and has not demonstrated clinical improvement, unless the licensee provides the patient with written notice, on or before the expiration of the third month, that the patient may need to seek a medical diagnosis from a licensed medical doctor or dentist before continuing with acupuncture, auricular detoxification therapy, or auricular therapy services, unless the patient was referred to the licensee by a licensed medical doctor or dentist.

Upon a finding of misconduct, the board may impose any sanction that the board is otherwise authorized to impose for misconduct under this chapter.

§ 40 – 47 – 770. Inspections.

The board or a person designated by the board may make unscheduled inspections of any office or facility employing an acupuncturist or auricular detoxification specialist.

§ 40 – 47 – 775. Display of license.

A person who holds a license issued in accordance with this article and who is engaged in the active practice of acupuncture, or the active practice of auricular therapy or the active practice of auricular detoxification, shall display the license in an appropriate and conspicuous location in the person's place of practice.

§ 40 – 47 – 780. Renewal of licenses.

(A) An acupuncture license issued under this article must be renewed biennially if the person holding the license:

(1) submits a completed license renewal application as prescribed by the board;

(2) submits the applicable fees provided for in Section 40 – 47 – 800;

(3) is not in violation of this article at the time of application for renewal;

(4) fulfills requirements for continuing education and professional development, as prescribed by the board in regulation;

(5) remains actively certified by the NCCAOM.

(B) An auricular therapist or auricular detoxification specialist license issued under this article must be renewed biennially if the person holding the license:

(1) submits a completed license renewal application prescribed by the board;

(2) submits the applicable fees provided for in Section 40 – 47 – 800;

(3) is not in violation of this article or any regulation promulgated under this article at the time of application for renewal;

(4) fulfills requirements for continuing education and professional development as prescribed by the board in regulation;

(5) remains active in the practice of auricular therapy or auricular detoxification.

§ 40 – 47 – 785. Request for inactive status.

Under procedures and conditions established by the board, a license holder may request that his or her license be declared inactive. The licensee may apply for active status at any time and, upon meeting the conditions established by the board in regulation, may be declared active.

§ 40 – 47 – 790. Licensee not to hold himself or herself out as authorized to practice medicine.

No person licensed under this article may advertise or hold himself or herself out to the public as being authorized to practice medicine under this chapter.

§ 40 – 47 – 800. Licensing fees.

Fees for acupuncturist, auricular therapist, and auricular detoxification specialist licensure must be established and adjusted biennially in accordance with Section $40 – 1 – 50(D)$ to ensure that they are sufficient but not excessive to cover expenses including the total of the direct and indirect costs to the State for the operations of the committee:

(1) initial licensing fee;

(2) renewal of license fee;

(3) late renewal fee;

(4) reactivation application fee.

§ 40 – 47 – 810. Third party reimbursement.

Nothing in this article may be construed to require third party reimbursement directly to an acupuncturist, auricular therapist, or auricular detoxification specialist for services rendered.

TENNESSEE

TENNESSEE CODE ANNOTATED

§ 63 – 6 – 1001. Definitions

As used in this part, unless the context otherwise requires:

(1) "ACAOM" means the Accreditation Commission for Acupuncture and Oriental Medicine;

(2) "Acupuncture" means a form of health care developed from traditional and modern oriental medical concepts that employs oriental medical diagnosis and treatment and adjunctive therapies and diagnostic techniques for the promotion, maintenance and restoration of health and the prevention of disease;

(3) "ADS" means an acupuncture detoxification specialist trained in, and who performs only, the five-point auricular detoxification treatment;

(4) "Board" means the Tennessee board of medical examiners;

(5) "NADA" means the National Acupuncture Detoxification Association;

(6) "NCCAOM" means the National Certification Commission for Acupuncture and Oriental Medicine; and

(7) "Practice of acupuncture" means the insertion of acupuncture needles and the application of moxibustion to specific areas of the human body based on oriental medical diagnosis as a primary mode of therapy. Adjunctive therapies within the scope of acupuncture may include acupressure, cupping, thermal and electrical treatment and the recommendation of dietary guidelines and supplements and therapeutic exercise based on traditional oriental medical concepts.

§ 63 – 6 – 1002. Application of part

(a) This part shall not apply to:

(1) Physicians licensed under this chapter or chapter 9 of this title, nor shall this part be construed so as to prevent the practice of acupuncture by such physicians or to prevent such physicians from using the title "acupuncturist";

(2) Registered nurses who are nationally certified as holistic nurses and who have successfully

completed an accredited education program in acupuncture; or

(3) Chiropractic physicians licensed under chapter 4 of this title, nor shall any part of this title be construed so as to prevent the practice of acupuncture by chiropractic physicians who have completed two hundred fifty (250) hours of an accredited acupuncture course and have passed the National Board of Chiropractic Examiners acupuncture exam.

(b) It is otherwise unlawful to practice acupuncture for compensation or gratuitously unless certified under this part. This restriction does not apply to the following:

(1) Students practicing acupuncture under the supervision of a certified acupuncturist as part of a course of study approved by the committee; or

(2) Individuals who do not otherwise possess the credentials required for the practice of acupuncture by this part or regulations promulgated hereunder by the board are granted limited certification as an ADS for the purpose of the treatment of alcoholism, substance abuse or chemical dependency if they meet the following conditions:

(A) Provide documentation of successful completion of a board-approved training program in auricular detoxification acupuncture that meets or exceeds standards of training set by NADA;

(B) Practice auricular detoxification treatment in a hospital, clinic or treatment facility that provides comprehensive alcohol and substance abuse or chemical dependency services, including counseling, under the supervision of a certified acupuncturist or medical director;

(C) Satisfy all appropriate ethical standards specified in § 63 − 6 − 1007; and

(D) Limit their practice to the five-point auricular detoxification treatment.

(c) A violation of this section is a Class C misdemeanor. A person who violates this section shall also be subject to the sanctions specified in § 63 − 6 − 1007.

§ 63 − 6 − 1003. Tennessee advisory committee for acupuncture; composition; duties; meetings

(a) To assist the board in the performance of its duties, there is hereby established the Tennessee advisory committee for acupuncture.

(b) The committee shall consist of five (5) members appointed by the governor. Three (3) of the members shall be certified acupuncturists, one (1) shall be an ADS practicing in Tennessee and one (1) shall be a consumer member who is neither employed in nor has any other direct or indirect affiliation with the health care profession or industry. The three (3) acupuncturists initially appointed need not be certified at the time of their appointments, but must meet all the qualifications for certification.

(c) (1) Notwithstanding § 3 − 6 − 304 or any other law to the contrary, and in addition to all other requirements for membership on the committee:

(A) Any person registered as a lobbyist pursuant to the registration requirements of title 3, chapter 6 who is subsequently appointed or otherwise named as a member of the committee shall terminate all employment and business association as a lobbyist with any entity whose business endeavors or professional activities are regulated by the committee, prior to serving as a member of the committee. This subdivision (c) (1) (A) shall apply to all persons appointed or otherwise named to the committee after July 1, 2010;

(B) No person who is a member of the committee shall be permitted to register or otherwise serve as a lobbyist pursuant to title 3, chapter 6 for any entity whose business endeavors or professional activities are regulated by the committee during such person's period of service as a member of the committee. This subdivision (c) (1) (B) shall apply to all persons appointed or otherwise named to the committee after July 1, 2010, and to all persons serving on the committee on such date who are not registered as lobbyists; and

(C) No person who serves as a member of the committee shall be employed as a lobbyist by any entity whose business endeavors or professional activities are regulated by the committee for one (1) year following the date such person's service on the committee ends. This subdivision (c) (1) (C) shall apply to persons serving on the committee as of July 1, 2010, and to persons appointed to the committee subsequent to such date.

(2) A person who violates this subsection (c) shall be subject to the penalties prescribed in title 3, chapter 6.

(3) The bureau of ethics and campaign finance is authorized to promulgate rules and regulations to effectuate the purposes of this subsection (c). All such rules and regulations shall be promulgated in accordance with the Uniform Administrative Procedures Act, compiled in title 4, chapter 5, and in accordance with the procedure for initiating and proposing rules by the ethics commission to the bureau of ethics and campaign finance as prescribed in § 4 – 55 – 103.

(d) In addition to all other requirements for membership on the committee, all persons appointed or otherwise named to serve as members of the committee after July 1, 2010, shall be residents of this state.

(e) Of the initial appointments to the committee, two (2) members shall be appointed for terms of three (3) years, two (2) members shall be appointed for terms of two (2) years and one (1) member shall be appointed for a term of one (1) year. All regular appointments thereafter shall be for terms of four (4) years. No person may serve more than two (2) consecutive full terms as a member of the committee. Each member shall serve on the committee until a successor is appointed. Vacancies shall be filled by appointment of the governor for the unexpired term.

(f) At the committee's first meeting each year after any new members have been appointed, the members shall choose one (1) member to chair the committee for the year and another to serve as co-chair. No person shall chair the committee for more than five (5) consecutive years.

(g) (1) The committee shall meet at least once each year within forty-five (45) days after the appointment of the new members. The committee shall meet at other times as needed to perform its duties.

(2) (A) Any member who misses more than fifty percent (50%) of the scheduled meetings in a calendar year shall be removed as a member of the committee.

(B) The committee's chair shall promptly notify, or cause to be notified, the appointing authority of any member who fails to satisfy the attendance requirement as prescribed in subdivision (g)(2)(A).

(h) Each member shall receive all necessary expenses incident to conducting the business of the committee and, in addition thereto, shall be entitled to a per diem of fifty dollars ($50.00) for each day's service in conducting the business of the committee. All reimbursement for travel expenses shall be in accordance with the comprehensive travel regulations promulgated by the department of finance and administration and approved by the attorney general and reporter.

(i) The committee shall receive from the division of health related boards of the department of health all administrative, investigatory and clerical services as provided for in § 63 – 1 – 101. Committee expenses shall be paid from funds generated by certification fees generated by acupuncturists and acupuncture detoxification specialists.

§ 63 – 6 – 1004.　Board duties

(a) The board, in consultation with the committee, shall:

(1) Establish the qualifications and fitness of applicants of certifications, renewal of certifications and reciprocal certifications;

(2) Establish grounds for revocation, suspension or denial of certification;

(3) Establish grounds for placing on probation a holder of a certificate;

(4) Establish the categories of fees and the amount of fees that may be imposed in connection with certification;

(5) Issue declaratory orders pursuant to the Uniform Administrative Procedures Act, compiled in title 4, chapter 5;

(6) If deemed necessary by the committee, establish standards of continuing education; and

(7) Adopt and use a seal to authenticate official documents of the committee.

(b) Any actions taken under this section shall only be effective after adoption of a majority vote of the members of the committee. The board, by a majority vote of its members at the next board meeting at which administrative matters are considered, may rescind any action taken by the committee.

§ 63 – 6 – 1005.　Certification requirements

(a) To receive certification to practice acupuncture from the board, a person must document:

(1) Either:

(A) Current active status as a diplomate in acupuncture of the NCCAOM; or

(B) Current state licensure in good standing by another state with substantially equivalent or higher standards;

(2) Successful completion of a three-year post secondary training program or acupuncture

college program that is ACAOM accredited or in candidacy status or that meets ACAOM's standards; and

(3) Successful completion of a NCCAOM-approved clean needle technique course.

(b) The committee shall waive the requirements of subsection (a) for an applicant residing in Tennessee upon July 1, 2001, who presents satisfactory evidence to the committee of successful completion of an approved apprenticeship or tutorial program that meets NCCAOM standards shall be granted certification by the board.

(c) The committee shall waive the requirements of subsection (a) and an applicant presenting satisfactory evidence to the committee that such applicant held a license in good standing from another state immediately prior to practicing in Tennessee and who has continually practiced in Tennessee since that time shall be granted certification by the board.

(d) ADSs who meet the requirements listed in § 63 – 6 – 1002 shall be issued a limited acupuncture certificate.

§ 63 – 6 – 1006. Certificate renewal

A certificate to practice acupuncture must be renewed every two (2) years. To renew a certificate, a person must submit proof of current active NCCAOM certification in acupuncture or document compliance with § 63 – 6 – 1005. To renew an ADS certificate, a person must submit proof of current active practice in auricular detoxification treatment, as determined by the committee.

§ 63 – 6 – 1007. Disciplinary actions

The board, in consultation with the committee, may deny, suspend or revoke certification, require remedial education or issue a letter of reprimand, if an applicant or certified acupuncturist:

(1) Engages in false or fraudulent conduct that demonstrates an unfitness to practice acupuncture, including:

(A) Misrepresentation in connection with an applicant for certification or an investigation by the committee;

(B) Attempting to collect fees for services that were not performed;

(C) False advertising, including guaranteeing that a cure will result from an acupuncture treatment; or

(D) Dividing or agreeing to divide a fee with anyone for referring the patient for acupuncture;

(2) Fails to exercise proper control over one's practice by:

(A) Delegating professional responsibilities to a person the acupuncturist knows or should know is not qualified to perform; or

(B) Failing to exercise proper control over uncertified personnel working with the practice;

(3) Fails to maintain records in a proper manner by:

(A) Failing to keep written records describing the course of treatment for each patient;

(B) Refusing to provide a patient, upon request, records that have been prepared for or paid for by the patient; or

(C) Revealing personally identifiable information about a patient, without consent, unless otherwise authorized by law;

(4) Fails to exercise proper care of a patient, including the exercising or attempting to exercise undue influence in the acupuncturist-patient relationship by making sexual advances or requests for sexual activity or making submission to such conduct a condition of treatment;

(5) Displays substance abuse or mental impairment to such a degree as to interfere with the ability to provide safe and effective treatment;

(6) Is convicted of or pleads guilty or no contest to any crime that demonstrates an unfitness to practice acupuncture;

(7) Negligently fails to practice acupuncture with the level of skill recognized within the profession as acceptable under such circumstances;

(8) Willfully violates any provision of this part or rule of the commission; or

(9) Has had a certificate or license denied, suspended or revoked in another jurisdiction for any reason that would be grounds for such action in Tennessee.

§ 63 – 6 – 1008.   Health practices

(a) All certified individuals under this part shall use only presterilized, disposable needles in their administration of acupuncture treatments. The use of staples in the practice of acupuncture is prohibited.

(b) Health practices shall include:

(1) Hands shall be washed with soap and water or other disinfectant before handling needles and between treatment of different patients;

(2) Skin in the area of penetration shall be thoroughly swabbed with alcohol or other germicidal solution before inserting needles; and

(3) Individuals shall pass a nationally recognized clean needle technique course before being allowed to practice acupuncture and related techniques.

§ 63 – 6 – 1009.   Fees

(a) The board, in consultation with the committee, shall set fees relative to the application, certification and renewal thereof in amounts sufficient to pay all of the expenses of certification and of the committee directly attributable to the performance of its duties under this part.

(b) All deposits and disbursements shall be handled in accordance with § 63 – 1 – 137.

§ 63 – 6 – 1010.   Titles

(a) The titles "licensed acupuncturist" or "ADS" may be used by persons certified under this part. No person who is not properly licensed to practice medicine or osteopathy shall use certification under this part to identify such person as a doctor or physician.

(b) Each person certified to practice acupuncture shall post the certificate in a conspicuous location at such person's place of practice.

TENNESSEE RULES AND REGULATIONS

0880 - 12 -.01. DEFINITIONS.

As used in these rules, the following terms and acronyms shall have the following meanings ascribed to them:

(1) ACAOM — The Accreditation Commission for Acupuncture and Oriental Medicine.

(2) Administrative Office — The office of the administrator assigned to the Board and the Committee located at 665 Mainstream Drive, Nashville, TN 37243.

(3) ADS — An acupuncture detoxification specialist trained in, and who performs only, the five (5) points auricular detoxification treatment.

(4) Board — Tennessee Board of Medical Examiners.

(5) Committee — The Advisory Committee for Acupuncture.

(6) Certificate or Certification — The document issued authorizing practice. Wherever these terms appear in this chapter of rules unless they are specifically designated by the language of the rule as applying only to limited certification, the terms apply to both limited and full certificate holders.

(7) Division — The Division of Health Related Boards, Tennessee Department of Health, from which the Committee receives administrative support.

(8) NADA — The National Acupuncture Detoxification Association.

(9) NCCAOM — The National Certification Commission for Acupuncture and Oriental Medicine.

0880 - 12 -.02. SCOPE OF PRACTICE.

(1) The scope of practice for all acupuncturists is governed by T.C.A. §§ 63 - 6 - 1001 (7).

(2) The scope of practice for all acupuncture detoxification specialists is governed by T.C.A. §§ 63 - 6 - 1001 (3) and 63 - 6 - 1002 (b) (2) (B) and (D).

0880 - 12 -.03. RESERVED.

0880 - 12 -.04. ACUPUNCTURE CERTIFICATION PROCESS.

To become certified in Tennessee a person must comply with one of the following sets of procedures and requirements:

(1) Grandfathering — Any person is eligible to receive a certificate upon compliance with all subparagraphs contained in paragraph (2) except subparagraphs (e), (i), and (j) and upon further showing satisfactory proof of one (1) of the following:

(a) Tennessee residency on January 1, 2001, and successful completion of an approved apprenticeship or tutorial program that meets NCCAOM standards.

1. Tennessee residency may be proven by submission of a copy of either a voter registration

card indicating residency in Tennessee on or prior to January 1, 2001, or a Tennessee driver license issued on or prior to January 1, 2001.

2. All documentation to support the apprenticeship or tutorial program and how it meets NCCAOM standards must be sent directly from the program or NCCAOM to the Administrative Office.

(b) Continuous practice of acupuncture in Tennessee since January 1, 2001, and having a license/certificate in good standing to practice acupuncture in another state immediately prior to practicing in Tennessee.

1. Continuous practice in Tennessee since January 1, 2001 may be proven by submission of either of the following:

(i) Photocopies of paycheck(s), paycheck stub(s), or Internal Revenue Service (IRS) Forms W-2, 1099-Misc., or Schedules C or C-EZ for IRS Form 1040 to verify proof of income from the practice of acupuncture; or

(ii) Notarized letters from two (2) individuals other than family members attesting to the applicant's continuous practice.

2. A certificate of licensure/certification in good standing in another state must be submitted directly from that state licensure/certification agency to the Administrative Office and show a date of issuance prior to the date on which the applicant commenced practice in Tennessee.

(2) Certification by diplomate status — An applicant for certification by diplomate status shall do the following:

(a) Request an application packet from the Administrative Office.

(b) Respond truthfully and completely to every question or request for information contained in the application form and submit it, along with all documentation and fees required by the form and rules, to the Administrative Office. It is the intent of this rule that activities necessary to accomplish the filing of the required documentation be completed prior to filing an application and that all documentation be filed simultaneously.

(c) Submit a clear, recognizable, recently taken bust photograph which shows the full head, face forward from at least the top of the shoulder up.

(d) Submit evidence of good moral character. Such evidence shall be two (2) recent (within the preceding 12 months) original letters from medical professionals, attesting to the applicant's personal character and professional ethics on the signator's letterhead.

(e) Have submitted directly from the NCCAOM to the Administrative Office proof of current diplomate status in acupuncture.

(f) Disclose the circumstances surrounding any of the following:

1. Conviction of any criminal law violation of any country, state or municipality, except minor traffic violations.

2. The denial of professional licensure/certification application by any other state or the

discipline of licensure/certification in any state.

3. Loss or restriction of licensure/certification.

4. Any civil suit judgment or civil suit settlement in which the applicant was a party defendant including, without limitation, actions involving malpractice, breach of contract, antitrust activity or any other civil action remedy recognized under the country's or state's statutory, common or case law.

5. Failure of any professional licensure or certification examination.

(g) An applicant shall cause to be submitted to the Committee's administrative office directly from the vendor identified in the Committee's certification application materials, the result of a criminal background check.

(h) Cause to be submitted the equivalent of a Tennessee Certificate of Endorsement (verification of licensure/certification) from each licensing/certifying board of each state or country in which the applicant holds or has ever held a license/certificate to practice any profession that indicates the applicant holds or held an active license/certificate and whether it is in good standing presently or was at the time it became inactive. It is the applicant's responsibility to request this information be sent directly from each such licensing/certifying board to the Administrative Office.

(i) Have proof of completion of a three (3) year post-secondary acupuncture training program or college acupuncture program sent directly from the training program or college to the Administrative Office. This proof must also include the following:

1. Proof that the college or training program either:

(i) holds ACAOM accreditation; or

(ii) is in ACAOM candidacy status; or

(iii) meets ACAOM standards.

2. Notation of successful completion or graduation from the acupuncture training program or college acupuncture program and carry the official seal of the institution.

(j) Have proof of successful completion of a NCCAOM-approved clean needle technique course sent directly from the course provider to the Administrative Office.

(k) Submit the fees required in Rule 0880 – 12 –.06.

(3) Certification by Reciprocity — To become certified in Tennessee based on licensure or certification in another state, an applicant must

(a) Comply with all the requirements of paragraph (2) of this rule except subparagraph (e); and

(b) Have proof of licensure or certification in a state that has licensure or certification requirements substantially equivalent, as determined by the Committee, to the requirements of T.C.A. §§ 63 – 6 – 1001, et seq., and this chapter of rules sent directly from the state licensing/certifying agency to the Administrative Office.

(4) Application review and certification decisions shall be governed by Rule 0880 – 12 –.07.

0880 – 12 –.05.   ADS CERTIFICATION PROCESS.

(1) To be issued a limited acupuncture certification as an ADS in Tennessee a person must comply with the following sets of procedures and requirements:

(a) Request an application packet from the Administrative Office.

(b) Respond truthfully and completely to every question or request for information contained in the application form and submit it, along with all documentation and fees required by the form and rules, to the Administrative Office. It is the intent of this rule that activities necessary to accomplish the filing of the required documentation be completed prior to filing an application and that all documentation be filed simultaneously.

(c) Submit a clear, recognizable, recently taken bust photograph which shows the full head, face forward from at least the top of the shoulder up.

(d) Submit evidence of good moral character. Such evidence shall be two (2) recent (within the preceding 12 months) original letters from medical professionals, attesting to the applicant's personal character and professional ethics on the signator's letterhead.

(e) Have submitted directly from the training program to the Administrative Office documentation of successful completion of a board-approved training program in auricular detoxification acupuncture. To become board-approved, the training program must meet or exceeds standards of training set by NADA.

(f) Disclose the circumstances surrounding any of the following:

1. Conviction of any criminal law violation of any country, state or municipality, except minor traffic violations.

2. The denial of professional licensure/certification application by any other state or the discipline of licensure/certification in any state.

3. Loss or restriction of licensure/certification.

4. Any civil suit judgment or civil suit settlement in which the applicant was a party defendant including, without limitation, actions involving malpractice, breach of contract, antitrust activity or any other civil action remedy recognized under the country's or state's statutory, common or case law.

5. Failure of any professional licensure or certification examination.

(g) An applicant shall cause to be submitted to the Committee's administrative office directly from the vendor identified in the Committee's certification application materials, the result of a criminal background check.

(h) Cause to be submitted the equivalent of a Tennessee Certificate of Endorsement (verification of licensure/certification) from each licensing/certifying board of each state or country in which the applicant holds or has ever held a license/certificate to practice any profession that indicates the applicant holds or held an active license/certificate and whether it is in good standing presently or was at the time it became inactive. It is the applicant's responsibility to request this information be sent directly from each such licensing/certifying board to the Administrative Office.

（i）Submit the fees required in Rule 0880 – 12 –.06.

（2）Application review and limited certification decisions shall be governed by Rule 0880 – 12 –.07.

（3）Prior to the commencement of practice as an ADS, an ADS certificate holder must provide the following documentation to the Committee's Administrative Office：

（a）Satisfactory written acknowledgement that the practice of auricular detoxification treatment will be in a hospital, clinic, or treatment facility which provides comprehensive alcohol and substance abuse or chemical dependency services including counseling, and

（b）Certification from the supervising licensed acupuncturist or medical director（a physician licensed under Chapter 6 or 9 of Title 63 of the Tennessee Code Annotated）of the institution, facility, or entity attesting to employment and acceptance of supervisory responsibility.

0880 – 12 –.06. FEES.

All fees provided for in this rule are non-refundable.

	Acupuncturist	Acupuncture Dextoxification Specialist
（1）Application fee to be submitted at the time of application.	$500.00	$75.00
（2）Initial certification fee to be submitted at the time of application.	$250.00	$25.00
（3）Biennial renewal fee to be submitted every two（2）years when certification renewal is due.	$300.00	$50.00
（4）Late renewal fee.	$100.00	$50.00
（5）Certification reinstatement and/or restoration fee.	$100.00	$50.00
（6）Duplication of Certificate fee.	$25.00	$10.00
（7）Biennial state regulatory fee to be submitted at the time of application.	$10.00	$10.00
（8）All fees may be paid in person, by mail or electronically by cash, check, money order, or by credit and/or debit cards accepted by the Division of Health Related Boards. If the fees are paid by certified, personal or corporate check they must be drawn against an account in a United States Bank, and made payable to the Advisory Committee for Acupuncture.		

0880 – 12 –.07. APPLICATION REVIEW, APPROVAL, AND DENIAL.

(1) Review of all applications to determine whether or not the application file is complete may be delegated to the Committee's administrator.

(2) A temporary authorization to practice, as described in T.C.A. § 63 – 1 – 142 may be issued to an applicant pursuant to an initial determination made by a Committee and Board designee who have both reviewed the completed application and determined that the applicant has met all the requirements for certification, renewal or reinstatement. The temporary authorization to practice is valid for a period of six (6) months from the date of issuance of the temporary authorization to practice and may not be extended or renewed. If the Committee or Board subsequently makes a good faith determination that the applicant has not met all the requirements for certification, renewal or reinstatement and therefore denies, limits, conditions or restricts certification, renewal or reinstatement, the applicant may not invoke the doctrine of estoppel in a legal action brought against the state based upon the issuance of the temporary authorization to practice and the subsequent denial, limitation, conditioning or restricting of certification.

(3) If an application is incomplete when received by the Administrative Office, or the reviewing Committee and/or Board member or the Committee's/Board's designee determine additional information is required from an applicant before an initial determination can be made, the Board administrator shall notify the applicant of the information required. The applicant shall cause the requested information to be received in the Administrative Office on or before the ninetieth (90th) day after the initial letter notifying the applicant of the required information is sent.

(4) If requested information is not timely received, the application file may be considered abandoned and may be closed by the administrator. If that occurs, the applicant shall be notified that the Committee and Board will not consider issuance of a certificate until a new application is received pursuant to the rules governing that process, including another payment of all fees applicable to the applicant's circumstances and submission of such new supporting documents as is required by the Committee and Board.

(5) If a reviewing Committee and/or Board member or Committee and/or Board designee initially determines that a completed application should be denied, limited, conditioned or restricted, a temporary authorization shall not be issued. The applicant shall be informed of the initial decision and that a final determination on the application will be made by the Committee and the Board at their next appropriate meeting. If the Committee and Board ratify the initial denial, limitation, condition or restriction, the action shall become final and the following shall occur:

(a) A notification of the denial, limitation, condition or restriction shall be sent by the Administrative Office by certified mail, return receipt requested, that contains the specific reasons for denial, limitation, condition or restriction, such as incomplete information, unofficial records, examination failure, or matters judged insufficient for certification, and such notification shall contain all the specific statutory or rule authorities for the denial, limitation, condition or restriction.

(b) The notification, when appropriate, shall also contain a statement of the applicant's right to request a contested case hearing under the Tennessee Administrative Procedures Act (T.C.A. §§ 4 - 5 - 301, et seq.) to contest the denial, limitation, condition or restriction and the procedure necessary to accomplish that action.

1. An applicant has a right to a contested case hearing only if the certification denial, limitation, condition or restriction is based on subjective or discretionary criteria.

2. An applicant may be granted a contested case hearing if the certification denial, limitation, condition or restriction is based on an objective, clearly defined criteria only if after review and attempted resolution by the Committee's Administrative Staff, the application can not be approved and the reasons for continued denial, limitation, condition or restriction present genuine issues of fact and/or law which are appropriate for appeal. Requests for a hearing must be made in writing to the Administrative Office within thirty (30) days of the receipt of the notice of denial, limitation, condition or restriction from the Committee and/or Board.

(6) If the Committee and/or Board finds it has erred in the issuance of a certification, it will give written notice by certified mail of its intent to revoke or cancel the certificate. The notice will allow the applicant the opportunity to meet the requirements for certification within thirty (30) days from the date of receipt of the notification. If the applicant does not concur with the stated reason and the intent to revoke or cancel the certification, the applicant shall have the right to proceed according to paragraph (5) of this rule.

0880 - 12 -.08. RESERVED.

0880 - 12 -.09. CERTIFICATION RENEWAL.

All certificates must be renewed to enable continued practice. Renewal is governed by the following:

(1) The due date for certification renewal is its expiration date which is the last day of the month in which a certificate holder's birthday falls pursuant to the Division of Health Related Boards "biennial birthdate renewal system" as provided in rule 1200 - 10 - 1 -.10.

(2) Methods of Renewal — Certificate holders may accomplish renewal by one (1) of the following methods:

(a) Internet Renewals — Individuals may apply for renewal via the Internet. The application to renew can be accessed at:

www.tennesseeanytime.org

(b) Paper Renewals — Certificate holders who have not renewed their authorization online via the Internet, will have a renewal application form mailed to them at the last address provided by them to the Committee. Failure to receive such notification does not relieve the individual of the responsibility of timely meeting all requirements for renewal.

(3) To be eligible for renewal an individual must submit to the Division of Health Related Boards on or before the expiration date the following:

(a) A completed and signed renewal application form; and

(b) The renewal and state regulatory fees as provided in Rule 0880 – 12 –.06; and

(c) Unless issued a certification under the grandfathering provisions of T. C. A. § 63 – 6 – 1005

1. For certified acupuncturists, proof of current, active NCCAOM certification.

2. For ADS certificate holders, proof of current active practice in auricular detoxification treatment.

(4) Any renewal application received after the certification expiration date but before the last day of the month following the certification expiration date must be accompanied by the Late Renewal Fee provided in Rule 0880 – 12 –.06.

(5) Any individual who fails to comply with the renewal rules and/or notifications sent to them concerning failure to timely renew shall have their certificate processed pursuant to rule 1200 – 10 – 1 –.10.

(6) Renewal of an Expired Certificate — Renewal of a certificate that has expired as a result of failure to timely renew in accordance with rule 1200 – 10 – 1 –.10 may be accomplished upon meeting the following conditions:

(a) For persons whose certificates have expired for less than (2) years:

1. Submit a completed reinstatement application; and

2. Submit the renewal and late renewal fees as provided in Rule 0880 – 12 –.06; and

3. For acupuncturists, submit along with the application, documentation of successful completion of the continuing education requirements provided in Rule 0880 – 12 –.12 for the two (2) calendar year (January 1 – December 31) period that the certificate was expired that precedes the calendar year during which the reinstatement is requested.

(b) For persons whose certificates have expired for two (2) years or more:

1. Submit a new application for certification pursuant to either Rule 0880 – 12 –.04 or. 05; and

2. Submit the application, initial certification, and certification reinstatement fees as provided in Rule 0880 – 12 –.06; and

3. For acupuncturists, submit along with the application, documentation of successful completion of the continuing education requirements provided in Rule 0880 – 12 –.12 for all the two (2) calendar year (January 1 – December 31) periods that the certificate was expired that precede the calendar year during which the reinstatement is requested.

(7) If derogatory information or communication is received during the renewal process, if requested by the Committee and/or Board or their duly authorized representative(s), the renewal

applicant must appear for an interview before the Committee and/or Board, a duly constituted panel of the Board, a Committee and/or Board member, a screening panel of the Board when the individual is under investigation or the Committee and/or Board Designee and/or be prepared to meet or accept other conditions or restrictions as the Board may deem necessary to protect the public.

(8) Renewal issuance decisions pursuant to this rule may be made administratively, or upon review by the Committee and Board or their designees.

0880 - 12 -.10. SUPERVISION.

All persons practicing with a limited certification as an ADS shall be under the supervision of a certified acupuncturist or a medical director of a hospital, clinic, or treatment facility which provides comprehensive alcohol and substance abuse or chemical dependency services, including counseling.

0880 - 12 -.11. RETIREMENT AND REACTIVATION OF CERTIFICATE.

(1) Certificate holders who wish to retain their certificates but not actively practice may avoid compliance with the renewal process by obtaining, completing, and submitting, to the Administrative Office, an affidavit of retirement form along with any documentation required by the form.

(2) Upon successful application for retirement with completion and receipt of all proper documentation to the Committee's and Board's satisfaction, the certificate shall be registered as retired. Any person who has a retired certificate may not practice in Tennessee.

(3) Reactivation — Any retired certificate may be reactivated by doing the following:

(a) Submit a written request for a Reactivation Application to the Administrative Office; and

(b) Complete and submit the Reactivation Application along with the renewal fee as provided in Rule 0880 - 12 -.06 to the Administrative Office. If reactivation was requested prior to the expiration of one (1) year from the date of retirement, the Board may require payment of the certificate restoration fee and past due renewal fees as provided in Rule 0880 - 12 -.06; and

(c) For acupuncturists, submit along with the application, documentation of successful completion of fifteen (15) points of continuing education pursuant to Rule 0880 - 12 -.12; and

(d) Submit any documentation which may be required by the form to the Administrative Office; and

(e) If requested, after review by the Committee and/or Board or a designated Committee and/or Board member, appear before either the Committee and/or Board, or a duly constituted panel of the Board, or another Committee or Board member, or the Committee and/or Board Designee for an interview regarding continued competence.

(f) In the event of retirement in excess of two (2) years or the receipt of derogatory information or communication during the reactivation process, the applicant should be prepared to meet or accept other conditions or restrictions as the Committee and/or Board may deem necessary to protect the public.

(g) If retirement was in excess of five (5) years, the applicant may be required to successfully complete whatever educational and/or testing requirements the Committee and/or Board feels necessary to establish current levels of competency.

(4) Certificate reactivation applications, review, and decisions shall be governed by Rule 0880 – 12 –.07.

0880 – 12 –.12.   CONTINUING EDUCATION.

All persons certified as acupuncturists must comply with the following continuing education rules as a prerequisite to certification renewal.

(1) All certified acupuncturists must obtain thirty (30) Professional Development Activity (PDA) points, as defined by NCCAOM, during the two (2) calendar year (January 1 – December 31) period that precedes the year in which certification is renewed.

(2) Continuing education for new certificate holders — Submitting proof of successful completion of all education and training requirements required for certification in Tennessee, pursuant to Rule 0880 – 12 –.04, shall be considered proof of sufficient preparatory education to constitute successful completion of continuing education requirements for the two (2) calendar year (January 1 – December 31) period in which such education and training requirements were completed.

(3) The approved hours of any individual course or activity will not be counted more than once in a two (2) calendar year (January 1 – December 31) period toward the required point total regardless of the number of times the course or activity is attended or completed by any individual.

(4) The Committee and/or Board may waive or otherwise modify the requirements of this rule in cases where there is illness, disability or other undue hardship that prevents a certificate holder from obtaining the requisite number of continuing education points. Requests for waivers or modification must be sent in writing to the Administrative Office prior to the expiration of the renewal period in which the continuing education is due.

(5) Acceptable Continuing Education Courses and Activities — The following professional courses and activities qualify for PDA points of continuing education:

(a) Courses — One (1) point for each hour of courses that directly enhance an acupuncturist's knowledge and/or practice of acupuncture. Points may be earned for courses in Oriental medical theory and techniques such as bodywork, nutrition, and herbology, as well as courses in western sciences that relate to the practice of Acupuncture. Points may also be earned for the study of tai chi and qi gong.

(b) Research — One point for every two (2) hours of documented research. Acceptable research projects include those that relate to knowledge and/or practice in acupuncture.

(c) Writing for Publication — Ten (10) points for each article; Thirty (30) points for a book or major work. Publications include articles, studies, reports, books, etc., that relate to knowledge and/or practice in acupuncture.

(d) Teaching/Clinic Supervision — One (1) point for each clock hour of instruction or supervision relating to acupuncture. Teaching or supervision refers to the ongoing responsibility for theoretical and/or practical education. Credit can be earned for a variety of teaching positions, including teaching or clinical supervision in a formal school or preceptorship, provided there is appropriate documentation.

(e) Supervised Clinical Experience — One and one-half (1½) points for each clock hour of supervised clinical experience under a senior acupuncturist who has a minimum of five years of experience in acupuncture and is an NCCAOM Diplomate in Acupuncture. The clinical experience may include observation, case discussion, and/or supervised practice.

(6) Proof of Compliance

(a) The due date for completion of the required continuing education is December 31st of the two (2) calendar year period that precedes the year in which certification is renewed.

(b) All acupuncturists must, on the certificate renewal form, enter a signature, electronic or otherwise, which indicates completion of the required continuing education obtained during the two (2) calendar year (January 1 – December 31) period that precedes the year in which certification is renewed.

(c) All acupuncturists must retain independent documentation of completion of all continuing education courses and activities. This documentation must be retained for a period of four (4) years from the end of the two (2) calendar year (January 1 – December 31) period in which the continuing education was acquired. This documentation must be produced for inspection and verification, if requested in writing by the Division during its verification process. Documentation verifying the acupuncturist's completion of the continuing education may consist of any one (1) or more of the following:

1. Courses — Dates, locations of continuing education courses, number of hours, course title/content and instructor's name, documented by notarized photocopies of original certificates of completion or original letters on official stationery from the course provider.

2. Research — Dates, location, and subject/title of research, documented by a notarized photocopy of an affidavit from a school, hospital, or other official agency detailing the activity.

3. Writing for Publication — Dates, titles, and names of publishers, documented by a photocopy of the title page.

4. Teaching Acupuncture Related Courses — Dates and locations of classes, syllabi, course titles and course hours, documented by catalogs, computer records, or notarized photocopies of certificates and other official statements that verify the activities and hours involved.

5. Preceptorship — Dates, hours, and locations of clinical or apprenticeship activity, documented by a notarized photocopy of an affidavit from the supervising practitioner.

(d) If a person submits documentation for continuing education that is not clearly identifiable as appropriate continuing education, the Committee and/or Board will request a written description of the education and how it applies to practice as an acupuncturist.

(7) Violations

(a) Any acupuncturist who falsely attests to completion of the required continuing education may be subject to disciplinary action pursuant to Rule 0880 – 12 –.15.

(b) Any acupuncturist who fails to obtain the required continuing education may be subject to disciplinary action pursuant to Rule 0880 – 12 –.15 and may not be allowed to renew certification.

(c) Continuing education obtained as a result of compliance with the terms of Committee and/or Board Orders in any disciplinary action shall not be credited toward the continuing education required to be obtained in any two (2) calendar year (January 1 – December 31) period.

0880 – 12 –.13. PROFESSIONAL ETHICS.

(1) All certificate holders shall comply with the Code of Ethics adopted by the NCCAOM except to the extent that they conflict with the laws of the state of Tennessee or the rules of the Committee and/or Board. If the NCCAOM Code of Ethics conflicts with state law or rules, the state law or rules govern the matter. Violation of the Code of Ethics or state law or rules may subject a certificate holder to disciplinary action pursuant to Rule 0880 – 12 –.15.

(2) A copy of the NCCAOM Code of Ethics may be obtained from NCCAOM at 11 Canal Center Plaza, Suite 300, Alexandria, VA 22314 or by phone at (703) 548 – 9004, or on the Internet at http://www.nccaom.org.

0880 – 12 –.14. RESERVED.

0880 – 12 –.15. DISCIPLINARY ACTIONS AND CIVIL PENALTIES.

(1) Upon a finding by the Committee and Board that a certificate holder has violated any provision of T.C.A. §§ 63 – 6 – 1001, et seq., or the rules promulgated pursuant thereto, the Committee and Board may take any of the following actions separately or in any combination which is deemed appropriate to the offense;

(a) Warning Letter — This is a written action issued for minor or near infractions. It is informal and advisory in nature and does not constitute a formal disciplinary action.

(b) Reprimand — This is a written action issued for one time and less severe violations. It is a formal disciplinary action.

(c) Probation — This is a formal disciplinary action which places a certificate holder on close scrutiny for a fixed period of time. This action may be combined with conditions that must be met before probation will be lifted and/or which restrict the individual's activities during the probationary period.

(d) Certificate Suspension — This is a formal disciplinary action that suspends the right to practice for a fixed period of time. It contemplates the re-entry into practice under the certificate previously issued.

(e) Revocation for Cause — This is the most severe form of disciplinary action which removes an individual from the practice of the profession and terminates the certificate previously issued. The Committee and/or Board, in their discretion, may allow reinstatement of a revoked certificate upon conditions and after a period of time which they deem appropriate. No petition for reinstatement and no new application for certification from a person whose certificate was revoked for cause shall be considered prior to the expiration of at least six (6) months from the effective date of the revocation order.

(f) Conditions — Any action deemed appropriate by the Committee and/or Board to be required of a disciplined certificate holder during any period of probation or suspension or as a pre-requisite to the lifting of probation or suspension or the reinstatement of a revoked certificate.

(g) Civil penalty — A monetary disciplinary action assessed by the Committee and Board pursuant to paragraph (5) of this rule.

(2) Once ordered, probation, suspension, revocation, assessment of a civil penalty, or any other condition of any type of disciplinary action may not be lifted unless and until the certificate holder petitions, pursuant to paragraph (3) of this rule, and appears before the Committee after the period of initial probation, suspension, revocation, or other conditioning has run and all conditions placed on the probation, suspension, revocation, have been met, and after any civil penalties assessed have been paid.

(3) Order of Compliance — This procedure is a necessary adjunct to previously issued disciplinary orders and is available only when a petitioner has completely complied with the provisions of a previously issued disciplinary order, including an uncertified practice civil penalty order, and wishes or is required to obtain an order reflecting that compliance.

(a) The Committee and Board will entertain petitions for an Order of Compliance as a supplement to a previously issued order upon strict compliance with the procedures set forth in subparagraph (b) in only the following three (3) circumstances:

1. When the petitioner can prove compliance with all the terms of the previously issued order and is seeking to have an order issued reflecting that compliance; or

2. When the petitioner can prove compliance with all the terms of the previously issued order and is seeking to have an order issued lifting a previously ordered suspension or probation; or

3. When the petitioner can prove compliance with all the terms of the previously issued order and is seeking to have an order issued reinstating a certificate previously revoked.

(b) Procedures

1. The petitioner shall submit a Petition for Order of Compliance, as contained in subparagraph (c), to the Committee's Administrative Office that shall contain all of the following:

(i) A copy of the previously issued order; and

(ii) A statement of which provision of subparagraph (a) the petitioner is relying upon as a basis for the requested order; and

(iii) A copy of all documents that prove compliance with all the terms or conditions of the previously issued order. If proof of compliance requires testimony of an individual(s), including that of the petitioner, the petitioner must submit signed statements from every individual the petitioner intends to rely upon attesting, under oath, to the compliance. The Committee's consultant and administrative staff, in their discretion, may require such signed statements to be notarized. No documentation or testimony other than that submitted will be considered in making an initial determination on, or a final order in response to, the petition.

2. The Committee authorizes its consultant and administrative staff to make an initial determination on the petition and take one of the following actions:

(i) Certify compliance and have the matter scheduled for presentation to the Committee and Board as an uncontested matter; or

(ii) Deny the petition, after consultation with legal staff, if compliance with all of the provisions of the previous order is not proven and notify the petitioner of what provisions remain to be fulfilled and/or what proof of compliance was either not sufficient or not submitted.

3. If the petition is presented to the Committee and Board the petitioner may not submit any additional documentation or testimony other than that contained in the petition as originally submitted.

4. If the Committee and Board finds that the petitioner has complied with all the terms of the previous order an Order of Compliance shall be issued.

5. If the petition is denied either initially by staff or after presentation to the Committee or Board and the petitioner believes compliance with the order has been sufficiently proven the petitioner may, as authorized by law, file a petition for a declaratory order pursuant to the provisions of T.C.A. § 4 – 5 – 223 and rule 1200 – 10 – 1 –.11.

(c) Form Petition

Petition for Order of Compliance Board of Medical Examiners Advisory Committee for Acupuncture

Petitioner's Name: _____

Petitioner's Mailing Address: _____

Petitioner's E-Mail Address: _____

Telephone Number: _____

Attorney for Petitioner: _____

Attorney's Mailing Address: _____

Attorney's E-Mail Address：_____

Telephone Number：_____

The petitioner respectfully represents, as substantiated by the attached documentation, that all provisions of the attached disciplinary order have been complied with and I am respectfully requesting：（circle one）

1. An order issued reflecting that compliance；or

2. An order issued reflecting that compliance and lifting a previously ordered suspension or probation；or

3. An order issued reflecting that compliance and reinstating a certificate previously revoked.

Note — You must enclose all documents necessary to prove your request including a copy of the original order. If any of the proof you are relying upon to show compliance is the testimony of any individual, including yourself, you must enclose signed statements from every individual you intend to rely upon attesting, under oath, to the compliance. The Committee's consultant and administrative staff, in their discretion, may require such signed statements to be notarized. No documentation or testimony other than that submitted will be considered in making an initial determination on, or a final order in response to, this petition.

Respectfully submitted this the ____ day of _____ , 20

_____ Petitioner's Signature

（4）Order Modifications — This procedure is not intended to allow anyone under a previously issued disciplinary order, including an uncertified practice civil penalty order, to modify any findings of fact, conclusions of law, or the reasons for the decision contained in the order. It is also not intended to allow a petition for a lesser disciplinary action, or civil penalty other than the one(s) previously ordered. All such provisions of Committee and Board orders were subject to reconsideration and appeal under the provisions of the Uniform Administrative Procedures Act（T.C.A. §§ 4 - 5 - 301, et seq.）. This procedure is not available as a substitute for reconsideration and/or appeal and is only available after all reconsideration and appeal rights have been either exhausted or not timely pursued. It is also not available for those who have accepted and been issued a reprimand.

（a）The Committee and Board will entertain petitions for modification of the disciplinary portion of previously issued orders upon strict compliance with the procedures set forth in subparagraph（b）only when the petitioner can prove that compliance with any one or more of the conditions or terms of the discipline previously ordered is impossible. For purposes of this rule the term "impossible" does not mean that compliance is inconvenient or impractical for personal, financial, scheduling or other reasons.

（b）Procedures

1. The petitioner shall submit a written and signed Petition for Order Modification on the form contained in subparagraph (c) to the Committee's Administrative Office that shall contain all of the following:

(i) A copy of the previously issued order; and

(ii) A statement of why the petitioner believes it is impossible to comply with the order as issued; and

(iii) A copy of all documents that proves that compliance is impossible. If proof of impossibility of compliance requires testimony of an individual (s), including that of the petitioner, the petitioner must submit signed and notarized statements from every individual the petitioner intends to rely upon attesting, under oath, to the reasons why compliance is impossible. No documentation or testimony other than that submitted will be considered in making an initial determination on, or a final order in response to, the petition

2. The Committee authorizes its consultant and administrative staff to make an initial determination on the petition and take one of the following actions:

(i) Certify impossibility of compliance and forward the petition to the Office of General Counsel for presentation to the Committee and Board as an uncontested matter; or

(ii) Deny the petition, after consultation with legal staff, if impossibility of compliance with the provisions of the previous order is not proven and notify the petitioner of what proof of impossibility of compliance was either not sufficient or not submitted.

3. If the petition is presented to the Committee and Board the petitioner may not submit any additional documentation or testimony other than that contained in the petition as originally submitted.

4. If the petition is granted a new order shall be issued reflecting the modifications authorized by the Committee and Board that it deemed appropriate and necessary in relation to the violations found in the previous order.

5. If the petition is denied either initially by staff or after presentation to the Committee or Board and the petitioner believes impossibility of compliance with the order has been sufficiently proven the petitioner may, as authorized by law, file a petition for a declaratory order pursuant to the provisions of T.C.A. § 4 – 5 – 223 and rule 1200 – 10 – 1 –.11.

(c) Form Petition

Petition for Order Modification Board of Medical Examiners Advisory Committee for Acupuncture

Petitioner's Name: _____

Petitioner's Mailing Address: _____

Petitioner's E-Mail Address: _____

Telephone Number: _____

Attorney for Petitioner: _____

Attorney's Mailing Address: _____

Attorney's E-Mail Address: _____

Telephone Number: _____

The petitioner respectfully represents that for the following reasons, as substantiated by the attached documentation, the identified provisions of the attached disciplinary order are impossible for me to comply with: _____

Note — You must enclose all documents necessary to prove your request including a copy of the original order. If any of the proof you are relying upon to show impossibility is the testimony of any individual, including yourself, you must enclose signed and notarized statements from every individual you intend to rely upon attesting, under oath, to the reasons why compliance is impossible. No documentation or testimony other than that submitted will be considered in making an initial determination on, or a final order in response to, this petition.

Respectfully submitted this the ____ day of ____, 20 ____.

____ Petitioner's Signature

(5) Civil Penalties

(a) Purpose — The purpose of this rule is to set out a schedule designating the minimum and maximum civil penalties which may be assessed pursuant to T.C.A. § 63 – 1 – 134.

(b) Schedule of Civil Penalties

1. A "Type A" Civil Penalty may be imposed whenever the Committee and Board find a person who is required to be licensed, certified, permitted, or authorized by the Committee and Board, guilty of a willful and knowing violation of T.C.A. §§ 63 – 6 – 1001, et seq., or regulations promulgated pursuant thereto, to such an extent that there is, or is likely to be, an imminent, substantial threat to the health, safety and welfare of an individual patient or the public. For purposes of this section, willfully and knowingly practicing as an acupuncturist or as an ADS without a permit, license, certificate, or other authorization from the Committee and Board is one of the violations for which a "Type A" Civil Penalty is assessable.

2. A "Type B" Civil Penalty may be imposed whenever the Committee and Board find the person required to be licensed, certified, permitted, or authorized by the Committee and Board is guilty of a violation of T.C.A. §§ 63 – 6 – 1001, et seq., or regulations promulgated pursuant thereto in such manner as to impact directly on the care of patients or the public.

3. A "Type C" Civil Penalty may be imposed whenever the Committee and Board find the person required to be licensed, certified, permitted, or authorized by the Committee and Board is guilty of a violation of T.C.A. §§ 63 – 6 – 1001, et seq., or regulations promulgated pursuant

thereto, which is neither directly detrimental to the patients or public, nor directly impacts their care, but has only an indirect relationship to patient care or the public.

(c) Amount of Civil Penalties.

1. "Type A" Civil Penalties shall be assessed in the amount of not less than $500 nor more than $1000.

2. "Type B" Civil Penalties may be assessed in the amount of not less than $100 and not more than $500.

3. "Type C" Civil Penalties may be assessed in the amount of not less than $50 and not more than $100.

(d) Procedures for Assessing Civil Penalties.

1. The Division of Health Related Boards may initiate a civil penalty assessment by filing a Memorandum of Assessment of Civil Penalty. The Division shall state in the memorandum the facts and law upon which it relies in alleging a violation, the proposed amount of the civil penalty and the basis for such penalty. The Division may incorporate the Memorandum of Assessment of Civil Penalty with a Notice of Charges which may be issued attendant thereto.

2. Civil Penalties may also be initiated and assessed by the Committee and Board during consideration of any Notice of Charges. In addition, the Committee and Board may, upon good cause shown, assess a type and amount of civil penalty which was not recommended by the Division.

3. In assessing the civil penalties pursuant to these rules the Committee and Board may consider the following factors:

(i) Whether the amount imposed will be substantial economic deterrent to the violator;

(ii) The circumstances leading to the violation;

(iii) The severity of the violation and the risk of harm to the public;

(iv) The economic benefits gained by the violator as a result of non-compliance; and

(v) The interest of the public.

4. All proceedings for the assessment of civil penalties shall be governed by the contested case provisions of Title 4, Chapter 5, T.C.A.

0880 – 12 –.16.   REPLACEMENT CERTIFICATES.

A Certificate holder whose "artistically designed" Certificate has been lost or destroyed may be issued a replacement document upon receipt of a written request in the Administrative Office. Such request shall be accompanied by an affidavit (signed and notarized) stating the facts concerning the loss or destruction of the original document and the fee required pursuant to Rule 0880 – 12 –.06.

0880 – 12 –.17.   CHANGE OF NAME AND/OR ADDRESS.

(1) Change of Name — Any certificate holder shall notify the Administrative Office in writing within thirty (30) days of a name change and will provide both the old and new names.

A name change notification must also include a copy of the official document involved and reference the individual's profession, committee/board, social security, and certificate numbers.

(2) Change of Address — Each person holding a certificate who has had a change of address shall file in writing with the Administrative Office his/her current address providing both the old and new addresses. Such requests must be received in the Administrative Office no later than thirty (30) days after such change is effective and must reference the individual's name, profession, social security number, and certificate number.

0880 − 12 −.18. RESERVED.

0880 − 12 −.19. COMMITTEE OFFICERS, CONSULTANTS, RECORDS, DECLARATORY ORDERS, AND SCREENING PANELS.

(1) The Committee shall annually elect from its members the following officers:

(a) Chair — who shall preside at all meetings of the Committee; and

(b) Co-Chair — who shall preside at meetings in the absence of the Chair and who along with the Committee Administrator shall be responsible for correspondence from the Committee.

(2) The Committee has the authority to select a Committee consultant who shall serve as a consultant to the Division and who is vested with the authority to do the following acts:

(a) Review complaints and recommend whether and what type disciplinary actions should be instituted as the result of complaints received or investigations conducted by the Division.

(b) Recommend whether and upon what terms a complaint, case or disciplinary action might be settled. Any matter proposed for settlement must be subsequently reviewed, evaluated and ratified by the Committee and Board before it becomes effective.

(c) Undertake any other matter authorized by a majority vote of the Committee and/or Board.

(3) Records and Complaints

(a) Minutes of the Committee meetings and all records, documents, applications and correspondence will be maintained in the Administrative Office.

(b) All requests, applications, notices, other communications and correspondence shall be directed to the Administrative Office. Any requests or inquiries requiring a Committee decision or official Committee action except documents relating to disciplinary actions or hearing requests must be received fourteen (14) days prior to a scheduled meeting and will be retained in the Administrative Office and presented to the Committee at the Committee meeting. Such documents not timely received shall be set over to the next Committee meeting.

(c) All records of the Committee, except those made confidential by law, are open for inspection and examination, under the supervision of an employee of the Division at the Administrative Office during normal business hours.

(d) Copies of public records shall be provided to any person upon payment of a fee.

(e) All complaints should be directed to the Division's Investigations Section.

(4) The Committee members or the Consultant are individually vested with the authority to do the following acts:

(a) Review and make determinations on certification, renewal and reactivation of applications subject to the rules governing those respective applications and subject to the subsequent ratification by the Committee and Board.

(b) Serve as Consultant to the Division to decide the following:

1. Whether and what type disciplinary actions should be instituted upon complaints received or investigations conducted by the Division.

2. Whether and under what terms a complaint, case or disciplinary action might be settled. Any proposed settlement must be subsequently ratified by the Committee and Board before it becomes effective.

(5) The Committee authorizes the member who chaired the Committee for a contested case to be the agency member to make the decisions authorized pursuant to rule 1360 – 4 – 1 –.18 regarding petitions for reconsideration and stays in that case.

(6) Requests for Verification of Licensure for an acupuncturist or an ADS desiring to practice in another state must be made in writing to the Administrative Office.

(7) Declaratory Orders — The Committee adopts, as if fully set out herein, rule 1200 – 10 – 1 –.11, of the Division of Health Related Boards and as it may from time to time be amended, as its rule governing the declaratory order process. All declaratory order petitions involving statutes, rules or orders within the jurisdiction of the Committee shall be addressed by the Committee pursuant to that rule and not by the Division. Declaratory Order Petition forms can be obtained from the Administrative Office.

(8) Screening Panels — The Committee adopts, as if fully set out herein, rule 1200 – 10 – 1 –.13, of the Division of Health Related Boards and as it may from time to time be amended, as its rule governing the screening panel process.

0880 – 12 –.20.   ADVERTISING.

(1) Policy Statement. The lack of sophistication on the part of many of the public concerning acupuncture, the importance of the interests affected by the choice of an acupuncturist and the foreseeable consequences of unrestricted advertising by acupuncturists which is recognized to pose special possibilities for deception, require that special care be taken by acupuncturists to avoid misleading the public. The acupuncturist must be mindful that the benefits of advertising depend upon its reliability and accuracy. Since advertising by acupuncturists is calculated and not spontaneous, reasonable regulation designed to foster compliance with appropriate standards serves the public interest without impeding the flow of useful, meaningful, and relevant information to the public.

(2) Definitions

(a) Advertisement. Informational communication to the public in any manner designed to attract public attention to the practice of an acupuncturist who is certified to practice in Tennessee.

(b) Certificate holder — Any person holding a certificate to practice acupuncture in the State of Tennessee. Where applicable this shall include partnerships and/or corporations.

(c) Material Fact — Any fact which an ordinary reasonable and prudent person would need to know or rely upon in order to make an informed decision concerning the choice of practitioners to serve her particular needs.

(d) Bait and Switch Advertising — An alluring but insincere offer to sell a product or service which the advertiser in truth does not intend or want to sell. Its purpose is to switch consumers from buying the advertised service or merchandise, in order to sell something else, usually for a higher fee or on a basis more advantageous to the advertiser.

(e) Discounted Fee — Shall mean a fee offered or charged by a person or product or service that is less than the fee the person or organization usually offers or charges for the product or service. Products or services expressly offered free of charge shall not be deemed to be offered at a "discounted fee."

(3) Advertising Fees and Services

(a) Fixed Fees. Fixed fees may be advertised for any service. It is presumed unless otherwise stated in the advertisement that a fixed fee for a service shall include the cost of all professional recognized components within generally accepted standards that are required to complete the service.

(b) Range of Fees. A range of fees may be advertised for services and the advertisement must disclose the factors used in determining the actual fee, necessary to prevent deception of the public.

(c) Discount Fees. Discount fees may be advertised if:

1. The discount fee is in fact lower than the certificate holder's customary or usual fee charged for the service; and

2. The certificate holder provides the same quality and components of service and material at the discounted fee that are normally provided at the regular, non-discounted fee for that service.

(d) Related Services and Additional Fees. Related services which may be required in conjunction with the advertised services for which additional fees will be charged must be identified as such in any advertisement.

(e) Time Period of Advertised Fees.

1. Advertised fees shall be honored for those seeking the advertised services during the entire time period stated in the advertisement whether or not the services are actually rendered or completed within that time.

2. If no time period is stated in the advertisement of fees, the advertised fee shall be

honored for thirty (30) days from the last date of publication or until the next scheduled publication whichever is later whether or not the services are actually rendered or completed within that time.

(4) Advertising Content. The following acts or omissions in the context of advertisement by any certificate holder shall constitute false or fraudulent conduct, and subject the licensee to disciplinary action pursuant to T.C.A. § 63 − 6 − 1007(1):

(a) Claims that the services performed, personnel employed, materials or office equipment used are professionally superior to that which is ordinarily performed, employed, or used, or that convey the message that one certificate holder is better than another when superiority of services, personnel, materials or equipment cannot be substantiated.

(b) The misleading use of an unearned or non-health degree in any advertisement.

(c) Promotion of professional services which the certificate holder knows or should know are beyond the certificate holder's ability to perform.

(d) Techniques of communication which intimidate, exert undue pressure or undue influence over a prospective client.

(e) Any appeals to an individual's anxiety in an excessive or unfair manner.

(f) The use of any personal testimonial attesting to a quality of competency of a service or treatment offered by a certificate holder that is not reasonably verifiable.

(g) Utilization of any statistical data or other information based on past performances for prediction of future services, which creates an unjustified expectation about results that the certificate holder can achieve.

(h) The communication of personal identifiable facts, data, or information about a patient without first obtaining patient consent.

(i) Any misrepresentation of a material fact.

(j) The knowing suppression, omission or concealment of any material fact or law without which the advertisement would be deceptive or misleading.

(k) Statements concerning the benefits or other attributes of acupuncture procedures or products that involve significant risks without including:

1. A realistic assessment of the safety and efficiency of those procedures or products; and

2. The availability of alternatives; and

3. Where necessary to avoid deception, descriptions or assessment of the benefits or other attributes of those alternatives.

(l) Any communication which creates an unjustified expectation concerning the potential results of any treatment.

(m) Failure to comply with the rules governing advertisement of fees and services, or advertising records.

(n) The use of "bait and switch" advertisements. Where the circumstances indicate "bait and switch" advertising, the Committee may require the certificate holder to furnish data or other evidence pertaining to those sales at the advertised fee as well as other sales.

(o) Misrepresentation of a certificate holder's credentials, training, experience, or ability.

(p) Failure to include the corporation, partnership or individual certificate holder's name, address, and telephone number in any advertisement. Any corporation, partnership or association which advertises by use of a trade name or otherwise fails to list all certificate holders practicing at a particular location shall:

1. Upon request provide a list of all certificate holders practicing at that location; and

2. Maintain and conspicuously display at the certificate holder's office, a directory listing all certificate holders practicing at that location.

(q) Failure to disclose the fact of giving compensation or anything of value to representatives of the press, radio, television or other communicative medium in anticipation of or in return for any advertisement (for example, newspaper article) unless the nature, format or medium of such advertisement make the fact of compensation apparent.

(r) After thirty (30) days of the certificate holder's departure, the use of the name of any certificate holder formerly practicing at or associated with any advertised location or on office signs or buildings. This rule shall not apply in the case of a retired or deceased former associate who practiced in association with one or more of the present occupants if the status of the former associate is disclosed in any advertisement or sign.

(s) Stating or implying that a certain certificate holder provides all services when any such services are performed by another licensee.

(t) Directly or indirectly offering, giving, receiving, or agreeing to receive any fee or other consideration to or from a third party for the referral of a patient in connection with the performance of professional services.

(5) Advertising Records and Responsibility

(a) Each certificate holder who is a principal partner, or officer of a firm or entity identified in any advertisement, is jointly and severally responsible for the form and content of any advertisement. This provision shall also include any licensed or certified professional employees acting as an agent of such firm or entity.

(b) Any and all advertisements are presumed to have been approved by the certificate holder named therein.

(c) A recording of every advertisement communicated by electronic media, and a copy of every advertisement communicated by print media, and a copy of any other form of advertisement shall be retained by the certificate holder for a period of two (2) years from the last date of broadcast or publication and be made available for review upon request by the Board or its designee.

(d) At the time any type of advertisement is placed, the certificate holder must possess and rely upon information which, when produced, would substantiate the truthfulness of any assertion, omission or representation of material fact set forth in the advertisement or public information.

(6) Severability. It is hereby declared that the sections, clauses, sentences and parts of these rules are severable, are not matters of mutual essential inducement, and any of them shall be rescinded if these rules would otherwise be unconstitutional or ineffective. If any one or more sections, clauses, sentences or parts shall for any reason be questioned in court, and shall be adjudged unconstitutional or invalid, such judgment shall not affect, impair or invalidate the remaining provisions thereof, but shall be confined in its operation to the specific provision or provisions so held unconstitutional or invalid, and the inapplicability or invalidity of any section, clause, sentence or part in any one or more instance shall not be taken to affect or prejudice in any way its applicability or validity in any other instance.

WEST VIRGINIA

ANNOTATED CODE OF WEST VIRGINIA

§ 30 – 36 – 1. License required to practice

In order to protect the life, health and safety of the public, any person practicing or offering to practice as an acupuncturist is required to submit evidence that he or she is qualified to practice, and is licensed as provided in this article. After the thirtieth day of June, one thousand nine hundred ninety-seven, it shall be unlawful for any person not licensed under the provisions of this article to practice acupuncture in this state, or to use any title, sign, card or device to indicate that he or she is an acupuncturist. The provisions of this article are not intended to limit, preclude or otherwise interfere with the practice of other health care providers working in any setting and licensed by appropriate agencies or boards of the state of West Virginia whose practices and training may include elements of the same nature as the practice of a licensed acupuncturist.

§ 30 – 36 – 2. Definitions

(a) Unless the context in which used clearly requires a different meaning, as used in this article:

(1) "Acupuncture" means a form of health care, based on a theory of energetic physiology, that describes the interrelationship of the body organs or functions with an associated point or combination of points.

(2) "Auricular acudetox" means auricular detoxification therapy, as approved by the board or as stipulated by the National Acupuncture Detoxification Association (NADA) for the treatment of substance abuse, alcoholism, chemical dependency, detoxification, behavioral therapy, or trauma recovery.

(3) "Board" means the West Virginia Acupuncture Board.

(4) "Certificate holder" means an authorization issued by the board to persons trained in auricular acudetox who meet the qualifications, established pursuant to this article and by board

rules, to be certified as an auricular detoxification specialist (ADS).

(5) "License" means a license issued by the board to practice acupuncture.

(6) "Moxibustion" means the burning of mugwort on or near the skin to stimulate the acupuncture point.

(7) "NADA" means the National Acupuncture Detoxification Association.

(8) "NADA protocol" means the National Acupuncture Detoxification Association protocol for auricular detoxification therapy.

(9) "Practice acupuncture" means the use of oriental medical therapies for the purpose of normalizing energetic physiological functions including pain control, and for the promotion, maintenance, and restoration of health.

(b) (1) "Practice acupuncture" includes:

(A) Stimulation of points of the body by the insertion of acupuncture needles;

(B) The application of moxibustion; and

(C) Manual, mechanical, thermal, or electrical therapies only when performed in accordance with the principles of oriental acupuncture medical theories.

§ 30 – 36 – 3.　Board established

There is hereby created a state board to be known and designated as the "West Virginia Acupuncture Board."

§ 30 – 36 – 4.　Board membership

(a) The board shall consist of five members appointed by the governor with the advise and consent of the Senate.

(1) Three shall be licensed acupuncturists appointed from a list submitted as provided in subsection (c) of this section;

(2) One shall be a member of the general public; and

(3) One shall be a physician licensed to practice medicine in the state of West Virginia.

(b) Each licensed acupuncturist shall:

(1) Be a resident of the state; and

(2) For at least three years immediately prior to appointment have been engaged in the practice of acupuncture in the state.

(c) For each vacancy of an acupuncture member, the board shall compile a list of names to be submitted to the governor in the following manner:

(1) The board shall notify all licensed acupuncturists in the state of the vacancy to solicit nominations to fill the vacancy;

(2) Each professional association of acupuncturists in the state shall nominate at least two persons for every vacancy; and

(3) Each educational institution that provides acupuncture training in the state shall nominate at least two persons for every vacancy.

(d) The member from the general public:

(1) May not be or ever have been an acupuncturist or in training to become an acupuncturist;

(2) May not have a household member who is an acupuncturist or in training to become an acupuncturist;

(3) May not participate or ever have participated in a commercial or professional field related to acupuncture;

(4) May not have a household member who participates in a commercial or professional field related to acupuncture; and

(5) May not have had within two years prior to appointment a substantial financial interest in a person regulated by the board.

(e) While a member of the board, the member from the general public may not have a substantial financial interest in a person regulated by the board.

(f) Before taking office, each appointee to the board shall take and subscribe to the oath prescribed by section 5, article IV of the constitution of this state.

(g) Tenure; vacancies.

(1) The term of a member is three years.

(2) The terms of members are staggered from the first day of July, one thousand nine hundred ninety-six. The terms of the members first appointed shall expire as designated by the governor at the time of the nomination, one at the end of the first year, two at the end of the second year, and two at the end of the third year. As these original appointments expire, each subsequent appointment shall be for a full three-year term.

(3) At the end of a term, a member continues to serve until a successor is appointed and qualifies.

(4) A member may not serve more than two consecutive full terms.

(5) A member who is appointed after a term has begun serves only for the rest of the term and until a successor is appointed and qualifies.

(h) The governor may remove any member from the board for neglect of any duty required by law or for incompetence or unethical or dishonorable conduct.

§ 30 – 36 – 5.   Officers

From among its members, the board shall elect officers in a manner and for terms that the board determines.

§ 30 – 36 – 6.   Quorum; meetings; reimbursement; staff

(a) A majority of the full authorized membership of the board constitutes a quorum.

(b) The board shall meet at least twice a year, at the times and places that it determines.

(c) Each member of the board is entitled to reimbursement of travel and other necessary expenses actually incurred while engaging in board activities. All reimbursement of expenses shall be paid out of the acupuncture board fund created by the provisions of this article.

(d) The board may employ such staff as necessary to perform the functions of the board, including an administrative secretary, and pay all personnel from the acupuncture board fund in accordance with the state budget.

(e) The board may contract with other state boards or state agencies to share offices, personnel and other administrative function as authorized under this article.

§ 30 – 36 – 7. Rule-making authority; miscellaneous powers and duties

(a) The board may propose for promulgation legislative rules to carry out the provisions of this article in accordance with the provisions of § 29A – 3 – 1 et seq. of this code.

(b) The board may adopt a code of ethics for licensure.

(c) In addition to the powers set forth elsewhere in this article, the board shall keep:

(1) Records and minutes necessary for the orderly conduct of business; and

(2) A list of each currently licensed acupuncturist.

(d) The board may propose emergency legislative rules upon the effective date of the reenactment of this article during the 2019 regular session of the Legislature to effectuate the provisions necessary to issue certificates to persons trained in auricular acudetox, and to establish fees for certificate holders pursuant to this article.

§ 30 – 36 – 8. Acupuncture board fund; fees; expenses; disposition of funds

(a) There is hereby established an acupuncture board fund in the state treasurer's office.

(b) The board may set reasonable fees for the issuance and renewal of licenses and its other services. All funds to cover the compensation and expenses of the board members or staff shall be generated by the fees set under this subsection.

(c) The board shall pay all fees collected under the provisions of this article to the state treasurer.

(d) The fund shall be used exclusively to cover the actual documented direct and indirect costs of fulfilling the statutory and regulatory duties of the board as provided by the provisions of this article. The fund is a continuing, nonlapsing fund. Any unspent portions of the fund may not be transferred or revert to the general revenue fund of the state, but shall remain in the fund to be used for the purposes specified in this article.

(e) The legislative auditor shall audit the accounts and transactions of the fund.

§ 30 – 36 – 9. License or certificate required; exemptions

(a) Except as otherwise provided in this article, an individual shall be licensed or certified by the board before he or she may practice acupuncture or auricular acudetox in this state.

(b) This section does not apply to:

(1) An individual employed by the federal government as an acupuncturist while practicing within the scope of that employment; or

(2) A student, trainee, or visiting teacher who is designated as a student, trainee, or visiting teacher while participating in a course of study or training under the supervision of a

licensed acupuncturist in a program that is approved by the board or the State Board of Education.

§ 30 – 36 – 10.　Qualifications of applicants for licensure; and qualifications for certificate holders

(a) To qualify for a license, an applicant shall:

(1) Be of good moral character;

(2) Be at least 18 years of age;

(3) Demonstrate competence in performing acupuncture by meeting one of the following standards for education, training, or demonstrated experience:

(A) Graduation from a course of training of at least 1,800 hours, including 300 clinical hours, that is:

(i) Approved by the national accreditation commission for schools and colleges of acupuncture and oriental medicine; or

(ii) Found by the board to be equivalent to a course approved by the national accreditation commission for schools and colleges of acupuncture and oriental medicine;

(B) Achievement of a passing score on an examination that is:

(i) Given by the national commission for the certification of acupuncturists; or

(ii) Determined by the board to be equivalent to the examination given by the national commission for the certification of acupuncturists;

(C) Successful completion of an apprenticeship consisting of at least 2,700 hours within a five-year period under the direction of an individual properly approved by that jurisdiction to perform acupuncture; or

(D) Performance of the practice of acupuncture in accordance with the law of another jurisdiction or jurisdictions for a period of at least three years within the five years immediately prior to application that consisted of at least 500 patient visits per year; and

(4) Achievement of any other qualifications that the board establishes in rules.

(b) Notwithstanding any other provisions of this code to the contrary, to qualify for a certificate as an auricular detoxification specialist, an applicant shall:

(1) Be at least 18 years old;

(2) Be authorized in this state to engage in any of the following:

(A) Physician assistant, pursuant to § 30 – 3E – 1 et seq. of this code;

(B) Dentist, pursuant to § 30 – 4 – 1 et seq. of this code;

(C) Registered professional nurse, pursuant to § 30 – 7 – 1 et seq. of this code;

(D) Practical nurse, pursuant to § 30 – 7A – 1 et seq. of this code;

(E) Psychologist, pursuant to § 30 – 21 – 1 et seq. of this code;

(F) Occupational therapist, pursuant to § 30 – 28 – 1 et seq. of this code;

(G) Social worker, pursuant to § 30 – 30 – 1 et seq. of this code;

(H) Professional counselor, pursuant to § 30 – 31 – 1 et seq. of this code;

(I) Emergency medical services provider, pursuant to § 16 – 4C – 1 et seq. of this code; or

(J) Corrections medical providers, pursuant to 15A – 1 – 1 et seq. of this code.

(3) Provide evidence of successful completion of a board-approved auricular acudetox program;

(4) Submit a completed application as prescribed by the board; and

(5) Submit the appropriate fees as provided for by legislative rule.

(c) A certificate may be issued to a retired or inactive professional as described in § 30 – 36 – 10(b) of this code: *Provided*, That the professional meets the qualifications for a certificate holder and the last three years of professional activity were performed in good standing: *Provided*, *however*, That a person who holds a certificate or its equivalent in another jurisdiction as an auricular detoxification specialist may be approved by the board to practice auricular acudetox during a public health emergency or state of emergency for a duration to be provided for in legislative rules of the board.

§ 30 – 36 – 11. Applications for license

To apply for a license, an applicant shall:

(a) Submit an application to the board on the form that the board requires; and

(b) Pay to the board the application fee set by the board.

§ 30 – 36 – 12. Issuance of license

The board shall issue a license to any applicant who meets the requirements of this article and the rules adopted by the board pursuant to this article.

§ 30 – 36 – 13. Scope of license

Except as otherwise provided in this article, a license authorizes the licensee to practice acupuncture while the license is effective.

§ 30 – 36 – 14. Term and renewal of licenses and certificates; restrictions; and advertisements

(a) Terms of license and certificate:

(1) The board shall provide for the term and renewal of licenses and certificates under this section;

(2) The term of a license or certificate may not be more than three years;

(3) A license or a certificate expires at the end of its term, unless the license or certificate is renewed for a term as provided by the board.

(b) Renewal notice. At least one month before the license or certificate expires, the board shall send to the licensee or certificate holder, by first-class mail to the last known address of the licensee, a renewal notice that states:

(1) The date on which the current license or certificate expires;

(2) The date by which the renewal application must be received by the board for the renewal

to be issued and mailed before the license or certificate expires; and

(3) The amount of the renewal fee.

(c) Applications for renewal. Before the license or certificate expires, the licensee or certificate holder periodically may renew it for an additional term, if the licensee or certificate holder:

(1) Otherwise is entitled to be licensed or certified;

(2) Pays to the board a renewal fee set by the board; and

(3) Submits to the board:

(A) A renewal application on the form that the board requires; and

(B) Satisfactory evidence of compliance with any continuing education requirements set under this section for license or certificate renewal.

(d) In addition to any other qualifications and requirements established by the board, the board may establish continuing education requirements as a condition to the renewal of licenses and certificates under this section.

(e) The board shall renew the license of and issue a renewal certificate to each licensee and certificate holder who meets the requirements of this section.

(f) A licensee may advertise only as permitted by rules adopted by the board.

(g) A certificate holder recognized as an auricular detoxification specialist is prohibited from needling any acupuncture body points beyond the scope of auricular acudetox, and may not advertise themselves as an acupuncturist: *Provided*, That nothing contained in this section prohibits a person from practicing within his or her scope of practice as authorized by law.

§ 30 - 36 - 15.　Reciprocal licensure of acupuncturists from other states or countries

(a) The acupuncture board may by reciprocity license acupuncturists in this state who have been legally registered or licensed acupuncturists in another state: Provided, That the applicant for such licensure shall meet the requirements of the rules for reciprocity promulgated by the board in accordance with the provisions of chapter twenty-nine-a of this code: Provided, however, That reciprocity is not authorized for acupuncturists from another state where that state does not permit reciprocity to acupuncturists licensed in West Virginia.

(b) The board may refuse reciprocity to acupuncturists from another country unless the applicant qualifies under such rules as may be promulgated by the board for licensure of foreign applicants.

(c) Applicants for licensure under this section shall, with their application, forward to the board the established fee.

§ 30 - 36 - 16.　Inactive status; reinstatement of expired license

(a) The board shall place a licensee on inactive status if the licensee submits to the board:

(1) An application for inactive status on the form required by the board; and

(2) The inactive status fee set by the board.

(b) The board shall issue a license to an individual who is on inactive status if the individual complies with the renewal requirements that exist at the time the individual changes from inactive to active status.

(c) The board shall reinstate the license of a former licensee who has failed to renew the license for any reason if the former licensee:

(1) Meets the renewal requirements of section fourteen of this article; and

(2) Pays to the board a reinstatement fee set by the board.

§ 30 – 36 – 17. Surrender of license by licensee or certificate by certificate holder

(a) Unless the board agrees to accept the surrender of a license or certificate, a licensee or certificate holder may not surrender the license or certificate nor may the license or certificate lapse by operation of law while the licensee or certificate holder is under investigation or while charges are pending against the licensee or certificate holder.

(b) The board may set conditions on its agreement with the licensee or certificate holder under investigation or against whom charges are pending to accept surrender of the license or certificate.

§ 30 – 36 – 18. Reprimands, probations, suspensions and revocations; grounds

The board, on the affirmative vote of a majority of its full authorized membership, may reprimand any licensee or certificate holder, place any licensee or certificate holder on probation, or suspend or revoke a license or certificate if the licensee or certificate holder:

(1) Fraudulently or deceptively obtains or attempts to obtain a license or certificate for the applicant or licensee or certificate holder or for another;

(2) Fraudulently or deceptively:

(A) Uses a license or certificate; or

(B) Solicits or advertises.

(3) Is guilty of immoral or unprofessional conduct in the practice of acupuncture or auricular acudetox;

(4) Is professionally, physically, or mentally incompetent;

(5) Provides professional services while:

(A) Under the influence of alcohol; or

(B) Using any narcotic or controlled substance, as defined in § 60A – 1 – 101 of this code, or other drug that is in excess of therapeutic amounts or without a valid medical indication;

(6) Knowingly violates any provision of this article or any rule of the board adopted under this article;

(7) Is convicted of or pleads guilty or nolo contendere to a felony or to a crime involving moral turpitude, whether or not any appeal or other proceeding is pending to have the conviction or plea set aside;

(8) Practices acupuncture or auricular detoxification therapy with an unauthorized person

or assists an unauthorized person in the practice of acupuncture or auricular detoxification therapy;

(9) Is disciplined by the licensing or disciplinary authority of this state or any other state or country or convicted or disciplined by a court of any state or country for an act that would be grounds for disciplinary action under this section;

(10) Willfully makes or files a false report or record in the practice of acupuncture or auricular detoxification therapy;

(11) Willfully fails to file or record any report as required by law, willfully impedes or obstructs the filing or recording of the report, or induces another to fail to file or record the report;

(12) Submits a false statement to collect a fee; or

(13) Refuses, withholds from, denies, or discriminates against an individual with regard to the provision of professional services for which the person is licensed and qualified to render because the individual is HIV positive, in conformity with standards established for treatment by physicians, dentists and other licensed health care professionals in cases of this nature.

§ 30 - 36 - 19. Due process procedure

(a) Upon filing with the board a written complaint charging a person with being guilty of any of the acts described in section sixteen of this article, the administrative secretary or other authorized employee of the board shall provide a copy of the complaint or list of allegations to the person about whom the complaint was filed. That person will have twenty days thereafter to file a written response to the complaint. The board shall thereafter, if the allegations warrant, make an investigation. If the board finds reasonable grounds for the complaint, a time and place for a hearing shall be set, notice of which shall be served on the licensee or applicant at least fifteen calendar days in advance of the hearing date. The notice shall be by personal service or by certified or registered mail sent to the last known address of the person.

(b) The board may petition the circuit court for the county within which the hearing is being held to issue subpoenas for the attendance of witnesses and the production of necessary evidence in any hearing before it. Upon request of the respondent or of his or her counsel, the board shall petition the court to issue subpoenas in behalf of the respondent. The circuit court upon petition may issue such subpoenas as it deems necessary.

(c) Unless otherwise provided in this article, hearing procedures shall be promulgated in accordance with, and a person who feels aggrieved by a decision of the board may take an appeal pursuant to, the administrative procedures in this state as provided in chapter twenty-nine-a of this code.

§ 30 - 36 - 20. Repealed by Acts 2010, c. 32, eff. June 11, 2010

WEST VIRGINIA CODE OF STATE RULES

Series 1.   Meetings of the Board of Acupuncture

§ 32 – 1 – 1.   General.

1.1. Scope. — This rule contains provisions for the time and place of all regularly scheduled meetings and the time, place and purpose of all special meetings of the Board.

1.2. Authority. — W. Va. Code § 30 – 36 – 7.

1.3. Filing Date. — August 3, 1998.

1.4. Effective Date. — September 2, 1998.

§ 32 – 1 – 2.   Application and Enforcement.

This procedural rule applies to the Board. The enforcement of this rule is vested with the president of the Board.

§ 32 – 1 – 3.   Definitions.

3.1. Board. — The West Virginia Board of Acupuncture.

3.2. President. — The Board member elected by the Board members to serve as president of the Board.

3.3. Vice President — Treasurer. — The Board member elected by the Board members to serve as vice president-treasurer of the Board.

3.4. Secretary. — The Board member elected by the Board members to serve as secretary of the Board.

3.5. Decision. — Any determination, action, vote or final disposition of a motion, proposal, resolution, order or measure on which a vote of the Board is required at any meeting at which a quorum is present.

3.6. Meeting. — The convening of the Board for which a quorum is required in order to make a decision or to deliberate toward a decision on any matter, but the term does not include

a. any meeting for the purpose of making an adjudicatory decision in any quasi-judicial administrative proceeding, or

b. any on-site inspection of any practitioner, clinic, or educational program of acupuncture or oriental medicine.

3.7. Quorum. — A simple majority of the constituent membership of the Board.

§ 32 – 1 – 4.   Meetings.

4.1. The president may call meetings of the Board, and the president shall call a meeting upon the written request of two (2) Board members.

4.2. The president shall notify Board members in writing at least seven (7) days in advance of a meeting setting forth the time and place of the meeting and the matters to be considered, except that the notice is not required if the time, the place and matters for consideration was fixed in a meeting where all the members were present.

4.3. The president shall notify the public and the news media by filing with the office of the Secretary of State a public notice of the meeting at least seven (7) days in advance. The public notice shall contain the time, the place and the matters to be considered.

4.4. The provisions of this section shall not apply in the event of an emergency requiring immediate official action by the Board.

4.5. Special meetings may be continued to a set time and place on the following workday by a majority vote of the Board members present and voting.

4.6. The president may cancel special meetings if no Board member objects.

§ 32 – 1 – 5.　Proceeding to Be Open; Exceptions; Executive Session Permitted.

5.1. All meetings of the Board shall be open to the public, except the Board may hold an executive session that is closed to the public during a regular, special or emergency meeting, after the presiding officer has identified the authorization under W. Va. Code § 6 – 9A – 4 for the holding of an executive session and has presented it to the Board and to the general public. The Board shall not make a decision in executive session.

5.2. The Board may hold an executive session only upon a majority affirmative vote of the Board members present for the reasons found in W. Va. Code § 6 – 9A – 4 et seq.

§ 32 – 1 – 6.　Minutes.

6.1. The Board shall provide for the preparation of written minutes of all its meetings. All minutes shall be available to the public within a reasonable time after the meeting and shall include the following information:

a. The date, time and place of the meeting;

b. The name of each Board member present or absent;

c. All motions, proposals, resolutions, orders, ordinances and measures proposed, the name of the person proposing them and their disposition; and

d. The results of all votes and, upon request of a member, the vote of each member, by name.

6.2. Minutes of executive sessions may be limited to material the disclosure of which is not inconsistent with the provisions listed in W. Va. Code § 6 – 9A – 4.

§ 32 – 1 – 7.　Majority Vote Required; Vote By Proxy Prohibited.

The vote of a majority of all members present at any meeting of the Board is necessary to take any action. Proxy voting is prohibited.

§ 32 – 1 – 8.　Records of the Board — Public.

Records of the Board are public records that may be inspected in accordance with W. Va. Code § 29B – 1 – 3 and copied at a charge of twenty-five cents ($.25) per page. Exceptions to this are those specified in W. Va. Code § 29B – 1 – 3.

Series 3.   Applications for Licensure to Practice Acupuncture

§ 32 – 3 – 1.   General.

1.1. Scope. — This rule governs the application process for acupuncture licensure.

1.2. Authority. — W. Va. Code § 30 – 36 – 7.

1.3. Filing Date. — May 21, 1999.

1.4. Effective Date. — May 21, 1999.

§ 32 – 3 – 2.   Application.

This legislative rule applies to applicants for licensure by the Board.

§ 32 – 3 – 3.   Definitions.

3.1. Apprenticeship. — A supervised course of study or tutorial program between one student and one instructor which is approved by the Board and which when successfully completed enables the applicant to meet the requirements of W. Va. Code § 30 – 36 – 10 for licensure as an acupuncturist.

3.2. CCAOM. — The Council of Colleges of Acupuncture and Oriental Medicine

3.3. Course of training. — A systematic course of study in acupuncture at a school or college of acupuncture or oriental medicine which leads to a degree or diploma in acupuncture or oriental medicine.

3.4. NACSCAOM. — The National Accreditation Commission for Schools and Colleges of Acupuncture and Oriental Medicine.

3.5. NCCA. — The National Commission for the Certification of Acupuncture or its successor organization the National Commission for the Certification of Acupuncture and Oriental Medicine.

§ 32 – 3 – 4.   Board Approval for Licensure.

4.1. The Board shall issue a license to practice acupuncture to an applicant who has submitted the required application form and supporting documentation for the Board Examination of Credentials if the applicant meets the requirements of W. Va. Code § 30 – 36 – 1 et seq. and rules promulgated by the Board.

4.2. If the Board determines that an applicant has met the requirements for acupuncture licensure, it shall issue to the applicant a license that is valid for a period of two years. The Board, at its discretion, may make a license provisional and may stipulate additional training, clinical experience, or the NCCAOM examination as requirements for licensure.

§ 32 – 3 – 5.   Licensure Qualifications.

5.1. An applicant for licensure shall:

5.1.1. Be of good moral character;

5.1.2. Be at least eighteen (18) years of age; and

5.1.3. Demonstrate competence in performing acupuncture.

5.2. An applicant shall demonstrate his or her good moral character by providing the Board with character references from three persons, each of whom can attest to the applicant's reputation for honesty and credibility. The character references shall include:

5.2.1. Two persons, who are not related to the applicant, and who have known the applicant for the five year period directly preceding application; and

5.2.2. One person who is a licensed acupuncturist or oriental medical doctor, who is not related to the applicant, and who has known the applicant for the three year period directly preceding application.

5.3. An applicant for licensure shall demonstrate his or her age to the Board by providing a certified copy of and official governmental document, passport or birth certificate which indicates the applicant's date of birth.

5.4. An applicant for licensure shall demonstrate his or her competence to perform acupuncture to the Board by providing documentation of training, apprenticeship, qualifying test scores, or licensure in another jurisdiction by submitting with his or her application:

5.4.1. An official transcript from his or her school or college of acupuncture or oriental medicine;

5.4.2. An official transcript from his or her supervising tutor of acupuncture or oriental medicine;

5.4.3. An official transcript from the NCCAOM of his or her qualifying test scores; or

5.4.4. An official copy of the applicants license from the licensing Board of another jurisdiction documenting previous licensure.

5.5. Applicants shall attach a current signed passport-size photograph to the application.

§ 32 – 3 – 6. Certification of Documentation.

Documentation submitted by or on behalf of the applicant shall be certified by the appropriate official or by governmental seal of authority, in cases of foreign trained applicants. The Board at its discretion may waive this requirement when it is determined that it cannot be obtained through the exercise of due diligence.

§ 32 – 3 – 7. Verification.

All statements submitted by or on behalf of an applicant shall be made under penalty of false swearing. An applicant or licensee who makes a false statement is subject to disciplinary action including, but not limited to, immediate revocation or suspension of the license.

§ 32 – 3 – 8. Translation Required.

All application documentation submitted in a language other than English shall be accompanied by a translation into English, certified by a translator other than the applicant, who shall attest to the accuracy of the translation under penalty of false swearing.

§ 32 – 3 – 9. Application Deadline.

9.1. A new applicant shall submit his or her application for licensure examination on a form provided by the Board, and shall attach all required statements and documents. All applications must be received in the Board's office at least 30 days prior to the date of the Board Examination of Credentials for which the application is made. The Board shall hold an examination of credentials twice per calender year.

9.2. A renewal applicant shall submit his or her application for renewal licensure on a form provided by the Board, and shall attach all required statements and documents. All applications must be received in the Board's office at least 30 days prior to the date of Board Examination of Credentials for which the renewal application is made.

9.3. All transcripts and supporting documents from qualifying education institutions and tutorial supervisors must be received in the Board's office at least 30 days prior to the date of the Board Examination of Credentials.

9.4. The Board, at its own discretion may waive the foregoing filing dates, if there are difficulties with the administration of the Board Examination of Credentials or other circumstances warrant the waiver.

§ 32 – 3 – 10. Review and Processing of Applications.

10.1. Within a reasonable time after receipt of an application, the Board shall inform the applicant whether the application is complete and accepted for the Board Examination of Credentials or is deficient and what specific information or documentation is required to complete the application.

10.2. Within a reasonable time after receipt of a completed application the Board shall notify the applicant of the date, time and location of his or her oral examination.

10.3. Within a reasonable time after completion of the Board Examination of Credentials and oral examination, the Board shall notify all applicants of their eligibility for licensure and upon payment of the specified fee for licensure found in the Board's Rule, Fees of the Board of Acupuncture, 32 CRS 4.

§ 32 – 3 – 11. Board Examinations of Credentials and Demonstration of Competency.

11.1. Board Examination of Credentials. — The Board shall review each applicant's credential documentation and the application form before it issues a license, pursuant to W. Va. Code § 30 – 36 – 12.

11.2. Location. — The Board shall give public notice of the times and locations of where the examination of credentials shall be held.

11.3. Languages. — The Board shall administer examination of credentials in English.

11.4. Content. — The examination of credentials shall consist of both a review of credential documentation and an oral examination. The oral examination shall test and review the applicant's knowledge and competency in the practice of oriental medicine through acupuncture.

11.5. Additional Training. — If the Board determines that an applicant has met the requirements for acupuncture licensure, it shall issue such license for a period of two years. The

Board, at its discretion, has the right to make a license provisional and to stipulate additional training, clinical experience, or the NCCAOM examination as requirements for licensure.

§ 32 - 3 - 12.　Documentation of Training.

12.1. Each applicant shall have completed the minimum educational or tutorial requirements set forth in the W. Va. Code § 30 - 36 - 10, as documented by the registrar of each school which the applicant attended or from the applicant's tutor, in the case of a tutorial or apprenticeship program.

12.2. All applicants who are graduates of an approved educational program who take the NCCA or NCCAOM examination as part of his or her licensure requirements shall have completed the course work and training set forth in W. Va. Code § 30 - 36 - 10.

12.3. All applicants applying for licensure shall meet the minimum educational or tutorial requirements set forth in W. Va. Code § 30 - 36 - 1 et seq. by the date of the Board Examination of Credentials for which the application has been made.

§ 32 - 3 - 13.　Abandonment of Applications.

The Board my deny an application without prejudice when an applicant does not exercise due diligence in the completion of his or her application, in furnishing additional information or documents required, or in the payment of any required fees.

§ 32 - 3 - 14.　Failure to Appear for Oral Examination-Withdrawal of Application.

An applicant for Board oral examination, who fails to appear for two oral examinations without a written explanation which is satisfactory to the Board shall have his or her application withdrawn by the Board. If the applicant subsequently decides to reapply for licensure, he or she shall file a new application and pay the full application fee.

§ 32 - 3 - 15.　Denial of Applications.

15.1. Any applicant whose application is denied, may submit within thirty (30) calendar days from the date of rejection, a written request that his or her application be presented to the Board for further evaluation at the Board's next regular meeting.

15.2. As part of this evaluation procedure, the Board may, in its discretion, request that the applicant be orally interviewed with respect to his or her qualifications for licensure.

15.3. Nothing in this section shall be constructed to deprive an applicant of his or her rights of appeal as afforded by other provisions of law.

§ 32 - 3 - 16.　Inactive License.

16.1. Any acupuncturist who is not actively engaged in the practice of acupuncture desiring an inactive license, W. Va. Code § 30 - 36 - 16, or to restore an inactive license to active status shall submit an application to the Board on a form provided by it (Active-Inactive License Application). The applicant need not submit his or her license or a copy of the license to the Board with the application.

16.2. In order to restore an inactive license to active status, the licensee shall complete a minimum of forty-eight (48) hours of approved continuing education within the two (2) years preceding application for return to active status, in compliance with the Board's Rule, Continuing Education Requirements, 32 CRS 9. If the license has been inactive less than one (1) year, a minimum of twenty-four (24) hours of continuing education is required.

16.3. The inactive status of any licensee shall not deprive the Board of its authority to institute or continue a disciplinary proceeding against a licensee upon any ground provided by law or to enter an order suspending or revoking a license or otherwise holding disciplinary action against the licensee on that ground.

Series 4.   Fees of the Board of Acupuncture

§ 32 – 4 – 1.   General.

1.1. Scope. — This rule establishes the fees relating to the Board.

1.2. Authority. — W. Va. Code § 30 – 36 – 7 and § 30 – 36 – 8.

1.3. Filing Date. — April 20, 2020.

1.4. Effective Date. — April 30, 2020.

1.5 Sunset Provision — This rule shall terminate and have no further force and effect upon the expiration of April 30, 2030.

§ 32 – 4 – 2.   Application.

This rule applies to all applicants, licensed acupuncturists, student acupuncturists, apprenticed acupuncturists, and continuing education instructors.

§ 32 – 4 – 3.   Fees.

3.1. Application fee. — The nonrefundable application fee is $75.

3.2. License fee. — The initial license fee for a period of two years is $425.

3.3. Renewal fee. — The renewal fee for a period of two years is $425.

3.4. Inactive license. — The biennial fee for an inactive license is $325.

3.5. Delinquency fee. — The delinquency fee for late filing is $50.

3.6. Duplicate license fee. — The fee for a duplicate or replacement engraved wall license is $25. The fee for a duplicate or replacement renewal receipt or pocket license is $10.

3.7. Endorsement fee. — The fee for a letter of endorsement is $10.

3.8. Auricular acudetox certificate fee. — The fee for a two-year certificate to perform auricular acudetox is $60. The certificate of authorization to practice auricular acudetox therapy shall be valid for two years from the month ending of the date of issuance.

3.9. Auricular acudetox certificate renewal fee. — The fee for a two-year renewal of a certificate to perform auricular acudetox is $50. A renewed certificate of authorization to practice auricular acudetox therapy shall be valid for two years from the month ending of the date of issuance.

3.10. Notwithstanding the fees set forth in this fee schedule, an applicant may seek a waiver of the initial licensing fees pursuant to 32 C.S.R. 15.

§ 32 - 4 - 4. Acupuncture Tutorials.

Acupuncture tutorial instructors and acupuncture tutorial students shall pay on annual registration renewal fee of $100 within 30 days of completion of one year of an approved acupuncture tutorial.

§ 32 - 4 - 5. Continuing Education Providers.

The annual fee for approval for each provider of continuing education is $50.

§ 32 - 4 - 6. Expired License Renewal.

A lapsed or expired license may be renewed at any time within three years after its expiration. The licensee shall pay all accrued and unpaid renewal fees, plus the delinquency fee with the application for renewal.

Series 5. Advertising by Licensed Acupuncturists

§ 32 - 5 - 1. General.

1.1. Scope. — This rule establishes standards for the advertising of acupuncture.

1.2. Authority. — W. Va. Code §§ 30 - 36 - 7 and 30 - 36 - 14 (f).

1.3. Filing Date. — May 21, 1999.

1.4. Effective Date. — May 21, 1999.

§ 32 - 5 - 2. Application and Enforcement.

This legislative rules applies to all licensed acupuncturists, all student acupuncturists and all apprenticed acupuncturists. The enforcement of these rules is vested with the Board.

§ 32 - 5 - 3. Recognized Titles.

Academic and professionally granted titles which may be used by acupuncturists practicing in W. Va. include, but are not limited to the following:

3.1. L.Ac. and Lic. Ac. — Licensed Acupuncturist

3.2. O.M.D. — Oriental Medical Doctor

3.3. MSOMed. — Master of Science in Oriental Medicine

3.4. D.Ac. — Doctor of Acupuncture

3.5. C.A. — Certified Acupuncturist

3.6. D.O.M. — Doctorate of Oriental Medicine

3.7. A.P. — Acupuncture Physician

§ 32 - 5 - 4. Advertising.

A Board licensed acupuncturist may advertise the provision of any acupuncture services to the public, which are within the scope of practice, authorized by W. Va. Code § 30 - 36 - 2. The advertising may not promote the excessive or unnecessary use of the services.

§ 32 - 5 - 5. Use of the Title Doctor.

5.1. An acupuncturist may use the title "Doctor" or the abbreviation "Dr." in connection with the practice of acupuncture when he or she possesses an earned doctorate degree from an accredited, approved or authorized educational institution in acupuncture, Oriental medicine or a biological science. The use of the title "Doctor" or the abbreviation "Dr." by an acupuncturist as authorized in this subsection without further indication of the type of license, certificate or degree which authorizes that use, constitutes unprofessional conduct.

5.2. An acupuncture doctor shall clearly explain to his or her patients, in writing and verbally, that he or she is not a physician licensed to practice medicne or surgery, unless he or she is licensed under W. Va. Code § 30 – 3 – 1 et seq or W. Va. Code § 30 – 14 – 1 et seq.

Series 6.   Standards of Practice of Acupuncture by Licensed Acupuncturists

§ 32 – 6 – 1.   General.

1.1. Scope. — This rule establishes the minimum standards of practice for acupuncture in this state.

1.2. Authority. — W. Va. Code § 30 – 36 – 7.

1.3. Filing Date. — May 21, 1999.

1.4. Effective Date. — May 21, 1999.

§ 32 – 6 – 2.   Application.

This legislative rule applies to all licensed acupuncturists, all student acupuncturists and all apprenticed acupuncturists.

§ 32 – 6 – 3.   Definitions.

3.1. Clean Needle Technique. — The standard protocol test as administered by the CCAOM.

3.2. CCAOM. — The Council of Colleges of Acupuncture and Oriental Medicine.

3.3. FDA. — The federal Food and Drug Administration.

3.4. OSHA. — The federal Occupational Safety and Health Administration.

§ 32 – 6 – 4.   Condition of Office.

4.1. Each acupuncture office, clinic, treatment center or institution shall be maintained in a clean and sanitary condition at all times, and shall have a readily accessible bathroom facilities for both male and female patients.

4.2. The Board or its representative may make announced or unannounced office inspections during regular business hours to insure that sanitary conditions are being maintained. The Board or its representative may inspect treatment as well as non treatment areas. Patient files and records shall be made available to any authorized inspection by the Board or its official representative.

§ 32 – 6 – 5.   Disposable Needles; Sterilization Equipment.

5.1. Disposable needles. — All acupuncture offices, clinics, treatment centers and institutions shall use only pre-sterilized disposable needles. A practitioner shall use pre-sterilized disposable needles according to "clean needle technique" and standards of practice established by the

CCAOM.

5.2. Sterilization Equipment. — All acupuncture offices, clinics, treatment centers and institutions shall have functioning sterilization equipment for sanitizing non-needle equipment which is used in the normal and regular treatment of patients, or they shall contract with a local hospital or medical service for the transportation and sterilization of the non-needle equipment. Sterilization equipment shall be inspected at least once every two years by W. Va. Department of Labor inspectors.

§ 32 − 6 − 6.   Treatment Procedures.

A licensed acupuncturist shall practice the standard protocols of the FDA and the CCAOM during treatments by adhering to the following procedures:

6.1. Hand washing. — The acupuncturist shall vigorously scrub his or her hands with soap and warm water immediately before examining patients or handling acupuncture needles and other instruments, and between patients.

6.2. Sterilization of Instruments. — All non-needle instruments shall be sterilized before use in a manner which will destroy all microorganisms. All needle trays which contain sterile needles shall also be sterile. Each time non-needle instruments are sterilized, the acupuncturist shall use a tape or strip indicator which shows that sterilization is complete.

6.3. Acupuncture needles. — A practitioner shall use only pre-packaged, pre-sterilized disposable needles for acupuncture treatments. Needles may not be reused on the same patient, even during the same treatment.

6.4. Acupuncture points. — The practitioner shall clean area of the patient's body where needles are to be inserted with an appropriate antiseptic before insertion of the needle.

6.5. Subcutaneous needle breakage. — In the event an acupuncture needle inserted in a patient breaks subcutaneously, the treating acupuncturist shall immediately consult a medical physician. An acupuncturist shall not sever or penetrate the tissues in order to excise the needle.

6.6. Medical treatment for complications. — An acupuncturist shall immediately refer any complications, including but not limited to, hematoma, peritonitis or pneumothorax arising out of an acupuncture treatment to a western medical doctor, osteopath or podiatrist, if appropriate, when immediate medical treatment is required.

6.7. Pointpuncture(aquapuncture). — A practitioner shall perform point-puncture injections using sterile disposable needles and sterile solutions.

6.8. Needle Disposal. — A practitioner shall dispose of all acupuncture needles, pointpuncture needles and instruments to be discarded into rigid biohazard containers. A practitioner shall discard needles in one of the two following ways:

6.8.1. They shall be sterilized and discarded in a sealed container; or

6.8.2. They shall be placed in a sealed unbreakable container marked "Hazardous Waste" and disposed of in a manner consistent with OSHA biohazardous waste regulations.

§ 32 – 6 – 7. Informed Consent.

The practitioner shall notify patients in writing and verbally, as any treatment requires, regarding any potential complications arising from the treatment plan.

§ 32 – 6 – 8. Treatments Outside the Office.

8.1. A practitioner who provides acupuncture treatment outside the office shall carry the required sterile needles and other instruments in a sterile airtight container.

8.2. A practitioner shall adhere to all standards of practice applicable to treatment when providing the treatment out of his or her office.

§ 32 – 6 – 9. Content and Retention Acupuncture Medical Records.

9.1. Acupuncturists shall maintain written medical records justifying the course of treatment of each patient. These records shall include for each patient at least the following:

9.1.1. The patient's medical history;

9.1.2. Acupuncture and Oriental Medical diagnosis;

9.1.3. Diagnostic testing and imaging procedures and laboratory results;

9.1.4. Points used and any treatment procedures administered at each visit;

9.1.5. The practitioner's prescriptions and recommendations; and

9.1.6. Patient treatment plan with progress notes.

9.2. The practitioner shall maintain all medical records for a period of five (5) years from the date of the last entry to the record.

§ 32 – 6 – 10. Financial Responsibility.

10.1. Financial Responsibility. — As a prerequisite for licensure or license renewal every acupuncturist shall maintain medical malpractice insurance or professional liability insurance and shall provide the Board with proof of that financial responsibility. Each licensee shall have one of the following:

10.1.1. Professional liability coverage in an amount not less that $10,000 per claim, with a minimum annual aggregate of not less than $30,000 from an authorized insurer.

10.1.2. An unexpired, irrevocable letter of credit in the amount not less than $10,000 per claim, with a minimum aggregate availability of credit of not less than $30,000. The letter of credit shall be payable to the acupuncturist as beneficiary upon presentment of a final judgement indicating liability and awarding damages to be paid by the acupuncturist or upon presentment of a settlement agreement signed by all parties to the agreement when the final judgement or settlement is a result of a claim arising out of the rendering of, or the failure to render, acupuncture services. The letter of credit shall be nonassignable and nontransferable. The letter of credit shall be issued by any bank or savings association organized under the W. Va. Code.

10.1.3. A surety bond in an amount not less than $10,000 per claim, with a minimum annual aggregate of not less than $30,000 written by a company licensed to do business in West Virginia.

10.2. Exemptions. — Upon application to the Board, the following licensees are exempt from the requirements of this section:

10.2.1. Any acupuncturist who practices exclusively as an officer, employee or agent of the federal government or of the state of West Virginia or its agencies or subdivisions. For the purposes of this rule, an agent of the State of West Virginia, its agencies or its subdivisions is a person who is eligible for coverage under any plan offered by the State of West Virginia;

10.2.2. Any licensee whose license has become inactive and who is not practicing in this state. Any licensee applying for reactivation of a license shall show either that the licensee maintained tail insurance coverage which provided liability coverage for incidents that occurred on or after January 1, 1998, or the initial date of licensure in West Virginia, whichever is later, and incidents that occurred before the date on which the license became inactive; or such licensee shall submit an affidavit stating that the licensee has no unsatisfied medical malpractice judgements or settlements at the time of application for reactivation;

10.2.3. Any licensee who practices only in conjunction with his or her teaching duties at an accredited school. That licensee may engage in the practice of acupuncture to the extent that the practice is incidental to and a necessary part of duties in connection with the teaching position in the school;

10.2.4. Any licensee holding an active license under W. Va. Code § 30 – 36 – 1 et seq. who is not practicing in West Virginia. If that person initiates or resumes practice in this state, he or she shall notify the Board of the activity and fulfill his or her obligation to obtain coverage; and

10.2.5. Any licensee who can demonstrate to the Board that he or she has no malpractice exposure in the State of West Virginia.

Series 7. Disciplinary and Complaint Procedures for Acupuncturists

§ 32 – 7 – 1. General.

1.1. Scope. — This rule establishes the due process procedure for disciplinary and complaint procedures for the Board. The Board is charged with these duties in W. Va. Code § 30 – 36 – 18.

1.2. Authority. — W. Va. Code §§ 30 – 1 – 8(a) and 30 – 36 – 1 et seq.

1.3. Filing Date. — April 16, 2008.

1.4. Effective Date. — April 16, 2008.

§ 32 – 7 – 2. Application and Enforcement.

This legislative rule applies to all licensed acupuncturists, student acupuncturists, and acupuncture trainees.

§ 32 – 7 – 3. Definitions.

3.1. "Board" means the West Virginia Board of Acupuncture.

3.2. "Licensee" means an acupuncturist who holds a license issued by the Board to practice acupuncture and oriental medicine.

3.3. "License" means a license issued by the Board.

3.4. "Practice of acupuncture and oriental medicine" means the practice of acupuncture as defined in W. Va. Code § 30 – 36 – 2 and includes licensed acupuncturists, student acupuncturists and acupuncture trainees.

3.5. "False and deceptive advertising" means a statement that includes a misrepresentation of fact, is likely to mislead or deceive because of a failure to disclose material facts, is intended or is likely to create false or unjustified expectations of favorable results or includes representations or implications that in a reasonable probability will cause an ordinary prudent person to misunderstand or be deceived.

3.6. "Adjudicatory hearing" means a formal administrative hearing before the Board or a designated hearing examiner, conducted to determine the truth and validity of complaints filed against a licensee.

3.7. "Probation" means imposing conditions and requirements upon a licensee for a period of time that the Board determines to be justified under any provision of law.

§ 32 – 7 – 4. Causes for Denial, Probation, Limitation, Discipline, Suspension or Revocation of Licenses of Acupuncturists.

4.1. The Board may deny an application for license, place a licensee on probation, suspend a license, limit or restrict a licensee or revoke any license issued by the Board, upon satisfactory proof that the licensee has:

4.1.1. Knowingly made, or presented or caused to be made or presented, any false, fraudulent or forged statement, writing, certificate, diploma or other material in connection with an application for a license;

4.1.2. Been or is involved in fraud, forgery, deception, collusion or conspiracy in connection with an examination for a license;

4.1.3. Become addicted to a controlled substance;

4.1.4. Become a chronic or persistent alcoholic;

4.1.5. Engaged in dishonorable, unethical or unprofessional conduct of a character likely to deceive, defraud or harm the public or member of the public;

4.1.6. Willfully violated a confidential communication;

4.1.7. Had his or her license to practice acupuncture or oriental medicine in any other state, territory, jurisdiction or foreign nation revoked, suspended, restricted or limited, or otherwise acted against, or has been subjected to any other disciplinary action by the licensing authority thereof, or has been denied licensure in any other state, territory, jurisdiction, or foreign nation;

4.1.8. Been or is unable to practice acupuncture or oriental medicine with reasonable skill and safety to patients by reason of illness, drunkenness, excessive use of alcohol, drugs, chemicals or any other type of material, or by any reason of any physical or mental abnormality;

4.1.9. Demonstrated a lack of professional competence to practice acupuncture or oriental medicine with a reasonable degree of skill and safety for patients. In this connection, the Board may consider repeated acts of an acupuncturist indicating his or her failure to properly treat a patient and may require the acupuncturist to submit to inquiries or examinations, written or oral, by members of the Board, by its agent, or designee, as the Board considers necessary to determine the professional qualifications of the licensee;

4.1.10. Engaged in unprofessional conduct, including, but not limited to, any departure from, or failure to conform to, the standards of acceptable and prevailing oriental medical practice, or the ethics of the oriental medical profession, or unprofessional conduct as presented in the Board's rule, Code of Ethics for Licensed Acupuncturist, 32CSR10 of the Boards Rules, irrespective of whether a patient is injured by the conduct, or has committed any act contrary to honesty, justice or good morals, whether the act is committed in the course of his or her practice or otherwise and whether committed within or without this State;

4.1.11. Been convicted of or found guilty of a crime in any jurisdiction which directly relates to the practice of acupuncture or oriental medicine or to the ability to practice acupuncture or oriental medicine. A plea of nolo contendere will be considered conviction for the purposes of this rule;

4.1.12. Advertised, practiced or attempted to practice under a name other than his or her own;

4.1.13. Failed to report to the Board any person whom the licensee knows is in violation of this rule or of provisions of the West Virginia Acupuncture Practice Act;

4.1.14. Aided, assisted, procured or advised any unlicensed person to practice oriental medicine contrary to this rule or the West Virginia Acupuncture Practice Act;

4.1.15. Failed to perform any statutory or legal obligation placed upon an acupuncturist;

4.1.16. Made or filed a report which the licensee knows to be false, intentionally or negligently failed to file a report or record required by state or federal law, willfully impeded or obstructed the filing or induced another person to do so. The reports or records will include only those which are signed in the capacity as a licensed acupuncturist;

4.1.17. Paid or received any commission, bonus, kickback or rebate, or engaged in any split-fee arrangement in any form whatsoever with an acupuncturist, organization, agency or person, either directly or indirectly, for patients referred to providers of health care goods and services, including, but not limited to, hospitals, nursing homes, clinical laboratories, ambulatory surgical centers or pharmacies. The provisions of this subdivision will not be construed to prevent an acupuncturist from receiving a fee for professional consultation service;

4.1.18. Exercised influence within a patient-practitioner relationship for purposes of engaging a patient in sexual activity;

4.1.19. Made deceptive, untrue or fraudulent representations in the practice of oriental medicine or employed a trick or scheme in the practice of oriental medicine when the trick or scheme fails to conform to the generally prevailing standards of treatment in the oriental medical community;

4.1.20. Solicited patients, either personally or through an agent, through use of fraud, intimidation, undue influence, or by overreaching or vexatious conduct. A solicitation is any communication which directly or implicitly requests an immediate response from the recipient;

4.1.21. Failed to keep written records justifying the course of treatment of the patient, including, but not limited to, patient histories, examination results and test results and treatment rendered, if any;

4.1.22. Exercised influence on the patient or client in such a manner as to exploit the patient or client for the financial gain of the licensee or of a third party, which includes, but not be limited to, the promoting or selling of services, goods, appliances or materia medica and the promotion or advertising on any prescription form of a pharmacy. For the purposes of this subdivision, prescribing, dispensing, administering, mixing or otherwise preparing materia medica, including all controlled and non-controlled substances, inappropriately or in excessive or inappropriate quantities, is not in the best interests of the patient and is not in the course of the acupuncturist or oriental medical practitioners professional practice, without regard to his or her intent;

4.1.23. Engaged in malpractice or failed to practice acupuncture or oriental medicine with that level of care, skill and treatment which are recognized by a reasonable, prudent, acupuncturist or an oriental medical practitioner engaged in the same or similar specialty as being acceptable under similar conditions and circumstances;

4.1.24. Performed any procedure or prescribed any therapy which, by the prevailing standards of oriental medical practice in the community, would constitute experimentation on a human subject, without first obtaining full, informed and written consent from the patient;

4.1.25. Practiced or offered to practice acupuncture beyond the scope permitted by the West Virginia Acupuncture Practice Act or accepted and performed professional responsibilities which the licensee knows or has reason to know he or she is not competent to perform;

4.1.26. Delegated professional responsibilities to a person whom the licensee knew or had reason to know was not qualified by training, experience or licensure to perform the responsibilities;

4.1.27. Violated or attempted to violate any law or rule of any jurisdiction, which relates to the practice of acupuncture.

4.1.28. Violated or failed to comply with a lawful order of the Board, or has violated an order of any court entered pursuant to any proceedings commenced by the Board;

4.1.29. Offered, undertaken or agreed to cure or treat disease by a secret method, procedure, treatment or medicine; or has treated for any human condition, by a method, means, or procedure which the licensee has refused to divulge upon demand of the Board;

4.1.30. Engaged in false or deceptive advertising. "False or Deceptive Advertising" means a statement that includes a misrepresentation of fact, is likely to mislead or deceive because of a failure to disclose material facts, is intended or is likely to create false or unjustified expectations of favorable results or includes representations or implications that in reasonable probability will cause an ordinary prudent person to misunderstand or be deceived; or

4.1.31. Engaged in advertising that is not in the public interest. Advertising that is not in the public interest includes the following:

4.1.31.a. Advertising that has the effect of intimidating or exerting undue pressure;

4.1.31.b. Advertising that uses testimonials;

4.1.31.c. Advertising which is false, deceptive, misleading, sensational or flamboyant;

4.1.31.d. Advertising which guarantees satisfaction or a cure;

4.1.31.e. Advertising which offers gratuitous services or discounts, the purpose of which is to deceive the public. This paragraph does not apply to advertising which contains an offer to negotiate fees, nor to advertising in conjunction with an established policy or program of free care for patients; and

4.1.31.f. Advertising which make claims of professional superiority which a licensee is unable to substantiate.

4.2. For the purposes of Section 4.1., acts declared to constitute dishonorable, unethical or unprofessional conduct of a character likely to deceive, defraud or harm the public or any member thereof includes, but is not limited to:

4.2.1. Prescribing or dispensing any "Controlled Substance" as defined in the W. Va. Code § 60A - 1 - 101 (d), except as defined in W. Va. Code § 30 - 36 - 2 when performed in accordance with the principles of oriental acupuncture medical theories;

4.2.2. Issuing or publishing in any manner whatsoever, representations in which grossly improbable or extravagant statements are made which have a tendency to deceive or defraud the public, or a member thereof, including, but not limited to:

4.2.2.a. Any representation in which the licensee claims that he or she is able to cure or treat manifestly incurable diseases, ailments or infirmities by any method, procedure, treatment or medicine which the licensee knows or has reason to know has little or no therapeutic value;

4.2.2.b. Represents or professes or holds himself or herself out as being able and willing to treat diseases, ailments or infirmities under a system or school of practice, except:

4.2.2.b.1. for which he or she holds a degree or diploma from a school otherwise recognized by the Board, or

4.2.2.b.2. Which he or she professes to be self-taught or self-developed.

4.2.3. A serious act, or a pattern of acts committed during the course of an acupuncture practice which, under the attendant circumstances, would be considered to be gross incompetence, gross ignorance, gross negligence or malpractice, including the performance of any unnecessary service or procedure;

4.2.4. Conduct which is calculated to bring or has the effect of bringing the acupuncture or oriental medical profession into disrepute, including, but not limited to, any departure from or failure to conform to the standards of acceptable and prevailing oriental medical practice within the State;

4.2.5. Any charges or fees for any type of service rendered within forty-eight (48) hours of the initial visit, if the licensee advertises free service, free examination or free treatment;

4.2.6. Failing to meet the standard of practice in connection with any supervisory and/or collaborative agreement with any category of health practitioner licensed under Chapter 30 of the W. Va. Code;

4.2.7. Charging or collecting an excessive or unconscionable fee. Factors to be considered as guides in determining the reasonableness of a fee include the following:

4.2.7.a. The time and effort required;

4.2.7.b. The novelty and difficulty of the procedure or treatment;

4.2.7.c. The skill required to perform the procedure or treatment properly;

4.2.7.d. Any requirements or conditions imposed by the patient or circumstances;

4.2.7.e. The nature and length of the professional relationship with the patient;

4.2.7.f. The experience, reputation, and ability of the licensee; and

4.2.7.g. The nature of the circumstances under which the services are provided.

4.2.8. In any case where it is found that an excessive, unconscionable fee has been charged, in addition to any actions taken under the provisions of section 4.3 of this rule, the Board may require the licensee to reduce or pay back the fee.

4.3. When the Board finds that any applicant is unqualified to be granted a license or finds that any licensee should be disciplined pursuant to the West Virginia Acupuncture Practice Act or rules of the Board, the Board may take anyone or more of the following actions:

4.3.1. Refuse to grant a license to an applicant;

4.3.2. Administer a public reprimand;

4.3.3. Suspend, limit or restrict any license for a definite period, not to exceed five (5) years;

4.3.4. Require any licensee to participate in a program of education prescribed by the Board;

4.3.5. Revoke any license;

4.3.6. Require the licensee to submit to care, counseling or treatment by physicians or other professional persons;

4.3.7. Require him or her to practice under the direction or supervision of another practitioner; or

4.3.8. Require the licensee to provide a period of free public or charitable service.

4.3.9. In addition to and in conjunction with these actions, the Board may make a finding adverse to the licensee or applicant, but withhold imposition of judgment and penalty, or it may impose the judgment and penalty but suspend enforcement of the penalty and place the acupuncturist on probation, which may be vacated upon the noncompliance with any terms imposed by the Board. In its discretion, the Board may restore and reissue a license under the West Virginia Acupuncture Practice Act, W. Va. Code § 30 - 36 - 1 et. seq, and as a condition it may impose any disciplinary or corrective measure provided for in this Rule or in the West Virginia Acupuncture Practice Act.

4.4. The Board has the authority to place a licensee in a probationary status and to apply varying conditions upon the licensee during the probationary period. Upon reaching the conclusion that a licensee to practice acupuncture should be placed on probation, the Board may impose anyone or more of the following conditions:

4.4.1. The Board may appoint one or more Board members to be responsible for having the probationary licensee report for interviews on a regular basis. These interviews may be set up on a periodic basis as determined by the Board and the appointed Board members will then report back to the Board at its regularly scheduled meeting on the progress of the licensee;

4.4.2. The Board may request the probationary licensee to appear before the Board at intervals determined by the Board order that the licensee may report on his or her progress. During these appearances by the probationary licensee, the Board may ask the probationary licensee questions so as to observe his or her behavior and progress;

4.4.3. The Board may select a physician or request the probationary licensee to select a physician who will be approved by the Board and the physician shall submit periodic progress reports on the probationary licensee as directed by Board;

4.4.4. The Board may appoint a medical consultant whose responsibility is to conduct interviews with the probationary licensee. The probationary licensee shall then report to the appointed medical consultant on a regular basis as determined by the Board, and the medical consultant shall report to the Board at intervals determined by the Board;

4.4.5. In cases of alcoholism and/or drug abuse, as a condition of probation, the Board may require that the probationary licensee submit periodic blood samples and/or urine drug screen samples;

4.4.6. The Board may require that the probationary licensee authorize his or her personal physician to submit to the Board, for review, the probationary licensee's medical history, both as to past medical history and any and all new medical history as may become available to the personal physician during the period of the probationary term;

4.4.7. The Board may require that the probationary licensee report all medications that he or she may be utilizing and that he or she make the reports to the Board, at intervals as directed by the Board from time to time;

4.4.8. The Board may require that prior to the termination of a probationary term, the probationary licensee appear at a regularly scheduled Board meeting and furnish the Board with information as it may request, and the Board may utilize subpoenas, subpoenas duces tecum and its investigators as it considers necessary to gather facts and evidence to determine compliance by the probationary licensee with the terms of probation; and

4.4.9. In those situations where indicated, the Board may impose additional terms of probation, restriction, or revocation upon a licensee who has initially been placed on probation. The period of probation shall not exceed five (5) years from its initiation date.

§ 32 – 7 – 5. Complaint Disposition.

5.1. Any person, medical peer review committee, firm, corporation, members of the Board or public officer may make a complaint to the Board which charges an acupuncturist with a violation of the W. Va. Code § 30 – 36 – 1 et seq., or of the Rules of the Board. The Board may provide a form for that purpose, but a complaint may be filed in any written form. In addition to describing the alleged violation which prompted the complaint, the complaint should contain the following:

5.1.1. The name and address of the individual against whom the complaint is lodged;

5.1.2. The date of care or other incident;

5.1.3. The name of individual who may have treated the patient after the alleged incident; and

5.1.4. The name of any health care institution in which the patient was an inpatient or outpatient after or during the alleged incident.

5.2. The Board may prepare forms for filing complaints and make them available upon request.

5.3. Any information regarding a complaint shall be sent by the Board to the practitioner concerned for his or her written comment and he or she will submit a written reply within twenty (20) days, or waive the right to do so.

§ 32 – 7 – 6. Appeal.

6.1. Any applicant for a license who has had his or her application denied by order of the Board may appeal the order within thirty (30) days of that action, in accordance with the contested case hearing procedure, W. Va. Code § 29A – 5 – 1 et seq., and rules of the Board: Provided, That the appeal shall not include cases in which the Board denies a license or certificate after an examination to test the knowledge or the ability of the applicant where the controversy concerns whether the examination was fair or whether the applicant passed the examination.

6.2. Any licensee practicing acupuncture and oriental medicine in this State, who has had his or her license denied, suspended, restricted, or revoked by order of the Board, may appeal the order within thirty (30) days of this action in accordance with the contested case hearing procedure, W. Va. Code § 29A – 5 – 1 et seq., and the rules of the Board.

Series 8.   Contested Case Hearing Procedure

§ 32 – 8 – 1.   General.

1.1. Scope. — This rule establishes procedures for the adjudication of contested case hearings before the Board.

1.2. Authority. — W. Va. Code §§ 30 – 36 – 1 et seq., 30 – 1 – 1 et seq. and 29A – 5 – 1 et seq.

1.3. Filing Date. — July 17, 2007.

1.4. Effective Date. — September 1, 2007.

§ 32 – 8 – 2.   Definitions.

The following words and phrases as used in these rules shall have the following meanings, unless the context otherwise requires:

2.1. "Board" means the West Virginia Board of Acupuncture.

2.2. The term "demanding party" means an individual who has been denied a license to practice acupuncture and oriental medicine by the Board and who, as a result, demands that a hearing be held before the Board on the issue of such denial.

2.3. The term "charged party" means an individual who holds a license to practice acupuncture and oriental medicine issued by the Board and who has been charged by the Board as described in subsection 3.4 of this rule.

2.4. The term "licensee" means an acupuncturist who holds a license issued by the Board to practice acupuncture and oriental medicine or a "trainee" who holds an educational training permit.

2.5. The term "license" means a license issued by the Board pursuant to W. Va. Code § 30 – 36 – 1 et seq.

2.6. "Practice of acupuncture and oriental medicine" means the practice of acupuncture and oriental medicine as defined in W. Va. Code § 30 – 36 – 1 et seq. and includes licensed acupuncturists, student acupuncturists and acupuncture trainees.

§ 32 – 8 – 3.   Hearing Procedures.

3.1. Any person denied a license or who has had their license/training permit suspended, restricted, or revoked by order of the Board and who believes such order was in violation of W. Va. Code §§ 30 – 1 – 1 et seq. and/or 30 – 36 – 1 et seq. shall be entitled to a hearing on the action.

3.2. Any person who desires a hearing for the reason described in subsection 3.1 of this section must present a written demand for such to the Board.

3.3. When the president of the Board or his or her authorized designee is presented with such a demand for a hearing, he or she shall schedule a hearing within forty-five (45) days of receipt by him or her of such written demand, unless postponed to a later date by mutual agreement.

3.4. Charges may be instituted against any licensed acupuncturist, student acupuncturist and acupuncture trainee by the Board when reasonable cause exists for believing that he or she may have engaged in conduct or be in such condition that his or her license should be suspended, revoked or otherwise disciplined for one or more of the grounds set forth in W. Va. Code § 30 − 36 − 1 et seq. or the Board's legislative rules. Charges may be based upon information received by way of a verified written complaint filed with the Board and further information gathered by the Board in the process of investigating such complaint. Charges may also be based upon information received solely through investigative activities undertaken by the Board.

3.5. Charges instituted against a licensee or trainee as described in subsection 3.4 of this section shall be set forth in a Complaint and Notice of Hearing issued in the name of the Board as the agency of the State regulating the practice of acupuncture and oriental medicine. Such Complaint and Notice of Hearing shall designate the Board as the "Complainant," and shall designate the licensed acupuncturist, student acupuncturist and acupuncture trainee involved in the proceeding as the "Respondent"; shall set out the substance of each offense charged with sufficient particularity to reasonably apprise the Respondent of the nature, time and place of the conduct or condition complained of therein; shall state the date, time and place for the hearing; and, shall contain a statement of intention by the Board to appoint a hearing examiner.

3.6. Upon receipt of a demand for a hearing described in subsection 3.1 and 3.2 of this section, the president or his or her designee shall provide the demanding party with a Complaint and Notice of Hearing issued in the name of the Board as the agency of the State regulating the practice of acupuncture and oriental medicine. Such Complaint and Notice of Hearing shall designate the demanding party as the "Complainant" and shall designate the Board as the "Respondent"; shall set out the substance of each and every reason that the Board has denied the demanding party a license with sufficient particularity to reasonably apprise the demanding party of the nature, time and place of the conduct or condition at issue therein; shall state the date, time and place for the hearing; and shall contain a statement of intention by the Board to appoint a hearing examiner.

3.7. The Board may amend the charges set forth in a Complaint and Notice of Hearing as it deems proper.

3.8. A Complaint and Notice of Hearing shall be served upon the demanding or charged party at least thirty (30) days prior to the date of hearing.

3.9. Upon written motion received by the Board no later than twenty (20) days prior to the date of hearing, a more definite statement of the matters charged or the reasons stated for denial of licensure shall be provided to the demanding or charged party or his or her counsel, at least fifteen (15) days prior to the hearing date.

3.10. Hearings shall be conducted as follows:

3.10.1. Any party to a hearing shall have the right to be represented by an attorney-at-law, duly qualified to practice law in the State of West Virginia.

3.10.2. The Board may be represented by the West Virginia Attorney General's Office.

3.10.3. Irrelevant, immaterial, or unduly repetitious evidence shall be excluded from the hearing. Furthermore, the rules of evidence as applied in civil cases in the circuit courts of this State shall be followed. However, when necessary to ascertain facts not reasonably susceptible of proof under those rules, evidence not admissible thereunder may be admitted, except where precluded by statute, if it is of a type commonly relied upon by reasonably prudent persons in the conduct of their affairs.

3.10.4. The rules of privilege recognized by the law of this State shall be followed.

3.10.5. Objections to evidentiary offers shall be noted in the record. Any party to the hearing may vouch the record as to any excluded testimony or other evidence.

3.10.6. Any party to a hearing may appear with witnesses to testify on his or her behalf; may be heard in person, by counsel or both; may present such other evidence in support of his or her position as deemed appropriate by the Board or its designated hearing examiner; and, when appropriate, may cross-examine witnesses called by the Board in support of the charges or in defense of its decision to deny licensure or educational training permit.

3.10.7. The hearing shall be held at such time and place as is designated by the Board, but no hearing shall be conducted unless and until at least thirty (30) days written notice thereof has been served upon the charged or demanding party and/or his or her attorney in person; or if he or she cannot be found, by delivering such notice at his or her usual place of abode, and giving information of its purport, to his wife or her husband, or to any other person found there who is a member of his or her family and above the age of sixteen (16) years; or if neither his wife or her husband nor any such person can be found there, and he or she cannot be found, by leaving such notice posted at the front door of such place of abode; or if he or she does not reside in this State, such notice may be served by the publication thereof once a week for three (3) successive weeks in a newspaper published in this State; or such notice may be served by registered or certified mail.

3.10.8. The hearing shall be open to the general public.

3.10.9. Members of the Board and its officers, agents and employees shall be competent to testify at the hearing as to material and relevant matters: Provided, that no member of the Board who testifies at such hearing shall thereafter participate in the deliberations or decisions of the Board with respect to the case in which he or she so testified.

3.10.10. The hearing may be conducted by one or more Board members or by a hearing examiner appointed by the Board.

3.10.11. A record of the hearing, including the complaint(s), if applicable, the notice of hearing, all pleadings, motions, rulings, stipulations, exhibits, documentary evidence, evidentiary depositions and the stenographic report of the hearing, shall be made and a transcript thereof maintained in the Board's files. Upon request, a copy of the transcript shall be furnished to any party at his or her expense.

3.10.12. Documentary evidence may be received in the form of copies or excerpts or by incorporation by reference.

3.10.13. Where a hearing is held upon the instance of the Board after charges have been brought against a licensee pursuant to subsections 3.4 and 3.5 of this section, the Board shall have the burden of proof and shall present its evidence and/or testimony in support of the charges first.

3.10.14. Where a hearing is held upon demand under the provisions of subsections 3.1, 3.2, 3.3, and 3.6 of this section, the demanding party shall have the burden of proof and shall therefore be required to present his or her evidence first. The Board may require the person demanding the hearing to give security for the costs thereof and if the demanding party does not substantially prevail, such facts may be assessed against them and may be collected in a civil action by other proper remedy.

3.10.15. Following the conclusion of the Board's presentation of evidence in accordance with subsection 3.10.13 of this section, the Respondent or charged party shall have the right to submit his or her evidence in defense.

3.10.16. Following the conclusion of the demanding party's presentation of evidence in accordance with subsection 3.10.14 of this section, the Board shall have the right to submit its evidence in defense.

3.10.17. The Board may call witnesses to testify in support of its decision to deny licensure or in support of the charges instituted against a licensee; may present such other evidence to support its position; and, may cross-examine witnesses called by the demanding party or charged party in support of his or her position.

3.10.18. All parties shall have the right to offer opening and closing arguments, not to exceed ten (10) minutes for each presentation.

3.10.19. Hearings held by the Board as a result of charges instituted against a licensee may be continued or adjourned to a later date or a different place by the Board or its designee by appropriate notice to all parties.

3.10.20. Motions for a continuance of a hearing may be granted upon a showing of good cause. Motions for continuance must be in writing and received in the office of the Board no later than seven (7) days prior to the hearing date. In determining whether good cause exists, consideration will be given to the ability of the party requesting the continuance to proceed effectively without a continuance. A motion for a continuance filed less than seven (7) days from the date of hearing shall be denied unless the reason for the motion could not have been ascertained earlier. Motions for continuance filed prior to the date of hearing may be ruled on by the Executive Secretary or Assistant Executive Secretary of the Board or designated hearing examiner. All other motions for continuance shall be ruled on by the Board member(s) or the hearing examiner presiding over the hearing.

3.10.21. All motions related to a case set for hearing before the Board, except motions for continuance and those made during the hearing, shall be in writing and shall be received in the office of the Board at least ten (10) days before the hearing. Prehearing motions shall be heard at a prehearing conference or at the hearing prior to the commencement of testimony. The Board member(s) or the hearing examiner presiding at the hearing shall hear the motions and the response for the non-moving party and shall rule on such motions accordingly.

§ 32 – 8 – 4. Transcription of Testimony and Evidence.

4.1. All testimony, evidence, arguments and rulings on the admissibility of testimony and evidence shall be recorded by stenographic notes and characters or by mechanical means.

4.2. All recorded materials shall be transcribed. The Board shall have the responsibility to make arrangements for the transcription of the recorded testimony and evidence.

4.3. Upon the motion of the Board or any party assigning error or omission in any part of any transcript, the Board or its appointed hearing examiner shall settle all differences arising as to whether such transcript truly discloses what occurred at the hearing and shall direct that the transcript be corrected and/or revised as appropriate so as to make it conform to the truth.

4.4. A transcript of the hearing shall be provided to all members of the Board for review at least ten (10) days before the vote is taken on its decision in any licensure or licensure disciplinary matter.

§ 32 – 8 – 5. Submission of Proposed Findings of Fact and Conclusions of Law.

5.1. Any party may submit proposed findings of fact and conclusions of law at a time and manner designated by the Board or its duly appointed hearing examiner.

§ 32 – 8 – 6. Hearing Examiner.

6.1. The Board may appoint a hearing examiner who shall be empowered to subpoena witnesses and documents, administer oaths and affirmations, examine witnesses under oath, rule on evidentiary matters, hold conferences for the settlement or simplification of issues by consent of the parties, cause to be prepared a record of the hearing so that the Board is able to discharge its functions and otherwise conduct hearings as provided in § 24 – 3 – 3.10 herein.

6.2. Hearing examiners appointed by the Board are not authorized or empowered to grant, suspend, revoke or otherwise discipline any license.

6.3. The hearing examiner shall prepare recommended findings of fact and conclusions of law for submission to the Board. The Board may adopt, modify or reject such findings of fact and conclusions of law.

§ 32 – 8 – 7. Conferences; Informal Disposition of Cases.

7.1. At any time prior to the hearing or thereafter, the Board, its designee or its duly appointed hearing examiner may hold conferences for the following purposes:

7.1.1. To dispose of procedural requests, prehearing motions or similar matters;

7.1.2. To simplify or settle issues by consent of the parties; or

7.1.3. To provide for the informal disposition of cases by stipulation or agreement.

7.2. The Board or its appointed hearing examiner may cause such conferences to be held on its own motion or by the request of a party.

7.3. The Board may also initiate or consider stipulation or agreement proposals with regard to the informal disposition of cases and may enter into such stipulations and/or agreements without conference.

§ 32 – 8 – 8.　Depositions.

8.1. Evidentiary depositions may be taken and read or otherwise included into evidence as in civil actions in the circuit courts of this State.

§ 32 – 8 – 9.　Subpoenas.

9.1. Subpoenas to compel the attendance of witnesses and subpoenas duces tecum to compel the production of documents may be issued by the Board or its Executive Secretary, and by the hearing examiner appointed by the Board. Such subpoenas shall be issued pursuant to W. Va. Code 29A – 5 – 1(b).

9.2. Written requests by a party for the issuance of subpoenas or subpoenas duces tecum as provided in subsection 9.1 of this section must be received by the Board no later than ten (10) days before a scheduled hearing. Any party requesting the issuance of subpoenas or subpoenas duces tecum shall see that they are properly served in accordance with W. Va. Code § 29A – 5 – 1(b).

§ 32 – 8 – 10.　Orders.

10.1. Any final order entered by the Board following a hearing conducted pursuant to these rules shall be made pursuant to the provisions of W. Va. Code §§ 29A – 5 – 3 and 30 – 1 – 8 (d). Such orders shall be entered within forty-five (45) days following the submission of all documents and materials necessary for the proper disposition of the case, including transcripts, and shall contain findings of fact and conclusions of law.

10.2. The findings of fact and conclusions of law must be approved by a majority of the Board either by a poll or vote at a regular meeting, before a final order is entered. A copy of the final order approved by a majority of the Board shall be served upon the demanding or charged party and/or his attorney of record, if any, within five (5) days after entry by the Board by personal service or by registered or certified mail.

§ 32 – 8 – 11.　Appeal.

11.1. An appeal from any final order entered in accordance with these rules shall comply with the provisions of W. Va. Code § 30 – 1 – 9.

§ 32 – 8 – 12.　Severability.

12.1. If any provision of this rule or the application thereof to any person or circumstance is held invalid, the invalidity shall not affect the provisions or application of this rule which can be given effect without the invalid provisions or application and to this end the provisions of this rule are declared to be severable.

Series 9.　Continuing Education Requirements

§ 32 - 9 - 1.　General.

1.1. Scope. — This establishes continuing education requirements for renewal of licensure pursuant to W. Va. Code § 30 - 36 - 14(d).

1.2. Authority. — W. Va. Code §§ 30 - 36 - 7(a) and 30 - 36 - 14(c).

1.3. Filing Date. — April 16, 2008.

1.4. Effective Date. — April 16, 2008.

§ 32 - 9 - 2.　Application.

This legislative rule applies to renewal licensees and instructors of continuing education courses.

§ 32 - 9 - 3.　Definitions.

3.1. Approved Provider. — Those persons or organizations offering continuing education in West Virginia, who are approved by the Board.

3.2. Course. — A systematic learning experience, at least one hour in length, which deals with and is designed for the acquisition of knowledge, skills and information relevant to the practice of acupuncture.

3.3. Hour. — A period of time spent in a course, lasting at least fifty (50) minutes, where participation in an organized learning experience occurs.

§ 32 - 9 - 4.　Criteria for Provider Approval.

4.1. In order to be an approved provider, a provider shall submit to the Board an application on a form provided by the Board accompanied by the fee required by Board of Acupuncture rules, Fees of the Board of Acupuncture 32 CSR 4 . All provider applications and documentation submitted to the Board shall be typewritten and in English.

4.2. The approval of the provider expires one (1) year after it is issued by the Board and may be renewed upon the filing of the required application and fee.

4.3. Acupuncture schools and colleges which have been approved by the Board, pursuant to the W. Va. Code § 30 - 36 - 10, are approved continuing education providers .

§ 32 - 9 - 5.　Approved Providers.

5.1. For the purpose of this rule a provider may only use the title "approved provider" when the person or organization has submitted a provider application form, remitted the appropriate fee and has been issued a provider number. Programs offered by the following organizations, or their successor organizations, will be considered "approved":

5.1.1. The West Virginia Association of Oriental Medicine (WVAOM);

5.1.2. The American Association of Acupuncture and Oriental Medicine (AAAOM);

5.1.3. The Council of Colleges of Acupuncture and Oriental Medicine (CCAOM);

5.1.4. The American Academy of Medical Acupuncturists (AAMA);

5.1.5. The National Acupuncture Teachers Association;

5.1.6. The National Acupuncture Detoxification Association; and

5.1.7. Accredited schools or colleges.

5.2. The Board shall assign only one provider number to a person or organization. When two or more approved providers co-sponsor a course, the course shall be identified by only one provider number and that provider shall assume responsibility for record keeping, advertising, issuance of certificates and instructor qualifications.

5.3. An approved provider shall keep the following records for a period of four years in one identified location:

5.3.1. Course outlines of each approved course given;

5.3.2. The record of time and places of each approved course given;

5.3.3. Course instructor curriculum vitae or resumes;

5.3.4. The attendance record for each approved course which shows the name, signature and license number of acupuncturists taking the course and a record of any certificates issued to them; and

5.3.5. Participant evaluation forms for each approved course given.

5.4. Within ten (10) days of completion of an approved course, the provider shall submit to the Board the following:

5.4.1. A copy of the attendance record showing the name, signature and license number of any licensed acupuncturists who attended the approved course; and

5.4.2. The participant evaluation forms of the approved course.

5.5. Approved providers shall issue, within 60 days of the conclusion of an approved course, to each participant who has completed the course a certificate of completion which contains the following information:

5.5.1. The provider's name and number;

5.5.2. The course title;

5.5.3. The participant's name and, if applicable, his or her acupuncture license number;

5.5.4. The date and location of the course;

5.5.5. The number of continuing education hours completed; and

5.5.6. A statement directing the acupuncturist to retain the certificate for at least four (4) years from the date of completion of the course.

5.6. An approved provider shall notify the Board of any changes to the date or location of an approved course. An approved provider shall not change to the date of an approved course prior to the date for which the course was approved if the new date would occur less than 45 days from receipt of the course request.

5.7. Any changes in the content of or instructor for an approved course requires prior approval of the Board. A request to change the content of or instructor(s) for an approved course shall be received by the Board at least ten (10) days before the course begins.

5.8. An approved provider shall notify the Board within 30 days of any changes in its organizational structure or the person responsible for the provider's continuing education course, including name, address, or telephone number changes.

5.9. Provider approval is non-transferable.

5.10. The Board may audit during reasonable business hours records, courses, instructors and related activities of an approved provider.

§ 32 - 9 - 6.　Approval Of Continuing Education Courses.

6.1. Only an approved provider may offer continuing education courses.

6.2. The content of all courses of continuing education shall be relevant to the practice of acupuncture and shall:

6.2.1. Be related to the knowledge and/or technical skills required to practice acupuncture; or

6.2.2. Be related to direct and/or indirect patient care. Courses in acupuncture practice management or medical ethics are also acceptable.

6.3. Each course shall include a method by which the course participants evaluate the following:

6.3.1. The extent to which the course met its stated objectives;

6.3.2. The adequacy of the instructor's knowledge of the course subject;

6.3.3. The utilization of appropriate teaching methods;

6.3.4. The applicability or usefulness of the course information; and

6.3.5. Other relevant comments.

§ 32 - 9 - 7.　Content of Courses Applicable for Continuing Education Credits.

7.1. License renewal requires a minimum of forty-eight hours of continuing education units or continuing medical education units from the following categories;

7.2. For each renewal period of two years, a licensee shall have a minimum of twenty-four hours of instruction in the area of acupuncture or oriental medicine from an approved provider, and;

7.3. For each renewal period of two years, a licensee may have up to twenty-four hours of instruction in western clinical sciences, medical practices, medical ethics, or medical research which are sponsored or accredited by, but not limited to, the following organizations, or their successor organizations:

7.3.1. The World Health Organization (WHO);

7.3.2. The National Institutes of Health (NIH);

7.3.3. The American Medical Association (AMA) ;

7.3.4. The American Osteopathic Association (AOA) ;

7.3.5. The American Nurses Association (ANA) ;

7.3.6. Local hospitals; or

7.3.7. Local colleges, and;

7.4. For each renewal period, a licensee may have no more than twelve (12) hours of training in accredited programs which will assist the licensee to carry out his or her professional management responsibilities, including, but not limited to:

7.4.1. Office, hospital, or administrative management;

7.4.2. Language training, such as Chinese or English as a foreign language; or

7.4.3. Education methodology, and;

7.5. An acupuncturist may obtain credit for any other programs which are pre-approved by the Board, at the Boards discretion.

§ 32 – 9 – 8.   Application for Course Approval.

8.1. In order to obtain approval for a course, an approved provider shall submit to the Board a request for course approval, in English, on a form provided by the Board or in a similar format which contains the following information:

8.1.1. The provider's name, provider number, address, telephone number and contact person;

8.1.2. Course title, date, location, and number of continuing education hours;

8.1.3. The type and method of instruction and educational objectives to be met;

8.1.4. A course outline, course description. and instructor information and qualifications; and

8.1.5. All proposed public advertisements which are intended to be used by the approved provider to advertise the course. Where the provider uses a public advertisement which is developed after the course has been approved and which was not provided to the Board with the course request, the provider shall mail a copy of that advertisement to the Board within ten (10) days after its publication.

8.2. An approved provider shall obtain Board approval for every course that is offered for continuing education credit. Where a previously approved course is to be repeated, the provider shall apply to the Board for approval of each subsequent administration of the course.

8.3. An approved provider shall submit all requests for course approval to the Board at least 45 days before the course is first offered.

§ 32 – 9 – 9.   Instructors.

9.1. It is the responsibility of each approved provider to use qualified instructors.

9.2. Instructors teaching approved continuing education courses shall have the following minimum qualifications:

9.2.1. An acupuncturist instructor, shall (A) hold a current valid license to practice acupuncture or be otherwise authorized to act as a guest acupuncturist in accordance with W. Va. Code § 30 - 36 - 9(b) and be free of any disciplinary order or probation imposed by the Board, and (B) be knowledgeable, current and skillful in the subject matter of the course as evidenced through:

1. holding a baccalaureate or higher degree from a college or university and written documentation of experience in the subject matter;

2. experience in teaching similar subject matter content within the two years preceding the course;

3. have at least one year's experience within the last two years in the specialized area in which he or she is teaching.

9.2.2. A non-acupuncturist instructor shall:

1. be currently licensed or certified in his or her area of expertise if appropriate;

2. show written evidence of specialized training, which may include, but not be limited to. a certificate of training or an advanced degree in the given subject area; and

3. have at least one year's teaching experience within the last two years in the specialized area in which he or she teaches.

§ 32 - 9 - 10.　Advertisements.

10.1. Information disseminated by approved providers publicizing continuing education shall be true and not misleading and shall include the following:

10.1.1. A clear, concise description of the course content and/or objectives;

10.1.2. The date and location of the course;

10.1.3. The provider's name and telephone number;

10.1.4. The statement "This course has been approved by the West Virginia Board of Acupuncture, Provider Number _____ , for _____ hours of continuing education"; and

10.1.5. The provider's policy on refunds for cases of non-attendance or cancellations.

10.2. A provider shall not describe a course as being Board approved until written confirmation of approval by the Board has been received by the provider. Where a provider is waiting for a determination by the Board on its request for course approval the provider may advertise that the course is "pending" approval. A provider which advertises that its course is pending approval shall assume all responsibility if a course is subsequently denied by the Board.

§ 32 - 9 - 11.　Denial, Withdrawal and Appeal of Approval.

11.1. The Board may withdraw its approval of a provider or deny a provider application for causes which include, but are not limited to, the following:

11.1.1. Conviction of crime substantially related to the activities of a provider; or

11.1.2. Failure to comply with any provision of the W. Va. Code § 30 - 36 - 1 et seq.

11.2. Any material misrepresentation of fact by a provider or applicant in any information required to be submitted to the Board is grounds for withdrawal of approval or denial of an application.

11.3. The Board may withdraw its approval of a provider or a course after giving the provider written notice setting forth its reasons for withdrawal and after giving the provider a reasonable opportunity to be heard by the Board or its designee.

11.4. Should the Board deny approval of a provider or a course request, the applicant may appeal the action by filing a letter stating the reason with the Board: The letter-of appeal shall be filed with the Board within twenty (20) days of the mailing of the applicant's notification of the Board's denial. The appeal shall be considered by the Board or its designee. In the event that the Board or its designee considers the appeal after the date of the course for which the appeal is being made, a retroactive approval may be granted.

§ 32 – 9 – 12.　Sanctions for Noncompliance.

12.1. Each acupuncturist at the time of license renewal shall sign a statement under penalty of false swearing that he or she has or has not complied with the continuing education requirements. The licensee shall submit photocopies of the documentation along with the approved renewal application form from the Board.

12.2. The Board may audit once each year a random sample of acupuncturists who have reported compliance with the continuing education requirement. No acupuncturist shall be subject to audit more than once every two (2) years.

12.3. It constitutes unprofessional conduct for any acupuncturist to misrepresent completion of the required continuing education.

12.4. Any acupuncturist selected for audit shall submit original documentation or records of continuing education course work he or she has taken and completed.

12.5. Each acupuncturist shall retain for a minimum of four (4) years records of all continuing education programs attended which indicate the provider's name, title of the course or program, date and location of course and the number of continuing education credits awarded.

12.6. Instructors of approved continuing education courses may receive a maximum of two (2) hours of continuing education credit per year. An instructor may claim credit only where the individual acts as an instructor of an approved course. In addition, one hour of credit shall be accrued for each classroom hour completed as an instructor of a Board approved continuing education course. Participation as a member of a panel presentation for an approved course shall not entitle the participant to earn continuing education credit as an instructor.

Series 10.　Code of Ethics for Licensed Acupuncturists

§ 32 – 10 – 1.　General.

1.1. Scope. — This rule establishes a code of ethics for acupuncture and oriental medicine in this state.

1.2. Authority. — W. Va. Code §§ 30 - 36 - 7 (a) and 30 - 36 - 7 (b).

1.3. Filing Date. — May 21, 1999.

1.4. Effective Date. — May 21, 1999.

§ 32 - 10 - 2.   Application.

This legislative rule applies to all licensed acupuncturists, student acupuncturists and apprenticed acupuncturists in the State.

§ 32 - 10 - 3.   Code of Ethics.

Licensed practitioners shall post the provisions of this section in each acupuncturist office, clinic, or treatment center:

3.1. The Acupuncture Practitioner's primary purpose is to restore, maintain and optimize health in human beings.

3.2. The Acupuncture Practitioner acts to restore, maintain and optimize health by providing individualized care, according to his or her ability and judgment, following the principles of Oriental Medicine.

3.3. The Acupuncture Practitioner shall endeavor to first, do no harm and provide the most effective health care available with the least risk to his or her patients at all times. (Primum Non Nocere)

3.4. The Acupuncture Practitioner shall recognize, respect and promote the self-healing power of nature inherent in each individual human being. (Vis Medicatrix Naturae)

3.5. The Acupuncture Practitioner shall strive to identify and remove the causes of illness, rather than to merely eliminate or suppress symptoms. (Tolle Causum)

3.6. The Acupuncture Practitioner shall educate his or her patients, inspire rational hope and encourage self-responsibility for health. (Practitioner as Teacher)

3.7. The Acupuncture Practitioner shall treat each person by considering all individual health factors and influences. (Treat the Whole Person)

3.8. The Acupuncture Practitioner shall emphasize the condition of health to promote well-being and to prevent disease for the individual, each community and our world. (Health Promotion, the Best Prevention)

3.9. The Acupuncture Practitioner shall acknowledge the worth and dignity of every person and therefore, shall not exclude anyone from treatment on the basis of ethnic, racial, gender, or sexual orientation.

3.10. The Acupuncture Practitioner shall safeguard the patient's right to privacy and only disclose confidential information when either authorized by the patient or mandated by law.

3.11. The Acupuncture Practitioner shall act judiciously to protect the patient and the public when the incompetent or unethical practices by any person adversely affect health care quality and safety.

3.12. The Acupuncture Practitioner shall maintain competence in Oriental Medicine and strive for professional excellence through assessment of personal strengths, limitations and effectiveness and by advancement of professional knowledge.

3.13. The Acupuncture Practitioner shall conduct his or her practice and professional activities with honesty, integrity and responsibility for individual judgment and actions.

3.14. The Acupuncture Practitioner shall strive to participate in professional activities to advance the standards of care, body of knowledge and public awareness of Oriental Medicine.

3.15. The Acupuncture Practitioner shall respect all ethical, qualified health care practitioners and cooperate with other health professions to promote health for individual's, the public and the global community.

3.16. The Acupuncture Practitioner shall strive to exemplify personal well-being, ethical character and trust worthiness as a health care professional.

§ 32 – 10 – 4. Ethics Regarding the Sale of Oriental Medicines in the Office.

4.1. The sale of medications within an acupuncturist's office shall be based on addressing the needs of the patient. The making of profit is always viewed as a secondary consideration. This is an extension of the code of ethics of the state and national associations governing the conduct of acupuncture physicians.

4.2. While the retail selling of medications could be construed as a conflict of interest on the part of the physician; as long as the underlying intention remains the patient's best interest and not to make profit, and no other source for the formulation and quality of the medication that the practitioner feels is adequate exists, this remains a legitimate and viable service.

4.3. Oriental medicines which may be prescribed by licensed acupuncturists include, but are not limited to:

4.3.1. Herbs, alone and in combinations;

4.3.2. Glandulars;

4.3.3. Minerals;

4.3.4. Vitamins; and

4.3.5. Chinese patent medicines.

4.4. The U. S. Food and Drug Administration rules regarding the sale of over the counter medications, herbs and materia medica shall be observed by licensees.

Series 11. Education Requirements

§ 32 – 11 – 1. General.

1.1. Scope. — This establishes the educational requirements for licensed acupuncture applicants who have graduated from a school or college of acupuncture or oriental medicine.

1.2. Authority. — W. Va. Code § 30 – 36 – 7.

1.3. Filing date. — May 21, 1999.

1.4. Effective date. — May 21, 1999.

§ 32 – 11 – 2.　Application.

This legislative rule applies to applicants for license who have graduated from a school or college of acupuncture or oriental medicine.

§ 32 – 11 – 3.　Definitions.

3.1. Accredited School or College. — An institution which has received accreditation or is a candidate for accreditation from the national accreditation commission for schools and colleges of acupuncture and oriental medicine (NACSSAOM).

3.2. NACSSAOM. — The national accreditation commission for schools and colleges of acupuncture and oriental medicine.

§ 32 – 11 – 4.　General Criteria for Approval of Acupuncture Training Programs.

4.1. The total number of hours of oriental medical theoretical training shall consist of a minimum of eighteen hundred (1,800) hours and the total number of hours of clinical instruction shall consist of a minimum of 300 hours. and the course work shall extend over a minimum period of four (4) academic years or, eight (8) semesters or, twelve (12) quarters or, nine (9) trimesters, or thirty-six (36) months.

4.2. Candidates for admission shall have successfully completed an approved high school course of study or have passed a standard equivalency test.

4.3. The course of training shall be located in a W. Va. State university or college, or an institution approved by the Board, or in the case of training programs located outside West Virginia, in an institution which is approved by the appropriate governmental accrediting authority or an accrediting agency recognized by the U.S. Department of Education.

4.4. The training program shall develop an evaluation mechanism to determine the effectiveness of its theoretical and clinical program.

4.5. Course work shall carry academic credit.

4.6. The director of the clinical portion of the training program shall be a licensed acupuncturist or other licensed practitioner authorized to practice acupuncture.

4.7. All instructors shall be competent to teach their designated courses by virtue of their education, training and experience.

4.8. Each approved course of training shall receive accreditation or approval for schools and colleges by an agency approved by the U. S. Department of Education or the approval of the course of training by the Board shall automatically lapse.

§ 32 – 11 – 5.　Specific Course Requirements for Approval of Acupuncture Training.

5.1. In order to be approved by the Board, pursuant to Code § 30 – 36 – 10 8 1 B an acupuncture course of training shall meet the following course curriculum criteria:

5.1.1. General biology, 8 semester hours;

5.1.2. Chemistry — including organic and biochemistry, 8 semester hours;

5.1.3. General physics — including a general survey of biophysics, 8 semester hours;

5.1.4. General psychology — including counseling skills, 8 semester hours;

5.1.5. Anatomy — a survey of microscopic, gross anatomy and neuroanatomy, 4 semester hours;

5.1.6. Physiology — a survey of basic physiology, including neurophysiology, endocrinology, and neurochemistry, 4 semester hours;

5.1.7. Pathology — a survey of the nature of disease and illness, including microbiology, immunology, psychopathology, and epidemiology, 4 semester hours;

5.1.8. Nutrition and vitamins, homeopathy and herbology, 4 semester hours;

5.1.9. History of medicine — a survey of medical history, including transcultural healing practices, 3 semester hours;

5.1.10. Medical terminology — fundamentals of English language medical terminology, 3 semester hours;

5.1.11. Clinical sciences — a review of internal medicine. pharmacology, neurology, surgery, obstetrics/gynecology, urology, radiology, nutrition and public health, 8 semester hours;

5.1.12. Clinical medicine-a survey of the clinical practice of medicine, osteopathy, dentistry, psychology, nursing, chiropractic, podiatry, and homeopathy to familiarize practitioners with the practices of other health care practitioners, 8 semester hours;

5.1.13. Western pharmacology, 8 semester hours;

5.1.14. Cardiopulmonary resuscitation (CPR), 8 contact hours;

5.1.15. Traditional Oriental medicine-a survey of the theory and practice of traditional diagnostic and therapeutic procedures, 8 semester hours;

5.1.16. Acupuncture anatomy and physiology — fundamentals of acupuncture. including the meridian system, special and extra loci, and auriculotherapy, 8 semester hours;

5.1.17. Acupuncture techniques — instruction in the use of needling techniques, moxibustion, and electroacupuncture, including precautions (e.g., sterilization of needles), contraindication and complications, 8 semester hours;

5.1.18. Acupressure techniques — instruction in the use of manual therapy pressure, 8 semester hours;

5.1.19. Breathing techniques — introductory course in Chi Kung, 4 semester hours;

5.1.20. Traditional Oriental exercise — introductory course in Tai Chi Chuan, 4 semester hours;

5.1.21. Traditional Oriental herbology including botany — a portion of the hours shall be given in a clinical setting, 12 semester hours, plus 100 clinical hours;

5.1.22. Practice management — instruction in the legal and ethical aspects of maintaining a professional practice, including record keeping, professional liability, patient accounts. and referral procedures, 3 semester hours; and

5.1.23. Ethics relating to the practice of acupuncture, 2 semester hours.

5.2. The curriculum shall include adequate clinical instruction, 75% of which shall be in a clinic which is operated by the course of training, which includes direct patient contact where appropriate in the following:

5.2.1. Practice Observation — supervised observation of the clinical practice of acupuncture with case presentations and discussions, 50 clinical hours;

5.2.2. Diagnosis and evaluation — the application of Eastern and Western diagnostic procedures in evaluating patients, 50 clinical hours; and

5.2.3. Supervised practice — the clinical treatment of a patient with acupuncture, 50 clinical hours

5.3. During the initial 100 hours of diagnosis evaluation and clinical practice the supervisor shall be physically present at all times during the diagnosis and treatment of the patient. Thereafter, for a second period of 100 hours the supervisor shall be physically present at the needling of the patient.

5.4. The supervisor shall otherwise be in close proximity to the location at which the patient is being treated during the clinical instruction. The student shall also consult with the supervisor before and after each treatment.

§ 32 – 11 – 6. Course of Training Evaluation.

6.1. Each training program in this State shall develop a mechanism to evaluate and award transfer credit to students for prior course work and experience which is equivalent to that course work and clinical instruction required in section 32 – 11 – 5 of this rule. The course of training's policies and procedures for evaluating and awarding transfer credit shall be set forth in writing and submitted to the Board. The policies and procedures shall include all of the following:

6.2. Credit shall only be awarded for actual course work or directly relevant experience received by the student. As used in this rule, 'experience' means academically relevant learning which involved the student directly in the area of the curriculum required in this section and includes integrated field and clinical internships, apprenticeships, tutorial programs and cooperative educational programs;

6.3. Where the course work and clinical instruction were completed at an acupuncture school not approved by the Board, the evaluation shall include an examination administered by the school in the subject area in which transfer credit may be awarded;

6.4. The outcome of the prior education and experience shall be equivalent to that of an average student who has completed the same subject in the training program and shall meet the curriculum standards and graduation requirements of the training program;

6.5. Transfer credit may be awarded for course work and clinical instruction completed successfully at another acupuncture school or college which is approved by the Board;

6.6. Up to 100% transfer credit may be awarded for courses completed successfully in biology, chemistry, physics, psychology, anatomy, physiology, pathology, nutrition and vitamins, history of medicine, medical terminology, clinical science, clinical medicine, Western pharmacology, cardiopulmonary resuscitation, practice management, and ethics at a school which is approved under or by an accrediting agency recognized by the U.S. Department of Education;

6.7. Credit for clinical course work and instruction in traditional oriental medicine, acupuncture anatomy and physiology, acupuncture techniques, acupressure. breathing techniques, traditional oriental exercise. or traditional oriental herbology completed successfully at a school which is not approved by the Board may be awarded by a school approved by the Board, provided that at least 50% of the course hours in these subject areas are completed successfully at a school approved by the Board;

6.8. The entire record of the training program's evaluation and award of the student's transfer credit shall be included in the student's academic file and shall be made an official part of the student's transcript which shall be filed with the Board upon request of the student; and

6.9. All students shall receive upon matriculation a copy of the training program's policies and procedures for evaluating and awarding transfer credit.

§ 32 – 11 – 7.   Documentation Required for Approval.

Educational institutions or programs seeking approval of an acupuncture training program shall provide the Board with any documents and other evidence as may be necessary for the Board to determine the actual nature and extent of the training offered, including but not limited to. catalogues, course description, curricula plans, and study bulletins.

§ 32 – 11 – 8.   Suspension or Revocation of Approval.

The Board may deny, place on probation. suspend or revoke the approval granted to any acupuncture training program for any failure to comply with W. Va. Code § 30 – 36 – 1 et seq. or this rule.

§ 32 – 11 – 9.   School Monitoring; Records; Reporting.

9.1. Every approved acupuncture school in W. Va. shall to submit the Board within sixty (60) days after the close of the school's fiscal year a current course catalog with a letter outlining the following:

9.1.1. Courses added or deleted or significantly changed from the previous year's curriculum;

9.1.2. Changes in faculty, administration, or the governing body;

9.1.3. Major changes in the school facility; and

9.1.4. A statement regarding the school's financial condition, which enables the committee to evaluate whether the school has sufficient resources to ensure the capability of the program for enrolled students.

9.2. If the Board determines it is necessary representatives of the Board shall make an on-site visit to the school to review and evaluate the status of the school. The school shall reimburse the Board for direct costs incurred in conducting the review and evaluation.

9.3. All student records shall be maintained in English.

9.4. Each approved acupuncture school shall report to the Board within 30 days any substantial changes to the facility or clinic, and curriculum required in this rule.

Series 12. Tutorial Education Requirements

§ 32 – 12 – 1. General.

1.1. Scope. — This section establishes the educational requirements for licensed acupuncture applicants completing a tutorial or apprenticeship program.

1.2. Authority. — W. Va. Code § 30 – 36 – 7.

1.3. Filing Date. — May 21, 1999.

1.4. Effective Date. — May 21, 1999.

§ 32 – 12 – 2. Application.

This legislative rule applies to applicants for licensure and applicants for tutorial programs.

§ 32 – 12 – 3. Definitions.

3.1. Acupuncture tutorial. — An acupuncture apprenticeship program which is approved by the Board pursuant to the Code which when successfully completed meets the requirements of W. Va. Code § 30 – 35 – 10 (3) for licensure as an acupuncturist.

3.2. Supervising acupuncturist. — A licensed acupuncturist who is approved by the Board to provide an acupuncture tutorial to a trainee who is registered with the Board.

3.3. Trainee. — A person who is registered with the Board in order to participate in an acupuncture tutorial under a supervising acupuncturist.

§ 32 – 12 – 4. Prior Approval to Practice as an Acupuncture Trainee.

A person shall obtain prior approval of the Board to practice in acupuncture tutorial.

§ 32 – 12 – 5. Prior Approval to Supervise an Acupuncture Trainee.

An acupuncturist shall obtain prior approval to supervise any acupuncture trainee in an acupuncture tutorial from the Board.

§ 32 – 12 – 6. Filing of Applications: Credit for Prior Training.

6.1. An applicant for acupuncture trainee shall file for approval on a form provided by the Board and accompanied by the required application fee, 32CRS4.

An applicant for supervisor shall file for approval on a form provided by the Board and accompanied by any necessary documents, including the training agreement and the required application fee, 32CRS4.

6.2. An acupuncture trainee with prior training and experience which meets the standards of the Board may reduce the required hours of theoretical and clinical training based on the prior training and experience. Evidence of the prior training and experience should be submitted to the Board for its review with the application for registration of the trainee.

§ 32 – 12 – 7. Requirements for Approval of an Acupuncture Tutorial.

7.1. The supervisor and the acupuncture trainee shall develop a written training agreement containing the required elements of the acupuncture tutorial. The agreement should provide a trainee with a structured learning experience in all the basic skills and knowledge necessary for the independent practice of acupuncture and should prepare the trainee for the Board's examination for acupuncture licensure.

7.2. The training agreement shall specify whether acupuncture tutorial is employment. Employment may be a full-time or part time.

7.3. An acupuncture tutorial shall provide formal clinical training with supplemental theoretical and didactic instruction. That training required in W. Va. Code § 30–36–10 from an approved acupuncture school or another post secondary educational institution which is accredited or approved under or is accredited by a regional accrediting agency authorized by the U.S. Department of Education.

7.4. The clinical training shall consist of a minimum of 300 hours in the following areas:

7.4.1. Practice observation;

7.4.2. History and physical examination;

7.4.3. Therapeutic treatment planning;

7.4.4. Preparation of the patient;

7.4.5. Sterilization, use and maintenance of sterilization equipment;

7.4.6. Moxibustion;

7.4.7. Electroacupuncture (AC and DC voltages);

7.4.8. Body and auricular acupuncture;

7.4.9. Treatment of emergencies, including cardiopulmonary resuscitation;

7.4.10. Pre- and post-treatment instruction to the patient; and

7.4.11. Contraindications and precautions.

7.5. The theoretical and didactic training for tutorials shall consist of a minimum of 2700 hours (approximately 270 semester units) in the following areas:

7.5.1. Traditional Oriental Medicine — a survey of the theory and practice of traditional diagnostic and therapeutic procedures.

7.5.2. Acupuncture anatomy and physiology — fundamentals of acupuncture, including the meridian system special and extra loci, and auriculotherapy.

7.5.3. Acupuncture techniques — instruction in the use of needling techniques, moxibustion, electroacupuncture, including precautions (e.g., sterilization of needles), contraindications and complications.

7.5.4. Clinical medicine — a survey of the clinical practice of medicine, osteopathy, dentistry, psychology, nursing, chiropractic, podiatry and homeopathy to familiarize acupuncture practitioners with the practices of other health care practitioners.

7.5.5. History of Medicine — a survey of medical history, including transcultural healing practices.

7.5.6. Medical terminology — fundamentals of English language medical terminology.

7.5.7. General sciences — a survey of general biology, chemistry, and physics.

7.5.8. Anatomy — a survey of microscopic and gross anatomy and neuroanatomy.

7.5.9. Physiology — a survey of basic physiology, including neurophysiology, endocrinology and neurochemistry.

7.5.10. Pathology — a survey of the nature of disease and illness, including microbiology, immunology, psychopathology, and epidemiology.

7.5.11. Clinical sciences — a review of internal medicine, pharmacology, neurology, surgery, obstetrics/gynecology, urology, radiology, nutrition and public health.

7.6. The acupuncture services provided by the tutorial trainee shall be done so in a manner which does not endanger the health and welfare of patients receiving the services. The tutorial trainee shall inform a patient that the services will be rendered by that trainee. The patient on each occasion of treatment shall be informed of the procedure to be performed by the tutorial trainee under the supervision of the supervising acupuncturist and shall consent in writing prior to performance of the acupuncture procedure by the tutorial trainee. These requirements shall also be applied to those instances where the trainee is to assist the supervisor in the rendering of acupuncture services.

7.7. The acupuncture tutorial training program shall be set forth in a written agreement signed by the supervisor and trainee which sets forth, but is not limited to, the training plan, length of training time, the method for providing the theoretical and didactic training and guidelines for supervision of the acupuncture services rendered by the trainee. A copy of the written agreement shall be submitted with the application for approval.

§ 32‑12‑8.　Supervising Acupuncturist's Responsibilities.

Supervising acupuncturists have the following duties and responsibilities:

8.1. A supervisor shall at all times be responsible for and provide supervision of the work performed by the trainee as required in this rule;

8.2. The supervisor shall only assign those patient treatments which can be safely and effectively performed by the trainee. The supervisor shall provide continuous direction and immediate supervision of the trainee when patient services are provided and shall be in close proximity during needle insertion and extraction;

8.3. The supervisor shall insure that patient informed consent is obtained when necessary;

8.4. The supervisor shall insure that the objectives of the submitted training plan are provided and met by the trainee;

8.5. The supervisor shall insure that the trainee complies with the standards of practice;

8.6. The supervisor shall file quarterly with the Board a progress report on a form provided by the Board which sets forth the schedules for theoretic and didactic training and for clinical training of the trainee;

8.7. The supervisor shall insure that when rendering services or otherwise engaging in professional activity the tutorial trainee always identifies himself or herself as an "acupuncture trainee"; and wears an identification badge stating his or her trainee status;

8.8. The supervisor shall not permit separate billing by the tutorial trainee;

8.9. The supervisor shall comply with the provisions of W. Va. Code § 30 – 36 – 1 et seq., applicable laws and rules governing wages and compensation paid to employees or apprentices, maximum hours and working conditions. Any overtime worked by the trainee shall not interfere with or impair the training program and shall not be detrimental to the health and safety of the trainee or patients.

§ 32 – 12 – 9.   Trainee's Responsibilities.

9.1. The tutorial trainee shall not provide acupuncture services without the required supervision or autonomously, and shall not provide any services for which he or she is not trained or competent to perform;

9.2. The tutorial trainee shall satisfactorily meet the objectives of the training plan submitted to the Board including the necessary theoretical training;

9.3. The tutorial trainee shall comply with the Board's rule Standards of Practice of Acupuncture by Licensed Acupuncturist, 32CRS6;

9.4. The tutorial trainee shall always identify himself or herself as an acupuncture trainee when rendering services or otherwise engaging in professional activity and shall wear an identification badge on an outer garment and in plain view which states the trainee's name and the title "Acupuncture Trainee";

9.5. The tutorial trainee shall report to the Board any delay, interruption or termination of the acupuncture tutorial not reported by the supervisor.

§ 32 – 12 – 10.   Termination or Modification of Tutorial.

10.1. The supervisor shall notify the Board in writing within ten (10) days of the termination of any acupuncture tutorial for any reason. At the time of the notification the Board shall cancel registration of both the supervisor and trainee shall be canceled. If the supervisor or trainee subsequently participate in an acupuncture tutorial, each shall file a new application for registration with the Board.

10.2. If the training plan of the acupuncture tutorial is substantially modified then the Board shall file a report of the modifications with the Board. There is no charge for filing the report.

10.3. If the supervisor is unable to complete the training, the Board at its discretion, may establish a plan to allow the tutorial trainee to complete the course of training. The Board may assign a new supervising acupuncturist.

§ 32 – 12 – 11.   Application for Examination of Credentials and Oral Examination.

At the completion of the tutorial the trainee may file an application for licensure.

§ 32 - 12 - 12. Denial. Suspension or Revocation of Registration as a Supervisor.

The Board may deny, issue subject to terms and conditions, suspend, revoke or place on probation a registration to supervise a trainee in an acupuncture tutorial for the following causes:

(a) Failure to comply with the provisions of the W. Va. Code § 30 - 36 - 1 et seq. or this Rule;

(b) Violation of the standards of practice, 32CRS5;

(c) The supervisor is the subject of a successful disciplinary action or has had charges in a disciplinary action filed against him or her;

(d) The registration was obtained by fraud or misrepresentation or false or misleading information was presented to the Board with respect to an acupuncture tutorial;

(e) Failure of the supervisor or the trainee to comply with patient informed consent; or

(f) The trainee has rendered acupuncture services in violation of this Rule within the setting of the acupuncture tutorial regardless of whether the supervising acupuncturist has knowledge of the acts performed.

§ 32 - 12 - 13. Denial, Suspension or Revocation of Registration as a Trainee.

The Board may deny, issue subject to terms and conditions, suspend, revoke or place on probation a registration as a trainee in an acupuncture tutorial for the following causes:

(a) Failure to comply with this Rule for approval and registration as a trainee;

(b) Violation of the W. Va. Code § 30 - 36 - 1 et seq. or the Board's Rules 32CRS1 et seq.;

(c) The registration was obtained by fraud or misrepresentation or false or misleading information was presented to the Board with respect to the acupuncture tutorial;

(d) Failure to comply with patient informed consent;

(e) The rendering of acupuncture services outside the approved acupuncture tutorial;

(f) Failure to identify oneself as an acupuncture trainee or failure to wear an appropriate identification badge when rendering acupuncture services; or

(g) Rendering acupuncture services under a supervising acupuncturist who is not approved as a supervisor by the Board or whose registration as a supervisor has been suspended.

Series 13. Formation and Approval of Professional Limited Liability Companies

§ 32 - 13 - 1. General.

1.1. Scope. — This legislative rule establishes the procedures for the formation and approval of professional limited liability companies for acupuncturists.

1.2. Authority. — W. Va. Code § 31B - 13 - 1304.

1.3. Filing Date. — May 21, 1999.

1.4. Effective Date. — May 21, 1999.

§ 32 – 13 – 2. Definitions.

2.1. Board. — The West Virginia Board of Acupuncture, established in W. Va. Code § 30 – 36 – 1 et seq.

2.2. Professional limited liability company. — A limited liability company organized under the W. Va. Code § 31B – 13 – 1 et seq. for the purpose of rendering a professional service.

2.3. Professional services. — The services rendered under W. Va. Code § 30 – 36 – 1 et seq., by acupuncturists.

§ 32 – 13 – 3. Procedures for Formation and Approval of Professional Limited Liability Companies for Acupuncturists. Fees.

3.1. Acupuncturists licensed to practice acupuncture in an active status in this State who desire to render acupuncture and oriental medical services as a limited liability company shall comply with the provisions of W. Va. Code § 31B – 13 – 1301 et seq. No professional limited liability company shall have as a member anyone other than a person who is duly licensed or otherwise legally authorized to render the professional services for which the professional limited liability company was organized.

3.2. The name of a professional limited liability company shall contain the words "professional limited liability company" or the abbreviation "P.L.L.C." or "Professional L. L. C."

3.3. Every professional limited liability company shall file with the Board at the time of formation, and on an annual basis on or before the first day of July, the names of its two or more members, and written documentation that the professional limited liability company carries at least one million dollars of professional liability insurance, together with an initial filing fee of $100.00 and annual renewal fee of $100.

3.3.a. The requirement of carrying one million dollars of professional liability insurance is satisfied if the professional limited liability company provides one million dollars of funds specifically designated and segregated for the satisfaction of judgements against the company members or any of its professional or nonprofessional services to patients or clients of the company, by:

3.3.a.1. Deposit in trust or in bank escrow of cash, a bank certificate of deposit or United States treasury obligations; or

3.3.a.2. A bank letter of credit or insurance company bond.

3.4. Every limited liability company shall file with the Board a copy of the annual report required to be filed with the Secretary of State under W. Va. Code § 31B – 2 – 211. The copy of the annual report, and a copy of any corrected annual report filed with the Secretary of State, shall be filed with the Board on or before the first day of July on an annual basis.

3.5. Every professional limited liability company in compliance with all the provisions of this rule shall be approved by and remain approved by the Board.

3.6. If any licensee ceases to be a member of any professional limited liability company, the company shall notify the Board in writing within twenty days therefrom that the licensee has ceased to be a member of a professional limited liability company. The fact that a licensee ceases to be a member of a professional limited liability company shall not affect the approval of such professional limited liability company by the Board, provided that the Board determines that the professional limited liability company remains in compliance with all the provision of this rule.

§ 32 - 13 - 4.   Notification of Non-compliance, Cessation of Rendering Professional Services.

4.1. If the Board determines that a professional limited liability company is not in compliance with all the provisions of this rule and should cease rendering professional services in the State, the Board shall notify the professional limited liability company in writing. Upon receipt of the written notice, the professional limited liability company shall cease rendering professional services in the State.

§ 32 - 13 - 5.   Practitioner-Patient Relationship.

5.1. The provisions of this rule shall not be construed to alter or affect the practitioner-patient relationship.

Series 14.   Auricular Detoxification Therapy Certificate

§ 32 - 14 - 1.   General.

1.1. Scope. — This rule establishes the application, certificate, qualification and terms for auricular acupuncture certificate holders pursuant to W. Va. Code § 30 - 36 - 10.

1.2. Authority. — W. Va. Code § 30 - 36 - 7(d) and § 30 - 36 - 10.

1.3. Filing Date. — April 20, 2020.

1.4. Effective Date. — April 30, 2020.

1.5. Sunset Provision — This rule shall terminate and have no further force or effect upon the expiration of April 30, 2030.

§ 32 - 14 - 2.   Application.

This legislative rule applies to application, issuance of a certificate, renewal, qualifications and terms for auricular acudetox certificate holders.

§ 32 - 14 - 3.   Definitions.

3.1. Auricular acudetox therapy — means therapy as approved by the board or as stipulated by the National Acupuncture Detoxification Association (NADA), for the treatment of substance abuse, alcoholism, chemical dependency, detoxification, behavioral therapy, or trauma recovery. Those persons certified as having successfully completed a course of study necessary to perform auricular detoxification therapy.

3.2. Certificate holder — means those persons issued an authorization by the board to persons trained in auricular acudetox who meet the qualifications to be certified as an auricular detoxification therapist or specialist (ADS).

3.3. National Acupuncture Detoxification Association (NADA protocol) — means the

National Acupuncture Detoxification Association protocol for auricular detoxification therapy.

§ 32 – 14 – 4. Application, Terms and Renewal for Certificate Holders.

4.1. A person seeking a certificate as an Auricular acudetox therapist or Auricular acudetox specialist shall apply to the board on a form prescribed by the board and pay the applicable board fee as established by the board by rule pursuant to Title 32, Series 4, Code of State Rules, Fees of the Board of Acupuncture.

4.2. The certificate of authorization to perform auricular acudetox therapy shall be valid for two years from month ending of the date of issuance by the board and such initial approval shall be communicated in writing to the applicable professional board listed in subsection 5.1.2. of this rule.

4.3. A certificate to perform auricular acudetox therapy shall be renewed by applying to the board for renewal on a form prescribed by the board, as required and accompanied with the payment of the applicable fee.

§ 32 – 14 – 5. Requirements for a Certificate.

5.1. To qualify for a certificate as an auricular detoxification specialist, an applicant shall:

5.1.1. Be at least 18 years old;

5.1.2. Be authorized in this state to engage in any of the following:

5.1.2.a. Physician assistant, pursuant to § 30 – 3E – 1 et seq. of this code;

5.1.2.b. Dentist, pursuant to § 30 – 4 – 1 et seq. of this code;

5.1.2.c. Registered professional nurse, pursuant to § 30 – 7 – 1 et seq. of this code;

5.1.2.d. Practical nurse, pursuant to § 30 – 7A – 1 et seq. of this code;

5.1.2.e. Psychologist, pursuant to § 30 – 21 – 1 et seq. of this code;

5.1.2.f. Occupational therapist, pursuant to § 30 – 28 – 1 et seq. of this code;

5.1.2.g. Social worker, pursuant to § 30 – 30 – 1 et seq. of this code;

5.1.2.h. Professional counselor, pursuant to § 30 – 31 – 1 et seq. of this code;

5.1.2.i. Emergency medical services provider, pursuant to § 16 – 4C – 1 et seq. of this code; or

5.1.2.j. Corrections medical provider, pursuant to § 15A – 1 – 1 et seq. of this code.

5.1.3. Provide evidence of successful completion of a board-approved auricular acudetox program;

5.1.4. Submit a completed application as prescribed by the board; and

5.1.5. Submit the appropriate fees as provided for by legislative rule.

5.2. A certificate may be renewed pursuant to the provision of this rule.

5.3. A certificate holder shall maintain and remain current in the professional competencies and authorizations as required pursuant to West Virginia Code § 30 – 36 – 10 and subsection 5.1.2. of this rule.

§ 32 - 14 - 6. Causes for Denial, Probation, Limitation, Discipline, Suspension or Revocation of Certificates for Auricular Acudetox.

6.1. The board may deny an application for a certificate, place a certificate holder on probation, suspend a certificate, limit or restrict a certificate or revoke any certificate issued by the Board, upon satisfactory proof that the certificate holder has:

6.1.1. Knowingly made, or presented or caused to be made or presented, any false, fraudulent or forged statement, writing, certificate, diploma or other material in connection with an application for a certificate;

6.1.2. Been or is involved in fraud, forgery, deception, collusion or conspiracy in connection with an application for certification;

6.1.3. Become addicted to a controlled substance;

6.1.4. Become a chronic or persistent alcoholic;

6.1.5. Engaged in dishonorable, unethical or unprofessional conduct of a character likely to deceive, defraud or harm the public or member of the public;

6.1.6. Willfully violated a confidential communication;

6.1.7. Had his or her license or other authorizations to practice in the professional capacity pursuant to West Virginia Code § 30 - 36 - 10 and subsection 5.1.2 of this rule, in this or any other state, territory, jurisdiction or foreign nation revoked, suspended, restricted or limited, or otherwise acted against, or has been subjected to any other disciplinary action by the licensing or governing authority thereof, or has been denied licensure or authorizations in this or any other state, territory, jurisdiction, or foreign nation;

6.1.8. Demonstrated a lack of professional competence in performing auricular acudetox with a reasonable degree of skill and safety for patients. In this connection, the Board may consider repeated acts of a certificate holder indicating his or her failure to properly treat a patient and may require the certificate holders to submit to inquiries or examinations, written or oral, by members of the Board, by its agent, or designee, as the Board considers necessary to determine the professional qualifications of the certificate holder;

6.1.9. Engaged in unprofessional conduct, including, but not limited to, any departure from, or failure to conform to, the standards of acceptable practice, pursuant to the guidelines established by the National Acupuncture Detoxification Association protocol for auricular detoxification therapy irrespective of whether a patient is injured by the conduct, or has committed any act contrary to honesty, justice or good morals, whether the act is committed in the course of his or her practice or otherwise and whether committed within or without this State;

6.1.10. With respect to existing certificate holders, been convicted of or found guilty of a crime in any jurisdiction which directly relates to the practice of auricular detoxification therapy or related to the professional or other authorizations as described pursuant to W.Va. Code § 30 - 36 - 10 and subsection 5.1.2. of this rule. A plea of nolo contender [FN1] will be considered conviction for purpose of this rule;

6.1.11. With respect to initial certification, been convicted of a crime in any jurisdiction that remains unreversed and bears a rational nexus to the practice of auricular detoxification therapy or to the professional or other authorizations as described pursuant to W.Va. Code § 30 – 36 – 10 and subsection 5.1.2. of this rule. A plea of nolo contendere will be considered conviction for purposes of this rule. In determining whether a conviction bears a rational nexus to the practice of auricular detoxification therapy or to the professional or other authorizations as described pursuant to W.Va. Code § 30 – 36 – 10 and subsection 5.1.2. of this rule, the board shall consider at a minimum:

6.1.11.a. The nature and seriousness of the crime for which the individual was convicted;

6.1.11.b. The passage of time since the commission of the crime;

6.1.11.c. The relationship of the crime to the ability, capacity, and fitness required to perform the duties and discharge the responsibilities of the profession or occupation; and

6.1.11.d. Any evidence of rehabilitation or treatment undertaken by the individual; and notwithstanding any other statutory provisions to the contrary, in the event that the applicant is disqualified from certification because of a prior criminal conviction the board shall permit a subsequent application in conformity with the W. Va. Code § 30 – 1 – 24.

6.1.12. Advertised, practiced or attempted to practice under a name other than his or her own;

6.1.13. Failed to report to the board any person whom the certificate holder knows is in violation of this rule, the of provisions of the West Virginia Acupuncture Practice Act, or in violation of any standard of professional conduct as described in § 30 – 1 – 1 et seq., of West Virginia Code;

6.1.14. Failed to perform any statutory or legal obligation placed upon a certificate holder;

6.1.15. Made or filed a report which the certificate holder knows to be false, intentionally or negligently failed to file a report or record required by state or federal law, willfully impeded or obstructed the filing or induced another person to do so. The reports or records will include only those which are signed in the capacity as a certificate holder;

6.1.16. Exercised influence within a patient-practitioner relationship for purposes of engaging a patient in sexual activity;

6.1.17. Made deceptive, untrue or fraudulent representations in the practice of auricular detoxification therapy or employed a trick or scheme in the practice of auricular detoxification therapy when the trick or scheme fails to conform to the generally prevailing standards of treatment in the oriental medical community;

6.1.18. Solicited patients, either personally or through an agent, through use of fraud, intimidation, undue influence, or by overreaching or vexatious conduct. A solicitation is any communication which directly or implicitly requests an immediate response from the recipient;

6.1.19. Performed any procedure or prescribed any therapy which, by the prevailing standards of auricular detoxification therapy in the community, that would constitute the experimentation on a human subject, without first obtaining full, informed and written consent from the patient;

6.1.20. Practiced or offered to practice auricular detoxification therapy beyond the scope permitted by the West Virginia Acupuncture Practice Act or accepted and performed professional responsibilities which the certificate holder knows or has reason to know he or she is not competent to perform;

6.1.21. Violated or failed to comply with a lawful order of the Board, or has violated an order of any court entered pursuant to any proceedings commenced by the Board; or

6.1.22. Failing to meet the standard of practice in connection with any supervisory and/or collaborative agreement with any category of health practitioner licensed under Chapter 30 of the W. Va. Code;

6.2. When the board finds that any applicant is unqualified to be granted a certificate or finds that any certificate holder should be disciplined pursuant to the West Virginia Acupuncture Practice Act or rules of the board, the board may take anyone or more of the following actions:

6.2.1. Refuse to grant a certificate to an applicant;

6.2.2. Administer a public reprimand;

6.2.3. Suspend, limit or restrict any certificate for a definite period, not to exceed five (5) years;

6.2.4. Require any certificate holder to participate in a program of education prescribed by the Board;

6.2.5. Revoke any certificate;

6.2.6. Require the certificate holder to submit to care, counseling or treatment by physicians or other professional persons;

6.2.7. Require the certificate holder to practice under the direction or supervision of another practitioner; or

6.2.8. In addition to and in conjunction with these actions, the board may make a finding adverse to the certificate holder or applicant, but withhold imposition of judgment and penalty, or it may impose the judgment and penalty but suspend enforcement of the penalty and place the auricular detoxification therapist on probation, which may be vacated upon the noncompliance with any terms imposed by the board. In its discretion, the board may restore and reissue a certificate under the West Virginia Acupuncture Practice Act, W. Va. Code § 30 – 36 – 1 et. seq., and as a condition it may impose any disciplinary or corrective measure provided for in this Rule or in the West Virginia Acupuncture Practice Act.

§ 32 – 14 – 7. Disciplinary and Complaint Procedures.

7.1 This rule establishes the same complaint process and procedures for an auricular acudetox certificate holder as referenced in Title 32 Legislative Rule Series 7 Disciplinary and Complaint Procedures for Acupuncturists. Once a final agency order or decision has been entered, the Board shall communicate this decision or order to the professional board listed in subsection 5.1.2. of this rule.

§ 32 – 14 – 8. Contested Case Hearing Procedure

8.1 This rule establishes the same contested case hearing procedures for an auricular acudetox certificate holder as referenced in Title 32 Procedural Rule Series 8 Contested Hearing Case Procedure.

Series 15. Application for Waiver of Initial Licensing Fees for Certain Individuals

§ 32 – 15 – 1. General.

1.1. Scope. — This rule establishes procedures for waiving the initial licensing fee for low income individuals and military personnel and their spouses.

1.2. Authority. — W. Va. Code § 30 – 1 – 23, and W. Va. Code § 30 – 36 – 7.

1.3. Filing Date. — April 20, 2020.

1.4. Effective Date. — April 30, 2020.

1.5. Sunset Provision. — This rule shall terminate and have no further force or effect upon the expiration of April 30, 2030.

§ 32 – 15 – 2. Definitions.

2.1. Board means the West Virginia Board of Acupuncture.

2.2. BoAcu-LIW means the Board of Acupuncture waiver form to request a waiver of the initial licensing fee for low income individuals as authorized by W. Va. Code subsection § 30 – 1 – 23.

2.3. BoAcu-MFW means the Board of Acupuncture waiver form to request a waiver of the initial licensing fee for military service members and their spouses as described in W. Va. Code subsection § 30 – 1 – 23.

2.4. "Initial" means obtaining a license in West Virginia for the practice of acupuncture for the first time.

2.5. "Local labor market" means every county in West Virginia, and any county outside of West Virginia if any portion of that county is within fifty miles of the border of West Virginia, pursuant to W.Va. Code § 21 – 1C – 2.

2.6. "Low-income individual" means an individual in the local labor market as defined in W. Va. Code § 21 – 1C – 2, whose household adjusted gross income is below 130 percent of the federal poverty line. This term also includes any person enrolled in a state or federal public assistance program including, but not limited to, the Temporary Assistance for Needy Families Program, Medicaid, or the Supplemental Nutrition Assistance Program.

2.7. "Military families" means any person who serves as an active member of the armed forces of the United States, the National Guard, or a reserve component as described in 38 U. S. C. § 101, honorably discharged veterans of those forces, and their spouses. This term also includes surviving spouses of deceased service members who have not remarried.

§ 32 – 15 – 3. Application for Waiver of Initial Licensure Fees.

3.1. The Board may issue a license to an applicant who meets the requirements of W. Va. Code § 30 – 36 – 3 et seq. and the rules promulgated by the Board, and the Board shall waive the initial licensure fee if the applicant qualifies as a "low-income individual" or as a member of one or more "military families" as defined in this rule.

3.2. Low-income individuals, as defined in this rule, may seek a low income waiver (LIW) of the initial licensure fee for licensure as a professional acupuncturist by submitting with their complete application a low-income waiver of initial licensure fee form, provided by the Board, and all required verification documents as prescribed by the Board. The Board shall review the application and issue a decision within 30 days of receipt of the complete application.

3.3. Military families, as defined in this rule, may seek a military family waiver (MFW) of the initial licensure fee for licensure as a professional acupuncturist by submitting with their complete application a military service verification form, provided by the Board and all required verification documents as prescribed by the Board. The Board shall review the application and issue a decision within 30 days of receipt of the complete application.

§ 32 – 15 – 4. Required Documentation for Waiver of Initial Licensure Fees

4.1. Individuals requesting a waiver of initial licensing fees for low income or military service personnel and their spouses, an applicant shall submit to the Board with the application for initial licensure waiver BoAcu-LIW or BoAcu-MFW form and the appropriate documentation as specified in this section.

4.2. To establish low income eligibility for an initial licensing fee waiver, an applicant shall submit to the Board evidence that the adjusted gross income of the household of the applicant is below 130% of the federal poverty level by submitting documentation of eligibility for:

4.2.1. Temporary Assistance for Needy Families Program;

4.2.2. Medicaid;

4.2.3. Supplemental Nutrition Assistance Program; or

4.2.4. A Federal Tax Return.

4.3. To establish military family eligibility for the initial licensing fee waiver, an applicant shall submit to the Board proof of qualifying military service and proof of eligibility as a qualifying spouse or surviving spouse, as follows:

4.3.1. A service members DD – 214 form;

4.3.2. A service members NGB – 22 form;

4.3.3. A service members DD – 1300 form; or

4.3.4. A copy of their current military orders; or

4.3.5. Other official military documentation, determined to be appropriate by the Board, demonstrating the service member's qualifying past or current military service; and

4.3.6. A copy of the marriage certificate with the qualifying service member where applicable, the death certificate of the service member if the surviving spouse is applying for the military family waiver and where applicable a notarized affidavit from the surviving spouse verifying the surviving spouse has not remarried.

4.4. Honorably discharged applicants shall submit to the Board a completed application and a DD – 214 form or an NGB – 22 form showing the applicant has been honorably discharged from military service.

Series 16. Consideration of Prior Criminal Convictions in Initial Licensure Determinations

§ 32 – 16 – 1. General.

1.1. Scope. — This rule establishes procedures for consideration of prior criminal convictions in initial licensure determinations.

1.2. Authority. — W. Va. Code § 30 – 1 – 24, and W. Va. Code § 30 – 36 – 7.

1.3. Filing Date. — April 20, 2020.

1.4. Effective Date. — April 30, 2020.

1.5. Sunset Provision. — This rule shall terminate and have no further force or effect upon the expiration of April 30, 2030.

§ 32 – 16 – 2. Definitions.

2.1. "Board" means the Board of Acupuncture established pursuant to W. Va. Code § 30 – 36 – 3.

2.2. "Initial license" means obtaining a license in West Virginia for the practice of acupuncture for the first time.

2.3. "License" or "licensure" means the official authorization by the board to engage in the practice of acupuncture.

2.4. "Unreversed", as that term refers to a criminal conviction, means that a conviction has not been set aside, vacated, pardoned, or expunged.

§ 32 – 16 – 3. Rational nexus to the practice of acupuncture.

3.1. The board may not disqualify an applicant from initial licensure because of a prior criminal conviction that remains unreversed unless that conviction is for a crime that bears a rational nexus to the practice of acupuncture. In determining whether a criminal conviction bears a rational nexus to the practice of acupuncture, the board shall consider at a minimum:

3.1.1. The nature and seriousness of the crime for which the individual was convicted;

3.1.2. The passage of time since the commission of the crime;

3.1.3. The relationship of the crime to the ability, capacity, and fitness required to perform the duties and discharge the responsibilities of a licensed acupuncturist; and

3.1.4. Any evidence of rehabilitation or treatment undertaken by the individual.

§ 32 - 16 - 4. Application after denial.

4.1. Notwithstanding any other provision of the West Virginia Code to the contrary, if an applicant has been denied licensure because of a prior criminal conviction, the board shall permit the applicant to apply for initial licensure if:

4.1.1. A period of five years has elapsed from the date of conviction or the date of release from incarceration, whichever is later;

4.1.2. The individual has not been convicted of any other crime during the period of time following the disqualifying offense; and

4.1.3. The conviction was not for an offense of a violent or sexual nature: *Provided*, That a conviction for an offense of a violent or sexual nature may subject an individual to a longer period of disqualification from licensure, to be determined by the board on a case by case basis.

§ 32 - 16 - 5. Petition for licensure eligibility determination.

5.1. An individual with a criminal record who has not previously applied for licensure may petition the board at any time for a determination of whether the individual's criminal record will disqualify the individual from obtaining a license.

5.2. The petition shall be submitted on an application form prescribed by the board and shall include sufficient details about the individual's criminal record to enable the board to identify the jurisdiction where the conviction occurred, the date of the conviction and the specific nature of the conviction.

5.3. The applicant may submit with the petition for licensure eligibility evidence of rehabilitation, letters of reference, and any other information the applicant deems relevant to show fitness and the ability to practice acupuncture.

5.4. The board shall provide the determination within 60 days of receiving the petition from the applicant.

GEORIGA

CODE OF GEORGIA ANNOTATED

§ 43 – 34 – 60. Short title

This article shall be known and may be cited as the "Acupuncture Act of Georgia."

§ 43 – 34 – 61. Legislative findings

The General Assembly finds and declares that the practice of acupuncture in Georgia affects the public health, safety, and welfare and that it is necessarily a proper subject of regulation and control.

§ 43 – 34 – 62. Definitions

As used in this article, the term:

(1) "Acupuncture" means a form of therapy developed from traditional and modern Oriental concepts for health care that employs Oriental medical techniques, treatment, and adjunctive therapies for the promotion, maintenance, and restoration of health and the prevention of disease.

(2) "Auricular (ear) detoxification therapy" means the insertion of disposable acupuncture needles into the five auricular acupuncture points stipulated by the National Acupuncture Detoxification Association protocol for the sole purpose of treatment of chemical dependency.

(3) "Board" means the Georgia Composite Medical Board.

(4) "Practice of acupuncture" means the insertion of disposable acupuncture needles and the application of moxibustion to specific areas of the human body based upon Oriental medical principles as a therapeutic modality. Dry needling is a technique of the practice of acupuncture. Adjunctive therapies within the scope of acupuncture may include manual, mechanical, herbal, thermal, electrical, and electromagnetic treatment and the recommendation of dietary guidelines and exercise, but only if such treatments, recommendations, and exercises are based on concepts of traditional Oriental medicine and are directly related to acupuncture therapy.

§ 43 – 34 – 63. Powers of Composite State Board of Medical Examiners

The board, in consultation with the advisory committee, shall have the power and responsibility to:

(1) Determine the qualifications and fitness of applicants for licensure and renewal of licensure;

(2) Adopt and revise rules consistent with the laws of this state that are necessary to conduct its business, carry out its duties, and administer this article;

(3) Examine for, approve, issue, deny, revoke, suspend, and renew the licenses of acupuncture applicants and licensed acupuncturists under this article and conduct hearings in connection with these actions;

(4) Conduct hearings on complaints concerning violations of this article and the rules adopted under this article and cause the prosecution and enjoinder of the violations;

(5) Establish application, examination, and licensure fees;

(6) Request and receive the assistance of state educational institutions or other state agencies and prepare information of consumer interest describing the regulatory functions of the board and the procedures by which consumer complaints are filed with and resolved by the board. The board shall make the information available to the public and appropriate state agencies; and

(7) Establish continuing education requirements.

§ 43 - 34 - 64. Requirements for licensure

(a) Each applicant for a license to practice acupuncture shall meet the following requirements:

(1) Be at least 21 years of age;

(2) Submit a completed application required by the board;

(3) Submit any fees required by the board;

(4) Be certified in acupuncture by a national certification agency accredited by the National Organization of Competency Assurance and approved by the board;

(5) Have successfully completed a nationally recognized clean needle technique course approved by the board;

(6) Have obtained professional liability insurance in the amount of at least $100,000.00/ $300,000.00;

(7) Have passed an acupuncture examination offered by an organization accredited by the National Organization of Competency Assurance and approved by the board; and

(8) Have successfully completed a degree in acupuncture or a formal course of study and training in acupuncture. The applicant shall submit documentation satisfactory to the board to show that such education or course of study and training was:

(A) Completed at a school that is accredited by the Accreditation Commission for Acupuncture and Oriental Medicine (ACAOM) or other accrediting entity approved by the board: or

(B) Completed by means of a program of acupuncture study and training that is substantially equivalent to the acupuncture education offered by an accredited school of acupuncture approved by the board.

(b) Reserved.

(c) Before any person licensed to practice acupuncture under this article, who has less than one year of postgraduate clinical experience, may practice on his or her own, such person must engage in one year of active practice under the supervision of a licensed acupuncturist with a minimum of four years active licensed clinical practice. Such supervising acupuncturist may be licensed in Georgia or any other state or country with licensing requirements substantially equal to Georgia's licensing requirements and may accumulate the required four years of active licensed clinical practice in any combination of states so long as the licensing requirements of such other states or countries are substantially equal to Georgia's licensing requirements.

(d) Each applicant for a license to perform auricular (ear) detoxification therapy as an auricular (ear) detoxification technician shall meet the following requirements:

(1) Be at least 21 years of age;

(2) Submit a completed application required by the board;

(3) Submit any fees required by the board;

(4) Have successfully completed a nationally recognized training program in auricular (ear) detoxification therapy for the treatment of chemical dependency as approved by the board; and

(5) Have successfully completed a nationally recognized clean needle technique course approved by the board.

(e) The practice of auricular (ear) detoxification therapy may take place in a city, county, state, federal, or private chemical dependency program approved by the board under the direct supervision of a licensed acupuncturist or a person authorized to practice acupuncture by the board who is also authorized to practice medicine under Article 2 of this chapter.

§ 43 – 34 – 65. Notice of acceptance or rejection of application for license

After evaluation of an application and other evidence submitted by an applicant, the board shall notify such applicant that the application and evidence submitted are satisfactory and accepted or unsatisfactory and rejected. If an application is rejected, the notice shall state the reasons for rejection.

§ 43 – 34 – 66. Surrender of license; display of license; change of address

(a) Any document evidencing licensure issued by the board is the property of the board and must be surrendered on demand.

(b) Every person who holds a license issued by the board in accordance with this article and who is engaged in the active practice of acupuncture or the active practice of auricular (ear) detoxification therapy as an auricular (ear) detoxification technician shall display the document evidencing licensure in an appropriate and public manner.

(c) Every person who holds a license issued by the board shall inform the board of any change of address.

§ 43 – 34 – 67.　Renewal of license; inactive status

(a) A license issued under this article shall be renewed biennially if the person holding such license is not in violation of this article at the time of application for renewal and if the application fulfills current requirements of continuing education as established by the board.

(b) Each person licensed under this article is responsible for renewing his or her license before the expiration date.

(c) Under procedures and conditions established by the board, a license holder may request that his or her license be declared inactive. The licensee may apply for active status at any time and, upon meeting the conditions set by the board, shall be declared active.

§ 43 – 34 – 68.　Informed consent

(a) Any person who undergoes acupuncture must consent to such procedure and shall be informed in general terms of the following:

(1) That the practice of acupuncture is based upon the Oriental arts and is completely distinct and different from traditional western medicine;

(2) That the acupuncturist cannot practice medicine, is not making a medical diagnosis of the person's disease or condition, and that such person should see a physician if he or she wants to obtain a medical diagnosis; and

(3) The nature and the purpose of the acupuncture treatment.

(b) The board shall develop a standard informed consent form to be used by persons licensed under this article. Such informed consent form shall include the information set forth in subsection (a) of this Code section as well as any other and additional information the board deems appropriate. The information set forth in the informed consent form shall be in language which is easy to read and readily understandable to the consuming public.

§ 43 – 34 – 69.　Prohibited conduct; sanctions

The board, in consultation with the advisory committee, may impose any sanction authorized under subsection (b) of Code Section 43 – 34 – 8 upon a finding of any conduct specified in subsection (a) of Code Section 43 – 34 – 8 or a finding that such conduct involved dividing or agreeing to divide a fee for acupuncture services with any person who refers a patient, notwithstanding that such board is not a professional licensing board.

§ 43 – 34 – 70.　Acupuncture advisory committee

The board shall appoint an acupuncture advisory committee. The advisory committee shall include members of the acupuncture profession licensed to practice acupuncture under this article, persons licensed to practice medicine under Article 2 of this chapter who are acupuncturists, and such members as the board in its discretion may determine. Members shall receive no compensation for service on the committee. The committee shall have such advisory duties and responsibilities as the board may determine. Acupuncture advisory committee members must be licensed pursuant to this article.

§ 43 – 34 – 71. Prohibited practices and representations; exceptions; penalties

(a) Unless licensed under this article or exempted under subsection (b) of this Code section, no person shall:

(1) Practice acupuncture or auricular (ear) detoxification therapy; or

(2) Represent himself or herself to be an acupuncturist or auricular (ear) detoxification technician who is licensed under this article.

(b) The prohibition in subsection (a) of this Code section does not apply to:

(1) Any person licensed to practice medicine under Article 2 of this chapter;

(2) The practice of acupuncture which is an integral part of the program of study by students enrolled in an acupuncture education program under the direct clinical supervision of a licensed acupuncturist with at least five years of clinical experience; or

(3) The practice of acupuncture by any person licensed or certified to perform acupuncture in any other jurisdiction that has requirements equivalent to or more stringent than this article where such person is doing so in the course of regular instruction in an approved educational program of acupuncture or in an educational seminar of an approved professional organization of acupuncture, provided that in the latter case the practice is supervised directly by a person licensed to practice acupuncture pursuant to this article or an acupuncturist who is licensed to practice medicine under Article 2 of this chapter.

(c) Any person violating subsection (a) of this Code section shall, upon conviction thereof, be guilty of a misdemeanor.

§ 43 – 34 – 72. Use of titles

(a) The titles "Licensed Acupuncturist" (L. Ac.) and "Acupuncturist" may only be used by persons licensed under this article.

(b) The title "Auricular Detoxification Technician" (A. D. T.) may only be used by persons licensed to practice auricular (ear) detoxification therapy under this article. Possession of a license to practice as an A.D.T. does not by itself entitle a person to identify himself or herself as an acupuncturist. An auricular (ear) detoxification technician is strictly limited to five ear points' treatment for detoxification for substance abuse, chemical dependency, or both.

(c) No person licensed under this article may advertise or hold himself or herself out to the public as being authorized to practice medicine under Article 2 of this chapter.

GEORGIA ADMINISTRATIVE CODE

360 – 6 –.01. Acupuncture. Purpose.

The purpose of these Rules is to implement the "Acupuncture Act of Georgia" ("Act") which authorizes the Composite State Board of Medical Examiners ("Board") to adopt rules and regulations and perform all acts necessary in carrying out the program of licensure for Acupuncture and Auricular Detoxification Therapy. These rules establish the standards for licensing persons to practice acupuncture and auricular (ear) detoxification therapy and for the enforcement of such standards through disciplinary action. These rules are also intended to inform all physicians, other allied health care professionals, and all persons who desire to become licensed about the Act and its requirements.

360 – 6 –.02. Definitions.

The terms used in these Rules, promulgated pursuant to the Act, are defined as follows:

(1) "ACAOM" means the Accreditation Commission for Acupuncture and Oriental Medicine which is a nationally recognized accreditation organization that accredits programs in acupuncture and oriental medicine.

(2) "Act" means the Acupuncture Act of Georgia, O.C.G.A. §§ 43 – 34 – 60 *et seq.*

(3) "Acupuncture" means a form of therapy developed from traditional and modern Oriental concepts for health care that employs Oriental medicine techniques, treatment, and adjunctive therapies for the promotion, maintenance, and restoration of health and the prevention of disease.

(4) "Advisory Committee" means the Acupuncture Advisory Committee of the Georgia Composite Medical Board.

360 – 6 –.03. Licensure Requirements for Acupuncture

(1) Each applicant for licensure as an acupuncturist must meet the requirements listed below.

(a) An affidavit that the applicant is a United States citizen, a legal permanent resident of the United States, or that he/she is a qualified alien or non-immigrant under the Federal Immigration and Nationality Act. If the applicant is not a U.S. citizen, he/she must submit documentation that will determine his/her qualified alien status. The Board participates in the DHS-USCIS SAVE (Systematic Alien Verification for Entitlements or "SAVE") program for the purpose of verifying citizenship and immigration status information of non-citizens. If the applicant is a qualified alien or non-immigrant under the Federal Immigration and Nationality Act, he/she must provide the alien number issued by the Department of Homeland Security or other federal immigration agency.

(b) Must be at least 21 years of age and of good moral character;

(c) Submit a completed application required by the Board. Said application shall not be considered completed until all fees have been paid and all required documents have been eceived[1] by the Board;

(d) Must submit three (3) acceptable references: one reference from a licensed United States physician either MD or DO in the jurisdiction where the applicant is practicing and who is familiar with the applicant's practice and two references from practicing acupuncturists familiar with the applicant's practice.

(e) Have successfully completed a degree in acupuncture or a formal course of study and training in acupuncture. The applicant shall submit documentation satisfactory to the board to show that such education or course of study and training was:

1. Completed at a school that is accredited by the Accreditation Commission for Acupuncture and Oriental Medicine (ACAOM) or other accrediting entity approved by the board; or

2. Completed by means of a program of acupuncture study and training that is substantially equivalent to the acupuncture education offered by an accredited school of acupuncture approved by the board.

(f) Have passed an acupuncture examination offered by an organization accredited by the National Organization of Competency Assurance and approved by the board;

(g) Submit proof of certification in acupuncture by the National Certification Commission for Acupuncture and Oriental Medicine;

(h) Completed successfully a clean needle technique course approved by the Board; and

(i) Submitted proof of having professional liability insurance of at least $100,000/ $300,000.

1. If the licensee changes liability carriers, is canceled by a liability carrier, or cancels liability coverage, the licensee must notify the Board within thirty (30) days of the date of change or cancellation.

2. Failure to maintain liability coverage, pursuant to the Act, may result in suspension of the license for acupuncture.

(i) [1] An applicant must submit all documentation required for the application process within twelve months from the date the Board receives the application.

(2) Every person who holds a license issued by the Board shall inform the Board of any change of address and any other change of information, including but not limited to professional liability coverage, for licensure by this Rule or the Act.

(3) The titles "Licensed Acupuncturist" and "Acupuncturist" shall only be used by persons licensed to practice acupuncture pursuant to the Act and these Rules.

360 - 6 -.04. Display of Name Tag and License for Acupuncture.

(1) A person licensed as an acupuncturist providing services in this state in a hospital, practice setting, nursing home, assisted living community or personal care home shall communicate the acupuncturist's specific licensure to all current and prospective patients and shall wear a clearly legible identification tag during all patient encounters with the licensee's name and the word "Acupuncturist."

(2) In all advertising that names a person in relation to his or her healthcare practice, a person licensed to practice as an acupuncturist in Georgia shall identify themselves as an acupuncturist.

(3) Every person who is licensed to practice acupuncture pursuant to the Act and these Rules and who is actively practicing acupuncture or the active practice of auricular (ear)

detoxification therapy as an auricular （ear） detoxification technician shall display the license issued by the Board in a public and appropriate manner.

（4）Any license or document evidencing licensure issued by the Board is the property of the Board and shall be surrendered on demand.

360 − 6 −.05. Supervised Practice of Acupuncture.

（1）Any person licensed to practice acupuncture under the Act （"practitioner"） who has less than one （1） year of postgraduate clinical experience may not practice on his or her own unless and until such person has completed one （1） year of active clinical practice under the supervision of a duly licensed acupuncturist. The supervising acupuncturist （"supervisor"） shall be currently licensed in Georgia and shall have four （4） years of active licensed clinical experience as an acupuncturist in Georgia or a combination of four （4）years experience in other states or countries as long as the other states or countries substantially equal or exceed Georgia's standards for licensure of acupuncturists.

（2）The supervision of postgraduate clinical practice of an acupuncture practitioner shall comply with the following provisions and guidelines.

（a）Definitions：

1. "Practitioner" is the person who is being supervised and monitored by the supervisor while performing acupuncture during postgraduate clinical practice.

2. "Supervisor" is the acupuncturist who meets the qualifications of this rule and the applicable statute who is responsible for the supervision of the practitioner during supervised postgraduate clinical practice.

3. "Supervised postgraduate clinical practice" is the practice of acupuncture performed by a practitioner under the direct supervision of an approved acupuncturist in facilities approved by the Georgia Composite Medical Board （"Board"）, in consultation with the Acupuncture Advisory Committee （"Advisory Committee"）, pursuant to the provisions of O.C.G.A. § 43 − 34 − 64 （c） and this rule.

（b）Supervisor：A supervisor shall be approved to supervise a practitioner by the Board, in consultation with the Advisory Committee. The supervisor must be licensed in Georgia as an acupuncturist and actively practicing in this state. The supervisor shall have no less than four （4） years of active licensed clinical experience as an acupuncturist. The four （4） years of active licensed clinical experience may be four （4） combined years of active licensed practice in Georgia or in other states or countries as long the standards for licensure of acupuncturists in said states or countries are substantially equivalent to or exceed the standards of licensure in Georgia.

（c）Supervision：The supervisor and practitioner who are engaged in supervised post clinical practice shall adhere to the following guidelines：

1. Plan of supervision：

（i）The supervisor shall submit a letter of intent and a written outlined plan of supervision to the Board, which shall be reviewed and approved by the Board, in consultation with the Advisory Committee, before supervised practice is begun.

(ii) The supervisor must be present on site and available at all times while the practitioner is seeing and treating patients. The practitioner shall practice in the same office with the supervisor.

(iii) A supervisor may not enter into a plan of supervision with more than two practitioners at a time.

2. Monitoring: The supervisor shall monitor no less than one (1) supervised patient treatment performed by the practitioner no less than every other week or bi-weekly. Monitoring shall include case review, supervision of safety procedures, clean needle technique, and assessment of professionalism of the practitioner.

3. Records:

(i) Patient treatment records: The supervisor shall keep written records of the supervised patient treatments by the practitioner and shall submit a summary of the patient treatment records along with quarterly reports to the Board for its review, in consultation with the Advisory Committee. The records shall include any information relevant to patient treatment that is included in the monitoring by the supervisor of the practitioner.

(ii) Practice records:

I. For supervisory purposes, practice is defined as performing a minimum of 500 acupuncture treatments on at least 100 different patients during a one (1) year or twelve (12) months supervised clinical period. Substance abuse or detoxification treatments are not acupuncture treatments for the purposes of supervised postgraduate clinical acupuncture practice.

II. Full and complete records with all relevant and supportive documentation are to be kept at the site of treatment at all times and made available to the Board for review and inspection. Records shall include, but not be limited to, appointment schedules, patient records, treatment records, receipts, and data pertaining to invoice and payment for acupuncture treatment.

4. Reports:

(i) Quarterly reports: Quarterly reports shall be submitted to the Board by the supervisor and shall include the performance, progress and understanding of basic skills of the practitioner. The report shall also include the number of patients that the practitioner has seen per month and the number of acupuncture treatments provided by the practitioner. Quarterly reports shall be filed with the Board and are due three, six, nine, and twelve months after provisional licensure issue date.

(ii) Final supervisory report: At the end of the probationary period, a final review from the supervisor shall be submitted about the practitioner's progress with a recommendation to the Board regarding fitness of the practitioner to practice acupuncture as a solo practitioner. The report shall be reviewed by the Advisory Committee and a recommendation made by the Advisory Committee concerning Board action.

(d) Provisions regarding supervised practice may also be used as guidelines for restrictions placed upon the practice of acupuncture by persons licensed by the Board as authorized by statute.

(e) Failure to adhere to guidelines regarding supervised postgraduate clinical practice may result in sanctions, restrictions, or disciplinary actions upon licensees by the Board.

360－6－.06. License Requirements for Auricular Detoxification Technician.

(1) Each applicant for a license to perform auricular (ear) detoxification therapy as an auricular (ear) detoxification technician must meet the requirements listed below. If an applicant does not meet all requirements for licensure stated in this Rule, the Board may, in its discretion, grant a license to an applicant upon the recommendation of the Advisory Committee.

(a) Be at least 21 years of age and of good moral character;

(b) Submit a completed application as required by the Board;

(c) Submit an application fee as required by the Board;

(d) Have successfully completed a nationally recognized training program in auricular (ear) detoxification therapy for the treatment of chemical dependence as approved by the Board; and

(e) Have successfully completed a nationally recognized clean needle technique course approved by the Board.

(f) Submit verification of applicant's coverage by employer's professional liability insurance.

(g) An applicant must satisfactorily complete all requirements for licensure within one year from the date the Board receives the application.

(2) The practice of auricular (ear) detoxification therapy may take place only in a city, county, state, federal or private chemical dependency program approved by the Board and under the direct supervision of a licensed acupuncturist or a person licensed to practice acupuncture by the Board who is also authorized to practice medicine in the State of Georgia.

(3) The title "Auricular Detoxification Technician (ADT)" may only be used by persons licensed pursuant to the Act and these rules who practice auricular (ear) detoxification therapy. Licensure as an ADT does not by itself entitle a person to use the title "Acupuncturist" or "Licensed Acupuncturist."

(4) Every person who holds a license issued by the Board shall inform the Board of any change of address or any other change of information, including but not limited to a change of employment, required for licensure pursuant to the Act and these Rules.

(5) A license for an Auricular Detoxification Technician (ADT) is limited to and only valid for the employer designated at time of licensure. The ADT licensee shall be covered by the professional liability insurance of the licensee's employer.

(a) If an ADT licensee changes employers, the licensee must file a "Request To Change Employers" form with the Board and must receive permission from the Board to change employers.

(b) If an ADT licensee terminates employment with the designated employer, the ADT license becomes automatically inactive until such time a new application is made.

(6) Every person who holds a license issued by the Board as an Auricular Detoxification Technician must wear an identification badge stating their name and title at all times while rendering therapy.

360 – 6 –.07. Display of License for Auricular Detoxification Technician.

(1) Every person who is licensed to practice auricular (ear) detoxification therapy pursuant to the Act and these Rules and who is actively practicing auricular (ear) detoxification therapy shall display the license issued by the Board in a public and appropriate manner.

(2) Any license or document evidencing licensure issued by the Board is the property of the Board and shall be surrendered on demand.

360 – 6 –.08. Unlicensed Practice of Acupuncture and Auricular Detoxification Therapy Prohibited. Exemptions.

(1) No person shall:

(a) Practice acupuncture or auricular detoxification therapy in Georgia without a license; or

(b) Represent himself or herself to be an Acupuncturist or Auricular Detoxification Technician if he or she is not licensed under the Act.

(2) The following persons are exempt from licensure by the Board to practice acupuncture or auricular detoxification therapy in Georgia:

(a) Students who practice acupuncture as an integral part of a program of study and who are enrolled in a Board-approved acupuncture education program under the direct clinical supervision of a licensed acupuncturist with at least five years of clinical experience; or

(b) Persons who are licensed or certified to perform acupuncture in any other jurisdiction where such persons are doing so in the course of regular instruction in a Board-approved educational program of acupuncture or in an educational seminar of a Board-approved professional organization of acupuncture; provided that in the latter case, the practice is supervised directly by a person licensed to practice acupuncture pursuant to the Act or an acupuncturist who is licensed to practice medicine under Georgia law.

360 – 6 –.09. Physicians.

Licensed physicians desiring to practice acupuncture in Georgia shall successfully complete a Board-approved 300 hour course and notify the Board in writing of their intent to practice acupuncture no less than thirty (30) days prior to incorporating such therapies into their medical practice. Physicians authorized by the Board to perform acupuncture are entitled to the same rights and privileges as those licensed to practice acupuncture and auricular detoxification therapy.

360 – 6 –.10. Composition and Responsibilities of the Acupuncture Advisory Committee.

(1) The intention and policy of the Board is to reflect the cultural diversity of the citizens of Georgia in the composition of the Acupuncture Advisory Committee ("Advisory Committee"). The Advisory Committee shall be comprised as follows:

(a) At least four (4) appointees, including one (1) individual who may be a lay person or a licensed acupuncturist, three (3) individuals who are licensed acupuncturists and representative of the acupuncture profession and other such individuals as the Board, in its discretion, may determine.

1. At time of appointment by the Board, such individuals shall be licensed to practice acupuncture;

2. All appointees to the Advisory Committee shall have on file with the Executive Director of the Board, or his/her designee, a resume and three (3) letters of recommendation, (one of which may be from a physician familiar with the appointee's practice of acupuncture);

3. In order to preserve continuity on the Advisory Committee, two (2) appointees shall serve a two year term and two (2) appointees shall serve a one year term which will be considered a partial term. At the time of appointment, each appointee will be notified in writing by the Executive Director of the Board as to the beginning and ending dates of their respective appointment terms. Each may reapply to the full Board to serve an additional term, but may not serve more than two consecutive terms;

4. In the event an Advisory Committee member is replaced during a term, the replacement member will serve the remaining time of that term as a partial term. An Advisory Committee member who serves a partial term will, after the completion of the partial term, be eligible to serve two consecutive two-year terms;

5. Appointees shall serve without compensation from the State of Georgia for their time and expenses;

(b) One (1) individual who is a licensed physician and who practices or teaches acupuncture who:

1. Shall serve a two year term and may be reappointed for an additional two year term by a majority vote of the Board, but may not serve more than two consecutive terms; and

2. Shall serve without compensation for time and expenses from the State of Georgia; and

(2) The Advisory Committee shall advise the Board on matters pertaining to the appointment of the Advisory Committee members and on all matters within the purview of the Act. The Board, in consultation with the Advisory Committee, shall:

(a) Determine the qualifications and fitness of applicants for licensure and renewal of licensure;

(b) Adopt and revise rules consistent with the laws of the State of Georgia that are necessary to conduct its duties and administer the Act; and

(c) Examine, approve, issue, deny, revoke, suspend and renew the license of applicants and licensees and conduct hearings in connection with all duties to be performed pursuant to the Act.

(3) Advisory Committee members, who are not members of the Board, must be available

to meet on an as needed basis and may not miss more than three (3) consecutive meetings of the Advisory Committee, or four (4) meetings in a calendar year, without an excused absence from either the Executive Director of the Board or the Board President.

(a) The Advisory Committee may recommend to the Board the removal of a member for violation of the attendance rule. Such a recommendation shall be by majority vote of the Advisory Committee.

(b) Upon receipt of a recommendation for removal, the Board may remove a member of the Advisory Committee by a majority vote.

(4) Advisory Committee vacancies may be filled by the Board upon recommendation from the Advisory Committee by advertising on the Board's web page or by any other appropriate means. All applicants must meet any deadline set by the Board and shall have on file with the Executive Director of the Board, or with his/her designee, a resume and three (3) letters of recommendation (one of which may be from a physician familiar with the applicant's practice of acupuncture).

360 – 6 –.11.　License Renewal

(1) All licenses issued pursuant to the Act shall be renewed on a biennial basis. The license will expire on the last day of the month in which the applicant's birthday falls.

(2) Failure to renew a license by the expiration date shall result in a penalty for late renewal as required by the Board.

(3) Licenses not renewed within three (3) months of expiration shall be administratively revoked for failure to renew and shall be posted to the public and posted on the Board's website.

(4) Notwithstanding the provisions of paragraph (3) of this Rule, any service member as defined in O.C.G.A. § 15 – 12 – 1 whose license expired while serving on active duty outside the state shall be permitted to practice in accordance with the expired license and shall not be charged with a violation relating to such practice on an expired license for a period of six (6) months from the date of his or her discharge from active duty or reassignment to a location within the state. Such service member shall be entitled to renew such expired license without penalty within six (6) months after the date of his or her discharge from active duty or reassignment to a location within this state. The service member must present to the Board a copy of the official military orders or written verification signed by the service member's commanding officer to waive any charges.

(5) To be eligible for renewal, a licensee must furnish satisfactory evidence of having met 40 hours of Board approved continuing education requirements, including a minimum of one hour concerning infectious disease.

(6) Licensees must certify on the renewal form that they have read, understand and are familiar with the Centers for Disease Control and Prevention (CDC) guidelines for preventing the transmission of the Human Immuno-deficiency virus, Ebola, Hepatitis B and C and other

infectious diseases.

(7) Licensees are subject to audit to determine compliance with the continuing education requirements as stipulated in rules promulgated by the Board.

(8) Failure to maintain continuing education requirements is a basis for non-renewal and revocation of license issued pursuant to the Act.

(9) All renewal applicants must provide an affidavit and a secure and verifiable document in accordance with O.C.G.A. 50 – 36 – 1 (f). If the applicant has previously provided a secure and verifiable document and affidavit of United States citizenship, no additional documentation of citizenship is required for renewal. If the applicant for renewal is not a United States citizen, he/she must submit documentation that will determine his/her qualified alien status. The Board participates in the DHS-USCIS SAVE (Systematic Alien Verification for Entitlements or "SAVE") program for purpose of verifying citizenship and immigration status information of non-U.S. citizens. If the applicant for renewal is a qualified alien or non-immigrant under the Federal Immigration and Nationality Act, he/she must provide the alien number issued by the Department of Homeland Security or other federal agency.

360 – 6 –.12. Disposal of Biohazard Material and Clean Needle Inventory Records and Used Needle Inventory Records.

(1) The practice of acupuncture and auricular (ear) detoxification is found to affect the public health, safety and welfare and is a proper subject of regulation.

(2) As acupuncture and auricular (ear) detoxification are prolonged invasive procedures of the human skin utilizing sharp instruments, all necessary precautions should be taken for the prevention of the transmission of the Human Immuno-deficiency Virus, (the virus known to cause Acquired Immune Deficiency Syndrome), Hepatitis B and C and other infectious diseases. Persons licensed under this Act and those exempt individuals practicing acupuncture should take all measures to conform to the most current recommendations of the Centers for Disease Control and Prevention (CDC) for preventing transmission of Human Immuno-deficiency Virus, Hepatitis B and C and other infectious diseases to patients during prolonged invasive procedures that are contained in the Morbidity and Mortality Weekly Report 1991; 40 (No. RR – 8) pages 1 – 9. It is the responsibility of all persons currently licensed by the Board to maintain familiarity with these recommendations, which are considered by the Board to be the minimum standards of acceptable and prevailing medical practice. Failing to meet these minimum standards will be considered by the Board to be unprofessional conduct and subject to review and disciplinary action by the Board.

(3) Disposable acupuncture needles are considered a biohazard waste material and must be disposed of in accordance with all applicable federal and state laws, rules and regulations. To further ensure the public health and safety of the citizens of Georgia, persons licensed under this Act and exempt individuals practicing acupuncture must keep accurate medical and office records

that reflect the following detailed information:

(a) Invoices for the purchase of disposable needles; and

(b) Documentive disposal of all needles and method of disposal.

(4) Records pertaining to needle purchase and needle disposal must be kept for a period of no less than five (5) years and are to be surrendered to the Board, when requested in writing by an authorized representative of the Board or requested by an agent of the Board, in reference to a complaint, allegation and/or investigation of the Board.

(5) All licensees licensed pursuant to this Act must file a notarized document, devised and approved by the Board, acknowledging that they have read, understand and are familiar with the Centers for Disease Control and Prevention (CDC) guidelines for preventing the transmission of the Human Immuno-deficiency virus, Hepatitis B and C and other infectious diseases. This document must be filed with the Board at the time of application and at each renewal cycle.

360 - 6 -.13. Temporary Permits.

Temporary permits for the license of acupuncturists and auricular (ear) detoxification technicians may be issued by the Board.

360 - 6 -.14. Chiropractors Must Meet Acupuncturists Licensure Requirements.

As stated in O.C.G.A. 43 - 9 - 16 and as amended by Section 1.1 of the Act, chiropractors who wish to practice acupuncture must meet the licensing requirements of the Act and the acupuncture rules promulgated by the Board. Chiropractor applicants must be licensed to practice as a chiropractor in the State of Georgia, have an active chiropractic license and be in good standing with the Georgia Board of Chiropractic Examiners. In compliance with the intent of the Georgia General Assembly, nothing in these rules shall be construed to prohibit a chiropractor who is licensed under Article 3 to perform acupuncture in Georgia from engaging in the practice of acupuncture. The Georgia Composite Medical Board, and no other examining board, shall have sole, exclusive and original jurisdiction over such chiropractors who have been granted a license to practice acupuncture in this State for the purpose of establishing standards for licensure of acupuncturists and for the enforcement of such standards of acupuncture through disciplinary action.

360 - 6 -.15. Unlicensed Practice.

(1) No person licensed under this Act may hold himself or herself out as licensed to practice medicine in the State of Georgia unless he or she is licensed by the Board to practice medicine.

(2) No person may advertise or hold himself out to the public as being a "Licensed Acupuncturist" or a licensed "Auricular Detoxification Technician" unless the person is licensed under this Act or otherwise exempt by law from licensure.

360 - 6 -.16. Informed Consent for Treatment.

(1) Any person who undergoes acupuncture must consent in writing prior to such a procedure

and shall be informed in general terms of the following:

(a) That an acupuncturist is not licensed to practice medicine in the State of Georgia;

(b) That an acupuncturist cannot practice medicine in the State of Georgia;

(c) That the acupuncturist is not making a medical diagnosis of the person's disease or medical condition;

(d) That, if the person wants to obtain a medical diagnosis, the person should see a licensed physician and seek medical advise from a licensed physician; and

(e) The nature and purpose of the acupuncture treatment being rendered.

(2) Any person who undergoes auricular (ear) detoxification must consent in writing prior to such a procedure and shall be informed in general terms of the following:

(a) That an Auricular (ear) Detoxification Technician is not licensed to practice medicine in the State of Georgia;

(b) That an Auricular (ear) Detoxification Technician cannot practice medicine in the State of Georgia;

(c) That an Auricular (ear) Detoxification Technician is not licensed to practice acupuncture in the State of Georgia;

(d) That an Auricular (ear) Detoxification Technician is not making a diagnosis of the person's disease or medical condition;

(e) That, if the person wants to obtain a medical diagnosis, the person should see a licensed physician and seek medical advice from a licensed physician; and

(f) The nature and purpose of the auricular (ear) detoxification therapy procedure being rendered.

(g) An Auricular (ear) Detoxification Technician is strictly limited to five ear points' treatment for detoxification for substance abuse, chemical dependency, or both.

(h) Persons licensed to practice acupuncture or auricular (ear) detoxification must use a Board approved, standardized "informed consent" form for each person treated. The form shall be signed and dated by both practitioner and patient prior to the rendering of services.

360 - 6 -.17. Imposition of Sanctions. Use of Referral Fees Prohibited.

The Board, in consultation with the Advisory Committee, may:

(1) Impose any sanction authorized under subsection (d) of O.C.G.A. 43 - 1 - 19 upon a finding of any conduct specified in subsection (a) of O.C.G.A. 43 - 1 - 19; or

(2) Make a finding that such conduct involved dividing or agreeing to divide a fee for acupuncture services with any person who refers a patient.

360 - 6 -.18. Inactive Status.

(1) A person who wishes to maintain his or her Acupuncturist license, but who does not intend to practice Acupuncture, may apply to the Board for inactive status by submitting an application and the fee.

(a) An individual with an inactive license may not practice as an Acupuncturist in this State.

(b) In order to reinstate an Acupuncturist license, the Board must receive a completed application and reinstatement fee. The applicant must be able to demonstrate to the satisfaction of the Board that he or she has maintained current knowledge, skill and proficiency in Acupuncture and that he or she is mentally and physically able to practice with reasonable skill and safety.

(2) A person who wishes to maintain his or her Auricular Detoxification Technician license, but who does not intend to practice auricular detoxification therapy, may apply to the Board for inactive status by submitting an application and the fee.

(a) An individual with an inactive license may not practice as an Auricular Detoxification Technician in this State.

(b) In order to reinstate a license to practice as an Auricular Detoxification Technician, the Board must receive a completed application and a reinstatement fee. The applicant must be able to demonstrate to the satisfaction of the Board that he or she has maintained current knowledge, skill and proficiency in Auricular Detoxification Therapy and that he or she is mentally and physically able to practice with reasonable skill and safety.

(3) Reinstatement of the license is within the discretion of the Board.